YOGA

FOR THE

BODY, MIND AND SOUL

*"The soul has been forgetful of God since eternity. True Yog
is that which unites the soul with the Supreme Divinity."*
Jagadguru Shree Kripaluji Maharaj

By

SWAMI MUKUNDANANDA

Second edition printed in 2015
Signature Book Printing, www.sbpbooks.com

Jagadguru Kripaluji Yog
7405, Stoney Point Dr
Plano, TX 75025
USA

Published by:
Jagadguru Kripaluji Yog
7405, Stoney Point Dr
Plano, TX 75025
USA

www.jkyog.org

ISBN: 978-0-9833967-1-0

Disclaimer:

1. It is an established principle of *Yog* that a participant must not perform exercises beyond the limits of his/her body. It is advisable to consult your family physician to find out if any special restrictions are applicable to you.

2. Any liability, loss, or damage in connection with any use of this program, included but not limited to any liability, loss, or damage resulting from the practice of *Yog* postures, exercises, lifestyle changes, advices, and information given in this book, is expressly disclaimed.

Dedication

This book is dedicated to my Spiritual Master, Jagadguru Shree Kripaluji Maharaj, the greatest of all Yogis, who is like the combined ocean of the Bliss of Devotion and the transcendental knowledge of the Vedas. He is illuminating the world with the sublime secrets of the most perfect system of Yog, imbued with the sweetness of Divine Love for God.

His desire to spread the teachings of the true Science of Yog to every part of the globe, for the spiritual and material well-being of all humankind, and to enlighten Yoga enthusiasts with its true meaning, has resulted in the establishment of the system of Jagadguru Kripaluji Yog.

I pray that by his blessings readers will be inspired to adopt the practices and techniques taught in this book to perfect their health, elevate their minds, enlighten their intellects, and unite their soul with God.

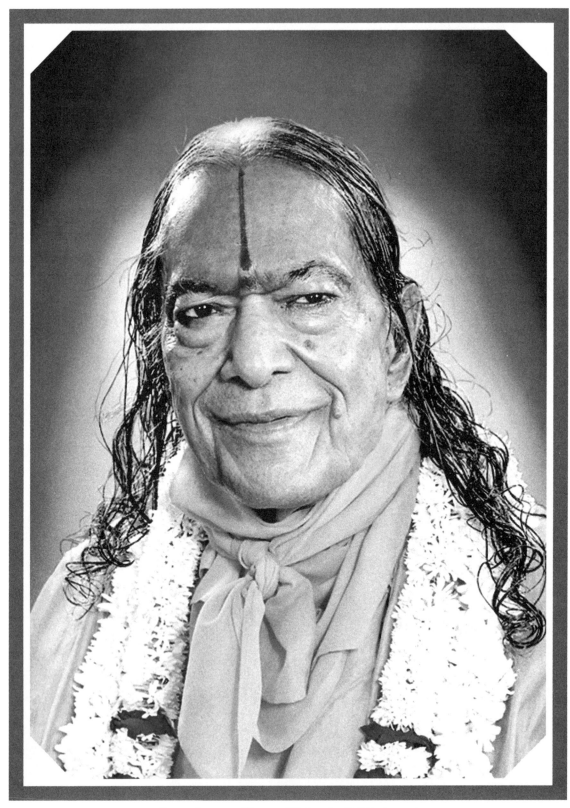

Jagadguru Shree Kripaluji Maharaj

Jagadguru Shree Kripaluji Maharaj

A Brief Introduction

Eternally liberated Divine personalities sometimes descend upon the earth for the welfare of humankind. Jagadguru Shree Kripalu Ji Maharaj is such a Divine personality. "Maharaj ji," as He is lovingly called by his devotees, was born on the auspicious night of Sharat Purnima in 1922, in the village Mangarh, near Allahabad.

Childhood and Youth

He spent his childhood in youthful fun, playing games and frolicking with his young friends. But at the same time, he would display intense gravity and excel effortlessly in his studies. Then at the age of 14, he left the village and attended three Universities, in Kashi, Chitrakoot, and Indore. There he covered a whole series of courses in the space of just two-and-a-half years.

Absorption in Divine Bliss

At the young age of 16, he suddenly gave up his studies and entered the dense forests of Chitrakoot. There he spent his time absorbed in intense of love for Radha Krishna. Often he would lose all external consciousness, and go without eating and drinking for many days at a stretch. For long intervals, he would remain in Mahābhāv, the highest stage of devotion that manifests in Radha Rani. These symptoms of Mahābhāv love had also manifested in Chaitanya Mahaprabhu, 500 years ago. He emerged from the forest after two years to begin his mission of revealing the glories of Radha Krishna devotion to the world.

Kīrtan Movement

He conducted satsangs that brought about a flood of Bhakti in the states of UP and Rajasthan in the 1940s and 50s. He would lead kīrtans imbued with intense devotion, which would continue throughout the night. These kīrtans, which he wrote himself, have been compared by scholars with those of Meerabai, Soordas, Tulsidas, and Ras Khan.

Jagadguru–Spiritual Master of the World

Divine personalities who displayed unparalleled mastery over all Vedic scriptures, and who brought about a spiritual revolution in the minds of the people by their unique explanation of Vedic knowledge, have traditionally been conferred with the title of Jagadguru, or Spiritual Master of the whole world.

In 1957, Kripaluji Maharaj expounded the true import of the scriptures, speaking in sophisticated Sanskrit language before the Kaśhī Vidvat Parishat, the supreme body of Vedic scholars in the country. After 10 days, when the entire body was convinced that his knowledge was deeper than the combined knowledge of all 500 of them put together, they honoured him with the title of "Jagadguru."

In the past 5000 years of the present age of Kali, only five personalities have been recognized as original Jagadgurus: Jagadguru Shankaracharya, who came about 2000 years ago, and propounded the philosophy of non-dualism; Jagadguru Nimbarkacharya, who came shortly after Shankaracharya, and preached the philosophy of dualistic non-dualism; Jagadguru Ramanujacharya, who appeared on the planet 800 years ago, and was the vigorous propagator of qualified non-dualism; and Jagadguru Madhvacharya, who appeared 700 years ago, and preached the philosophy of dualism.

Kripaluji Maharaj is the fifth original Jagadguru in history. Further, the Kāśhī Vidvat Parishat declared that Kripaluji Maharaj was Jagadguruttam, or Supreme amongst the Jagadgurus. Seeing his absorption in the devotion of Radha Krishna, they also accorded on him the title of "Bhakti-Yog Rasavatar," or the Descension of the Bliss of Divine Love.

Scriptural Discourses

After accepting the title of Jagadguru, Kripaluji Maharaj travelled throughout the country for 14 years. He would deliver month-long discourses in each city, in which he would unravel the mysteries of the scriptures before the public. Tens of thousands of people would throng to these discourses, and listen spellbound while he tantalized them with humour, worldly examples, practical instructions, and chastisement. It was a unique experience as he made the deepest scriptural truths accessible to everyone in the simplest language.

Devotional Literature

Kripaluji Maharaj has written thousands of verses, revealing the Divine pastimes of Radha Krishna. His style of writing is unique: he begins the chanting of a pada or kīrtan, and then keeps adding lines to it, as it goes along.

Worldwide Mission

To enable the worldwide spread of his teachings, Kripaluji Maharaj began training preachers and sending them to different parts of the globe. He also created a formal organization and began the construction of huge āśhrams, to provide facilities for devotees who wished to practically apply the teachings in their lives. This organization is today known as the Jagadguru Kripalu Parishat. It is a huge umbrella organization that has sister and branch organizations in various states of India, and many countries of the world. Jagadguru Kripaluji Yog is one such organization that has been established for the propagation of "Yog" around the world, in its true and complete form.

About the Author

Swami Mukundananda is a world-renowned spiritual teacher from India, and is the senior disciple of Jagadguru Shree Kripaluji Maharaj. He is the founder of the Yogic system called "Jagadguru Kripaluji Yog."

Swamiji is a unique sanyāsī (in the renounced order of life), who has a distinguished technical and management educational background as well. He completed B.Tech. from the world-renowned Indian Institute of Technology (IIT), Delhi. He then did MBA from the equally distinguished Indian Institute of Management (IIM), Kolkata. After that, he worked for some time with one of India's topmost industrial houses.

However, distinguished material education and a promising corporate career did not quench his thirst for knowing the Absolute Truth. The longing for God was so strong that he renounced his career and travelled throughout India as a sanyāsī. During these travels, he got the opportunity to closely associate with many elevated Saints of India, read the writings of the great Āchāryas of the past, and resided in many famous holy places.

Ultimately his search took him to the lotus feet of his Spiritual Master, Jagadguru Shree Kripaluji Maharaj (who is lovingly called "Maharajji" by his devotees). He was overawed by the unfathomable scriptural knowledge and ocean of Divine love that he saw manifest in his Spiritual Master. About this first meeting, Maharajji later remarked, "He recognized me as one would recognize his mother."

Under the guidance of Shree Maharajji, he practiced intense sādhanā while residing at the āshram. He also extensively studied the Vedic scriptures, and the Indian and Western systems of philosophy. Upon completion of his studies, his Guru entrusted him with the key task of propagating the ancient knowledge of the Eternal Truth the, world over.

Swamiji was first introduced to yogasans and Hatha Yog meditational techniques in childhood, and he continued its practice while growing up. As he transitioned to Bhakti Yog, he changed his meditational techniques, but continued with his daily practice of yogasans. Seeing his interest in Yog, Kripaluji Maharaj asked him to teach a holistic system of Yog, to correct the anomaly in the Western world, where Yoga was being taught as a mere physical science. On his Spiritual Master's instructions, Swamiji visited reputed Yoga Universities all over India, studying their yogic techniques. He then incorporated the best practices of Hatha Yog, and amalgamated it with Bhakti Yog, to formulate the system of "Jagadguru Kripaluji Yog."

For the last quarter of a century, Shree Swamiji has been traveling far and wide, awakening hundreds of thousands of seekers. Wherever Swamji goes, he attracts huge audiences. Hearing the profound secrets of the Vedas from him is a rare privilege, for he is able to explain the ancient esoteric knowledge with rigourous scientific logic, in the modern context. Using perfect logic, and a simple-yet-scientific approach, Swamiji offers new ways of understanding and applying the knowledge of the scriptures in our daily lives. The hallmark of his lectures is the ease with which he dispels various myths and misnomers associated with the various paths of God-realization, and his ability to penetrate even the toughest minds and convince them with the depth of understanding and scriptural veracity.

Swamiji's lectures cover the teachings of the Vedas, Upanishads, Shreemad Bhagavatam, Purānas, Bhagavad Geeta, Ramayan, and other Eastern scriptures and Western philosophies. Like the true Disciple of a true Master, Swamiji masterfully quotes from the scriptures of all the great religions, to satisfy even the most discerning of knowledge-seekers. He also reveals the simple and straightforward path to God-realization that can be practiced by anyone.

Although Swamiji started preaching in India two decades ago, he now preaches both— in India and abroad. He has inspired innumerable devotees in Singapore, Malaysia, and Hong Kong, where his visit is always anxiously awaited. Since 2008, on the instruction of Shree Maharajji, Swamiji has increasingly begun spending more time in the USA, where his educational background and command over the English language make his programs particularly charming to the intelligentsia, professionals, and academicians.

Shree Swamiji has founded many organizations in India with permanent centres and āshrams, such as Jagadguru Kripaluji Yog Trust, India, Radha Govind Dham, Delhi, Radha Krishna Bhakti Mandir, Cuttack, Radha Govind Dham, Berhampur, Shyama Shyam Dham, Jajpur, Radha Govind Dham, Parla Khemundi, Radha Govind Dham, Karanjia, etc.

In the USA, Swamiji has inspired the formation of Jagadguru Kripaluji Yog, a 501(c) (3) non-profit organization. In the space of a few years, JKYog centers have opened throughout the length and breadth of the USA.

Swamiji cares deeply about imparting Hindu cultural and religious values to the younger generation, especially in the West. Toward this end, he has conceived a special Personality Development program for children and young adults. This program is called "The Bal-Mukund Playground for Vedic Wisdom." It includes character building, Yog, meditation, devotional singing, and religious training. Many Bal-Mukund centres have been started for the benefit of children, both in the USA and in India.

Shree Swamiji has a God-gifted ability to keep all kinds of audiences enthralled and entertained through wisdom filled anecdotes, humorous stories, and irrefutable logic. He has inspired innumerable people, of all ages, toward the path of God-realization, the world over. Swamiji's warmth and humility touch all those who have the fortune to have his association. In fact, his very presence radiates grace and Bliss.

Acknowledgements

This book has been written because of the inspiration received from my Spiritual Master, Jagadguru Shree Kripaluji Maharaj, who is the topmost exponent of the science of Bhakti Yog in the last 5000 years. I offer my humble obeisance at his lotus feet for gracing me with the opportunity to render service in the form of teaching Yog to seekers around the world.

The Supreme Master of all yogis is Yogeshwar Shree Krishna, who bestowed the unparalleled Divine knowledge of the Bhagavad Geeta to humankind. I prostrate before His lotus feet, and pray that He may bless the readers of this book with success in Yog. I also offer my respects to the Divine Mother, Shree Radha Rani, who by a mere glance of Her Grace bestows success in the practice of Yog.

The techniques of the various branches of the Science of Yog revealed in this book are not new. They have been taught and practiced by true yogis in India for many centuries. Thus, I respectfully offer my gratitude to all the great yogis in the history, who practiced and propagated the science of Yog in the past, and whose priceless contributions in the form of their books, instructions, disciples, etc. have continued to inspire future generations of Yog enthusiasts. The speciality of this book is that you will find the authentic scriptural form of the various techniques taught by these great yogis — yogasans, pranayam, meditation, subtle-body relaxation, and the science of proper diet — all in one place.

The publishing of "Yoga for the Body, Mind and Soul" was a huge project, which was only made possible by the dedication, sincerity, hard work, and expertise of the JKYog team in India. Our two Yogacharyas, Tara Prasad Paudyal and Krishna Chapagain, researched hundreds of books and personally tried various combinations of asans for many hours every day, to help me finalize the set for this book. They also worked with the artist to perfect the illustrations for each posture. I would also like to express my appreciation to Shree Maheshwar Maharana, the artist, who toiled for many months to create over six hundred illustrations for this book.

I am thankful to Shailee Adhikari, the master designer of our team, for providing the cover design. Jashu Bhai Patel of Ahmedabad did the initial proofreading and editing.

Pragnyan Vaidya spent many months in editing the book and doing the laborious work of typing the diacriticals and Hindi fonts. He also worked tirelessly to help finalize the glossary of Hindi terms. The typesetting and composition was meticulously done by Tara Prasad. Shreya Bhat of Dallas offered invaluable suggestions, as always. Pankaj Verma from our publication team did the grueling work of overseeing the printing process. My heartfelt gratitude to the entire team!

SWAMI MUKUNDANANDA

Guide to Hindi Pronunciation

अ	*a*	as *u* in b*u*t
आ	*ā*	as *a* in f*a*r
इ	*i*	as *i* in p*i*n
ई	*ī*	as *i* in mach*i*ne
उ	*u*	as *u* in p*u*sh
ऊ	*ū*	as *o* in m*o*ve
ए	*e*	as *a* in ev*a*de
ऐ	*ai*	As *a* in m*a*t; sometimes as *ai* in *ai*sle with the only difference that a should be pronounced as *u* in b*u*t, not as *a* in f*a*r.
ओ	*o*	as *o* in g*o*
औ	*au*	as *o* in p*o*t, or as *aw* in S*aw*
ऋ	*ṛi*	as *r* in *Kṛiṣhṇa*
:	*ḥ*	it is a strong aspirate; also lengthens the preceding vowel and occurs only at the end of a word. It is pronounced as a final *h* sound
.	*ṁ*	nasalizes and lengthens the preceding vowel and is pronounced as *n* in the French word B*on*
क	*ka*	as *k* in *k*ite
ख	*kha*	as *kha* in E*ckha*rt
ग	*ga*	as *g* in *g*oat
घ	*gha*	as *gh* in Di*gh*ard
ङ	*ṅa*	as *n* in fi*n*ger
च	*cha*	as *cha* in *cha*ir
छ	*chha*	as *chh* in staun*chh*eart
ज	*ja*	as *j* in *j*ar
झ	*jha*	as *dgeh* in He*dgeh*og
ञ	*ña*	as *n* in lu*n*ch
ट	*ṭa*	as *t* in *t*ub

ठ	*ṭha*	as *th* in hot*h*ead
ड	*ḍa*	as *d* in *d*ivine
ढ	*ḍha*	as *dh* in Re*dh*ead
ण	*ṇa*	as *n* in bur*n*t
त	*ta*	as *t* in French word ma*t*ron
थ	*tha*	as *th* in e*th*er
द	*da*	as *th* in ei*th*er
ध	*dha*	as *dh* in Bud*dh*a
न	*na*	as *n* in *n*o
प	*pa*	as *p* in *p*ink
फ	*pha*	as *ph* in U*ph*ill
ब	*ba*	as *b* in *b*oy
भ	*bha*	as *bh* in a*bh*or
म	*ma*	as *m* in *m*an
य	*ya*	as *y* in *y*es
र	*ra*	as *r* in *r*emember
ल	*la*	as *l* in *l*ight
व	*va*	as *v* in *v*ine, as *w* in s*w*an
श	*śha*	as *sh* in *sh*ape
स	*sa*	as *s* in *s*in
ष	*ṣha*	as *sh* in *sh*ow
ह	*ha*	as *h* in *h*ut
क्ष	*kṣha*	as *ksh* in frea*ksh*ow
ज्ञ	*gya*	as *gy* in bi*gy*oung
ड़	*ṛa*	There is no sign in English to represent the sounds ड़ and ढ़. They have been written as *ṛa* and *ṛha*.

Table of Contents

I. What is *Yog*?

One of the most ancient treasures of Indian culture, tradition, and heritage is the science of *Yog*. *Yog* is mentioned in the Upanishads—the later part of the Vedas—that form the philosophical foundation of *Yogic* science. This Divine science of *Yog* has been practiced in India for thousands of years.

The word "*Yog*" means "to unite" and is derived from the Sanskrit word "*yuj*," which means "to join." So, the aim of *Yog* is to yoke the *jīva* (individual soul) with *Bhagavān* (Supreme Soul). Union with the Absolute frees the soul from the veil of Maya, allowing it to realize its true nature. The *Garuḍ Purāṇa* defines *Yog* as follows:

संयोगो योग इत्युक्तो जीवात्मा परमात्मनो:॥ (गरुड़ पुराण)

sanyogo yog ityukto jīvātmā paramātmanoḥ (Garuḍ Purāṇa)

"The Union of the soul with the Supreme is called *Yog*." A similar idea has been mentioned in the *Yāgyavalkya Sanhitā* and the *Devī Bhāgavat Purāṇa*. The same concept of the uniting of the *jīva* with *Paramātmā* has been mentioned in the following verse of the *Yāgyavalkya Sanhitā*:

ऐवयं जीवात्मनोराहुर्योगं योगविशारदा:॥ (याज्ञवल्क्य संहिता)

aivayaṁ jīvātmanorāhuryogaṁ yogaviśhāradāḥ (Yāgyavalkya Sanhitā)

Yog incorporates the science of healthy and righteous living into our daily life. It works on all aspects of an individual—physical, mental, emotional, and spiritual. It takes into purview—the mind, the body, and the soul of a *jīva* in its aim of reaching the Absolute. *Yog* has the power of integrating the physical, mental, and spiritual dimensions of a *jīva*. The body must be purified and strengthened through various practices. The mind must be cleansed of all gross factors and turn both—inward and toward—the Absolute in order to attain unmitigated peace, satisfaction, and bliss. This requires the collective development of various facets of our personality. Therefore, we must learn the art of attaining perfect health of body, mind, intellect, and soul. For this, we need a judicious blend of spiritual and material sciences.

Our intellect is subject to certain weaknesses that are universal in the materially bound state. *Avidyā*—lack of knowledge, *asmitā*—pride due to identification with the designations of the body, *rāg*—longing and attachment for sensory objects and affections, *dveṣh*—dislike for objects and persons, and *abhiniveśh*—the fear of death. These are the five flaws of the intellect that must be rooted out. *Yog* helps to eradicate these mental flaws. *Yog* is a practical discipline that teaches us how to attain permanent bliss. It makes us free from worries, anxieties, and depressions.

Yog has no age barrier. Whether one is on the threshold of life, or in the spring of youthfulness, or has become old—anybody can practice it as there are no restrictive factors. Irrespective of cultural and religious background, *Yog* practice possesses the capacity of tuning the body and mind to the laws of nature and the infinite Divinity, and forges an integrated personality of the practitioner. *Yog* is a rational discipline with powerful tools for conquering the stormy mind and harnessing the physical and mental energies. It greatly helps an aspirant rapidly move toward Divinity. The greatness of *Yog* is also discussed by Lord Shree Krishna in the Bhagavat Geeta:

तपस्विभ्योऽधिको योगी ज्ञानिभ्योऽपि मतोऽधिकः।
कर्मिभ्यश्चाधिको योगी तस्माद्योगी भवार्जुन॥ (भगवद् गीता ६.४६)

tapasvibhyo 'dhiko yogī gyānibhyo 'pi mato 'dhikaḥ
karmibhyaśhchādhiko yogī tasmādyogī bhavārjuna (Bhagavad Geeta 6.46)

"The *Yogī* is greater than the ascetics, he is greater than even the wise or *Gyānī*; he is greater than a man of actions or rituals; become thou a *Yogī*, O Arjun!" Further, the *Yāgyavalkya Smṛiti* states:

इज्याचारदमाहिंसादानस्वाध्यायकर्मणाम्।
अयं तु परमो धर्मो यद्योगेन आत्मदर्शनम्॥ (याज्ञवल्क्य स्मृति १.१.८)

ijyāchāradamāhinsādānasvādhyāyakarmaṇām
ayaṁ tu paramo dharmo yadyogena ātmadarśhanam (Yāgyavalkya Smṛiti 1.1.8)

"Among sacrifices, customs, refreshment of the senses, non-violence, charity, and *Vedāntic* practices, the most important is the realization of the Supreme through *Yog*."

The Sage Patanjali also defines *Yog* as:

योगश्चित्तवृत्तिनिरोधः। (पतञ्जलि योग सूत्र १.२)
yogaśhchittavṛittinirodhaḥ (Patañjali Yog Sūtra 1.2)

"*Yog* is the restriction of the perturbations of the mind." The word *chitta* denotes the mind, which is composed of three elements—*manas*, or the mind associated with the senses, which has got the power of attention, selection, and rejection; *buddhi*, or intellect; and *ahankār,* or ego. The *chitta*, or mind, is constantly in flux since it is operated through inputs from all its three parts. In normal life, it is hardly possible to be free from these inputs and they become the sources of diversion because of which the mind is never quiet. Unfortunately, a stormy mind can never be drawn toward the Divine. In this way, one is unable to see oneself and others as parts of God.

Yog pacifies the vacillations of the mind that divert it from the Absolute. According to St. Augustine, "Our heart is restless, O Lord! And it shall continue to remain restless until it comes to rest in Thee." Therefore, it is *Yog* that uplifts us to the level of the Supreme and makes us Blissful like Him.

Yog harmonizes, balances, purifies, and strengthens the body, mind, and soul of the practitioners. It shows the right way to perfect health, complete mind control, and total peace with one's self, the world, the nature, and God. Highlighting the importance of *Yog*, Sri Aurobindo also said, "*Yog* is the process of all round development of a man."

A healthy body and a sound mind are the building blocks for attaining our goal in this life. Without their support, life itself will become a painful and tedious experience. No matter how perfect and successful we are in our fields of work, if the body is ill and the mind is fluctuating or distressed, we will always remain unhappy and hopeless in our lives. So, our most priceless possession is not our riches and gold, but our own body and mind.

Yog is an exercise for moral and mental cultivation that generates *ārogya* (good health), and contributes to *chirāyu* (longevity).

Those who practice *Yog* should maintain moderation in everything such as diet, sleeping, waking, speaking, etc., so that they do not feel disturbed during the period of *sādhanā*. Highlighting the "moderate approach" in everything, Shree Krishna says in the Bhagavad Geeta:

नात्यश्नतस्तु योगोऽस्ति न चैकान्तमनश्नतः।
न चाति स्वप्नशीलस्य जाग्रतो नैव चार्जुन॥
युक्ताहारविहारस्य युक्तचेष्टस्य कर्मसु।
युक्तस्वप्नावबोधस्य योगो भवति दुःखहा। (भगवद् गीता ६.१६-१७)

nātyaśhnatastu yogo 'sti na chaikāntamanaśhnataḥ
na chāti svapnaśhīlasya jāgrato naiva chārjuna
yuktāhāravihārasya yuktacheṣhṭasya karmasu
yuktasvapnāvabodhasya yogo bhavati duḥkhahā (Bhagavad Geeta 6.16-17)

"O Arjun! This *Yog* is not attained by one who overeats, nor by one who fasts. Nor by those who keep awake or sleep too much. To achieve *Yog*, you must eat, play, work, sleep, and relax in moderation; thereby you will overcome miseries." Contemplating upon the above verses, a *Yogī* should control the mind in dieting, fasting, sleeping, speaking, etc., and spend time and effort to learn the science of healthy living (*Yogic* practices) for physical, mental, and spiritual well-being.

Arms of Yog and Its Benefits

Yog usually includes the following aspects: *asans* (postures), *pranayam* (breath control), Subtle Body Relaxation, *dhyan* (meditation), and *ṣhaṭkarm* (six purification processes). *yogasans* are the physical stretches or postures. They consist of standing, sitting, and inverted exercises, which help in improving suppleness, flexibility, and posture. They also stretch the muscles, and produce stamina and strength in the body, along with soothing the wavering mind.

The next aspect, *pranayam*, is the various breathing exercises, especially designed to control the movements of *prāṇ* within us. The practice of *pranayam* enhances lungs' capacity, resulting in oxygenating and energizing the body, and improves the blood circulation. Like the *asans*, *pranayam* also soothes the mind, helping its practitioner experience a feeling of tranquility and emotional well-being, because it is practiced over a period of time.

Dhyan techniques allow us to become aware of how our mind works, thus enabling us to accept ourselves. We become more single-minded, our concentration improves, and we give up deleterious thought patterns—to become focused, self-confident, open-minded, and honest with ourselves and others. The fixation of mind on the Divine realm helps cleanse the mind and approach the goal of Divine Bliss very easily. Similarly, other aspects of *Yog*—*ṣhatkarm* and Subtle Body Relaxation—contribute in cleansing both—the body and the mind, and thus result in the development of a healthy overall personality.

A sincere and regular practice of *Yog* offers many benefits to the body, the mind, and soul. As a form of isometric exercises, the prolonged holding of *Yog* postures tones and strengthens the muscles and internal organs. They also stretch and lengthen muscles, tendons, and ligaments—making them more flexible. Especially deep breathing during *Yog* practice opens the chest and strengthens the diaphragm. Attentively making bodily-momements—while maintaining awareness of the body and breath—develops focus, attention, and concentration.

When the gentle stretching, deep breathing, *dhyan*, and guided relaxation are integrated, the bodily tension disappears, and the nervous system and emotions become calm, and there is a sense of renewal in the body, the mind, and spirit. *Yog* builds internal and external awareness when it is practiced along with awareness on synchronizing the breath and the Divine Names. Thus, *Yog* builds awareness of the body and experiences, along with increasing awareness of the needs of others. Besides, exercising the mind and muscles, *Yog* exercises and massages the glands and organs, and increases circulation throughout the body, resulting in improved digestion, elimination of toxins, and promotion of overall health.

Historical Aspect of *Yogasans*

Historians respect the Vedas as the oldest books in the world. However, "oldest" is not a sufficient description of their antiquity. The Vedas are the knowledge of God, and they are eternal like God Himself. Each time He creates the world, He manifests the Vedas; and at the time of dissolution, the Vedas merge back into His Divine body. Thus, the system of *Yog*—described in the eternal Vedas—is called *Sanātan Dharm*, or "Eternal Religion." God manifests this eternal knowledge in the world either by taking an Avatar Himself, or by inspiring the knowledge in the hearts of the God-realized Saints.

In this cycle of creation, the first teacher of *yogasans* (the physical aspect of *Yog*), was Lord Shiv Himself. It is said that Lord Shiv first practiced *yogasans* and taught them to Mother Parvati, Who became the first pupil. Manifold seals and statues excavated at the prehistoric places—chiefly in India—reveal that the *yogasans* being performed in India many millennia prior to the beginning of western history. Even at present, one can obtain myriad statues and idols in the Indus Valley at Harappa and Mohenjo-daro of deities of Lord Shiv and Mother Parvati doing different postures and sitting in meditation. The secrets of *yogasans* were handed over from Guru to disciple orally. Through personal experience, the *Yogīs* guided their disciples on the path very clearly and systematically.

Between 400 BC and 200 BC, a great hermit, Patanjali, wrote a dissertation on *Yog* in pithy aphorisms, in a system that is called *Aṣhṭāṅg Yog*. The eight steps to *Yog* that he delineated through 185 terse aphorisms are: *yam*, *niyam*, *asan*, *pranayam*, *pratyāhār*, *dhāraṇā*, *dhyan*, and *samādhi*. The word *yam* means self-restraints; *niyam* means self-observances; *asan* means postures of the body; *pranayam* means organized way of breathing; *pratyāhār* denotes disassociation of consciousness from the external surrounding; *dhāraṇā* means concentration; *dhyan* means meditation, and *samādhi* refers to experiencing oneself with the pure consciousness.

The Buddha came around 6th century BC, and preached the techniques of meditation and ethics like non-violence, truth, etc. differently to the world, but sidelined the path of *yogasans*. After Him, Yogi Matsyendranath emphasized that the body should be purified prior to the performance of meditation. His renowned disciple, Gorakhnath, also wrote the treatises on the *Haṭha Yog*, both—in the local and Hindi language. Subsequently, Swami Swatmarama, one of the authoritative writers on the *Haṭha Yog*, wrote a renowned book, the "*Haṭha Yog Pradīpikā*," or "The Light on *Haṭha Yog*." Despite the fact that he incorporated several ideas on *Yog*, he did not lay much emphasis on *yam* and *niyam*, due to which beginners of *Yog* find it very comfortable and easy to practice. Unlike in Patanjali's *Yog Sutra*, Swatmarama in his treatise, at first, focused on the body and then only, self-control and self-discipline after maintaining the stability of the mind.

Indispensability of *Yog* in the Present Times

The vast technological and scientific advancements made in the current decade have made our day-to-day life very intricate and hectic. Most aspects of the average modern lifestyle move at a rapid pace. In the era of wi-fi networks, internet, cell phones, beepers, and excessive burden of work, people do not have time for even eating and resting properly. Due to cut-throat competition and the rat-race, stress has filled their lives, making them frustrated, tense, and miserable. Therefore, stress-relief is the first and foremost motivation for the practice of *Yog* in the current time. In such a critical situation of stress and anxiety, *Yog* has proved itself as a panacea by giving a welcome relief to stress-stricken people.

Yogasans reduce the over-stimulation of the nervous system and activate the "rest and repair" of the parasympathetic nervous system. The science of *Yog* benefits all through practical lifestyle tips like vegetarian diet, positive thinking, and meditative practices—thus assisting in rooting out stressful conditions. Hence, *Yog* has been a remedying key to such self-created mental stress in people's lives.

Although many people learn *Yog* to fight with stress and multifarious maladies, they start reaping the fruits of spiritual bliss that comes from within as they begin to realize themselves as the soul and an eternal fragment of God. Indisputably *Yog's* main purpose is to bring a soul to the attainment of the Supreme. Nevertheless, the *Yogic* practices such as *asans*, *pranayam*, *dhyan*, *ṣhaṭkarm*, etc. also yield several bodily and mental benefits.

There are many other systems that people follow in order to develop their personality, health, and fortune. Nonetheless, personal experience tells us that these practices have not helped us develop the spiritual side of our personality. In this 21ˢᵗ century, we are still plagued by mental afflictions such as desire, anger, lust, jealousy, and an inflated ego. True happiness has evaded us, although the eagerness to search for it has not diminished. Thus, it is only *Yog* which can abolish all these unwanted evils of the mind through its spiritual knowledge and techniques.

A healthy body and a composed mind are the building blocks for attaining our goal in this life. In this regard, *Yog* has been a successful alternative therapy in the diseases like asthma, high blood pressure, constipation, spondylitis, etc., where even the modern allopathy has not succeeded. The regular practice of various *Yogic* methods has shown many positive results even in cases of cancer, HIV AIDS, diabetes, etc., by reducing their detrimental effects, by working at the cellular level, and increasing the resistance power of each cell in the body.

Apart from benefitting individuals, *Yogic* practices like *asans* and *dhyan* done with God's Name and His Form help uproot social disorders and chaos. In this way, *Yog* can establish the forgotten past values and norms among the people in modern time. It can also spread the message of harmony, order, non-violence, truth, charity, integrity, and spirituality among all, by bestowing incredible advantages of inner peace to the ones who do it sincerely and regularly.

In conclusion, *Yog* is not only a matter of theory, but its substratum also lies in practicality and action. For this reason, the present generation should learn it in order to hone their lives materially, mentally, and spiritually. Through its sincere practice, people can realize that true *Yog* is established within oneself and not externally, and that the rich source of inner evolution must be searched within, turning back from the outer world. People can then realize themselves as not a physical body, but an eternal soul, which is naturally an eternal servant of God.

Guidelines for Radhey Krishna Yogasans

Place

The place for *yogasans* should be neat and clean. Preferably, there should not be any noise of vehicles, factories, or loud speakers. If you practice *yogasans* in a room, it should be adequately ventilated with plenty of oxygen supply, allowing you to breathe freely. It should not be stuffy or suffocating. A good lawn with trees or a garden is very suitable. You should not practice in a place with strong winds, out in the cold, or in a polluted atmosphere.

Time

The most suitable time for practicing *asans* is the morning hours, especially after emptying your bowels. However, *asans* can be done in the evening too, if your stomach is empty. If you are unable to manage time in the morning or evening, you can do it even during the day time, either four hours after a heavy meal or two hours after a light meal.

Dress

Yogasans should be performed with the minimum of clothes on the body depending upon the season. It is better to wear a loose, light, and clean dress that enables free movement of your body. Also, remove your wrist watch, ornaments, chains, spectacles, etc. prior to doing *asans*.

Duration

It is advisable to do *asans* from 15 minutes to an hour every day. After that, you should not eat anything for at least half an hour. Always do Shavasan or other relaxing *asans* like Balasan, Relaxing Makarasan, Matsya Kreedasan, etc., for about 5-10 minutes after the completion of *asans* to gain maximum benefit.

Breathing

The general rule for breathing during the practice of *yogasans* is to breathe in (chanting "Radhey") while bending backward, and breathe out (chanting "Krishna") while bending forward and sideward, to match the natural expansion and contraction of the lungs throughout the *asan*. However, for each *asan*, you should carefully note its particular system of breathing as per the bodily movements.

Chanting the Divine Names

Always remember God's Name along with each movement and breath. In your mind, chant or remember "Radhey" as you breathe in and "Krishna" as you breathe out. You can also chant or remember any other Divine Names of God.

Note: It is always advisable to consult your doctor before starting *yogasans*. You should not practice them while carrying or recovering from injuries and/or post-surgery without consulting a certified doctor.

General Precautions

Those suffering from hernia and colitis should not perform backward bending *asans*. Those suffering from backache or sciatica should not perform forward bending *asans*. Those who have high blood-pressure or heart ailments should not perform the *asans* in which excessive effort is required.

While selecting *asans* suitable for yourself, you should also keep in your mind age and physical condition. Similarly, the number of repetitions of the *asans* should not be overdone. Repeat them only for as long as your mind copes with them and finds comfortable. It is also worth noting that while performing *asans*, your physical movements and breathing should be gentle and smooth; wild and thrusty movements or breathing may trigger physical and/or mental harms. Take for example, those who have got any fracture in the past should not perform the *asans* that exert pressure on their bone(s), until the fractures get fully healed.

Yogasans should be perfomed, according to one's flexibility, stamina, strength, and energy level. A practitioner is not advised to cross such limits, although he might gradually try to increase them.

Yogasans are not a subject matter for a competition or wager; such things tend to defeat the very purpose of *yogasans*. In case you feel tired or exhausted, stop the *asans* for a while, lie down in any of the relaxing poses like Shavasan, Relaxing Makarasan, Balasan, Matsya Kreedasan, etc., and while breathing deeply, bring your body back to the normal condition.

II. About Jagadguru Kripaluji Yog (JKYog)

Jagadguru Kripaluji Yog is a complete system of *Yog* that incorporates both—material and spiritual knowledge—for the physical, mental, intellectual, and spiritual health of humankind. It is based upon the timeless wisdom of the Vedic scriptures. They are the authentic scriptural form of the various techniques for mind-management and exemplary physical health. There are five arms of Jagadguru Kripaluji Yog:

1. **Radhey Krishna Yogasans.** These are physical postures and exercises practiced along with the remembrance of God.

2. **Radhey Krishna Pranayams.** These are breathing exercises done with the chanting/remembering of the Holy Names of God.

3. **Subtle Body Relaxation.** This is a technique for removing all tension and anxiety from the mind and the body, and bringing it to a state of complete relaxation.

4. *Roop Dhyan* **Meditation**. This is a Divine system of meditation on the all-attractive Form of God.

5. **Science of Healthy Diet.** It is the science of understanding the impacts of different foods on our body and mind and eating proper foods to develop a *sāttvic* nature, in accordance with the famous proverb: "You are what you eat."

For anyone yearning to learn the holistic science of healthy living, sincere practice of these techniques will definitely bring about a complete well-being from within.

The techniques of Jagadguru Kripaluji Yog are not something new; they have been practiced by "true *Yogīs*" in India for centuries. They are described in the Vedas, and are taught in varying degrees around the world. Nonetheless, in their study and practice, the role of the mind is invariably ignored. The most shocking revelation is that most *Yog* therapists and practitioners of India and abroad instruct and perform *Yog* only as a form of physical exercises. They rarely pay adequate heed to the mind-dimension and soul-diminsion. For this reason, *Yog* enthusiasts are deprived of the experience of the Bliss of Devotion. Whatever benefit is obtained while improving health, is only transient, due to ignoring the mind. The maladies of the mind, such as lust, anger, greed, envy, and illusion, can only be cured through remembrance of the Supreme God. The *Pañchadaśī* states:

मन एव मनुष्याणां कारणं बन्ध मोक्षयोः। (पञ्चदशी)

mana eva manuṣhyāṇāṁ kāraṇaṁ bandha mokṣhayoḥ (Pañchadaśī)

"The mind alone is the reason for bondage and liberation." If the mind is overlooked, then any science of *Yog* will be incomplete and only partially beneficial. In fact, without reining our turbulent and fluctuated mind, there can be no true *Yog*. The Shreemad Bhagavatam states:

एतावान् योग आदिष्टो मच्छिष्यैः सनकादिभिः।

सर्वतो मन आकृष्य मय्यद्धावेश्यते यथा। (श्रीमद् भागवतम् ११.१३.१४)

etāvān yoga ādishṭo machchhiṣhyaih sanakādibhih
sarvato mana ākriṣhya mayyaddhāveśhyate yathā

(Shreemad Bhagavatam 11.13.14)

"True *Yog* means removing the mind from all objects of material attachment, and fixing it completely on the Supreme."

Almost in every town of every nation of the world, *Yog* institutions have been established. Their way of training practitioners is completely different from the way mentioned in the Vedic scriptures. In Vedic literature, the precise word is "*Yog*" and not "Yoga." The real *Yog* is the fusion of the soul with the Absolute. Its body oriented aspects (*asans*) are aimed to increase physical health and stability. Nevertheless, the absolute *Yog* is not only about the body, but also about the mental, intellectual, and spiritual dimensions. Unless we rectify our minds with constant *dhyan* on Him, we cannot get rid of even the physical diseases.

Unfortunately, most publications and *Yog* institutes at present, rarely focus on the mental aspect of *Yog*. Rather they train the practitioners just in physical exercises and incomplete meditation techniques in the name of "Yoga." Hence, unless and until we emphasize the major problems that afflict our minds, real happiness will continue to elude us. Practicing penance, austerity, and *yogasans* will never bring us the real peace or bliss that we have been seeking. Certainly, *yogasans* can ensure a very healthy body, but cannot treat the disorders and turmoils of the mind. *Dhyan*, if practiced in accordance with the system of the Vedic scriptures, can usher us to the right path and give us its true benefit. Without the total immersion of the mind in Divine Love, true "*Yog*" can't be achieved. For this reason, the mind needs to be fixed on God for any of these *Yogic* techniques to be effective.

In the *Yog Sūtras*, Patanjali mainly highlights the mind and its modifications. He emphasizes on the training of the mind to achieve Union with the Divinity. The aim of *Patañjali Yog* is to set a *jīva* free from the cage of matter. As mind is a subtler form of matter, a person who releases his or her consciousness from this mesh of *chitta* or *ahankar* (mind or ego) becomes a pure being.

The *Patañjali Yog Darshan* mentions eight steps to *Yog*, in which *yam*, and *niyam*, or self-control and rules, come before *asans*. *Niyam* are five:

शौच संतोष तप: स्वाध्यायेश्वर प्रणिधानानि नियमा:।

(पतञ्जलि योग सूत्र २.३२)

śhaucha santoṣha tapah svādhyāyeśhvara praṇidhānāni niyamāh

(Patañjali Yog Sūtra 2.32)

"The *niyam*, or rules, are five: cleanliness, contentment, austerity, contemplation, and surrender to God." Amongst these five rules, surrender to God is the most essential one. This submission to God is the foundation of Jagadguru Kripaluji Yog.

In Jagadguru Kripaluji Yog, in place of mere *asans*, Radhey Krishna Yogasans have been incorporated, i.e. *asans* along with the mental chanting or recalling of the Names of God. This practice offers dual benefits of remembering the Divine Names and enhances flexibility and strength of the body. In the same way, there is Radhey Krishna Pranayam that is performed by synchronizing the breaths along with the mental chanting of the Sacred Names of God. Instead of the mechanical process of *yog nidrā*, there is Subtle Body Relaxation technique, in which practitioners learn the superb art of relaxing their minds along with simultaneous and constant fixation of their minds on the Divine Pastimes of God with great ease and comfort. As the mind is attached to the Divine realm, it becomes cleansed by constant meditation on God. From the physical perspective too, Subtle Body Relaxation is many more times advantageous as compared to all the *yogasans* and *pranayams* put together. Unlike fixing the mind on worldly areas through different types of meditation techniques taught in different parts of the world, *Roop Dhyan* Meditation of JKYog imparts to the aspirants the art of meditating on the Names, Forms, Virtues, Pastimes, Abodes, and Associates of God. This helps them come closer to the Divinity by developing an affinity for Him.

Jagadguru Shree Kripaluji Maharaj, the Supreme Spiritual Master of this age, has revealed the true knowledge of *Yog* to the world. He explains that achievement of a sound mind in a sound body needs a conglomeration of both—material and spiritual knowledge. The body—which is formed by five material elements and sustained by what we eat and drink—has to be kept in good shape with the help of material sciences. Simultaneously, the mind must be cleansed and elevated through the spiritual science.

Some spiritual practitioners sometimes incorrectly proclaim that since we are the soul and not the material body, we must only promote the spirit, ignoring the body aspect. However, if the body falls sick, the mind has to suffer from the sensation of physical pain, resulting in zero contemplation about God. We should not forget that a healthy body is our boat for crossing the ocean of material existence. Conversely, materialists often consider spiritual science as waste of time and an impediment to material progress. This is also naïve, for without spiritual cognition, material science has no means of mitigating the negative inclinations of the mind. We may facilitate ourselves through modern technology and multiply our bodily comforts, but how will we overcome the forces of our internal nature, such as lust, anger, greed, envy, and illusion?

Sincere and regular practice of all the aforementioned five disciplines of Jagadguru Kripaluji Yog is a simple and sure means to achieve the inner peace and tranquility. With the aforesaid five simple and time-tested techniques, JKYog is aimed at empowering people to conquer the negative aspects like stress, anxiety, strife, tension, sorrow, etc., very easily. The greatest benefit that you can reap from JKYog is the Divine essence of the eternal path to God-realization and getting closer to the Divinity, irrespective of wherever you are and whoever you are.

Physically, the practice of *asans* prescribed by JKYog assists our body to be stronger and more flexible; it also assists in developing, building, and strengthening the muscles, bones, and joints.

The *yogasans* chiefly comprise of stretching of the muscles and the bodily/physical movements from pose to pose. These exercises help us balance our weight by burning fats from the cells of the body. The ability to focus on breathing, while practicing various physical poses is of great significance in uprooting tensions, stress, anxiety, distress, depression, etc.

However, most of the *Yog* institutes of the world halt at the level of the physical *asans*, ignoring management of the mind. A holistic system of *pranayams*, called Radhey Krishna Pranayams, are practiced along with the mental uttering and/or remembering of the Divine Names of God. This act of chanting and remembering has the effect of transporting the mind to the Divine realm.

Subtle Body Relaxation is a mind controlling technique, and is one of the cheif disciplines of Jagadguru Kripaluji Yog. Its practice offers complete relaxation to both—the gross and subtle bodies. Along with calming down the stressed and tense minds, the practitioners are also instructed to embark on a spritual jounery, in which they have opportunity to see, meet, talk, share, etc. with both—Shree Krishna and Shree Radha Rani. Resultantly, such Divine activities help cleanse their minds rapidly. In this way, Subtle Body Relaxation contributes for the true "*Yog*" or union with God, which is the main target of *Yog*.

Thus, the mind is naturally purified and imbued with Divine consciousness. JKYog offers time-tested techniques of *dhyan* that enable us to relish the Bliss of Divinity with ease and simplicity. In order to elevate the mind, we learn in JKYog about meditation on the Divine and also about synchronizing the chanting of God's Name with every breath. When proper meditation is practiced along with the other four sciences of JKYog, it leads to true enlightenment from within.

Everbody knows that health is the foundation of all other aspects and has a meaning provided that health is in proper state. It is a great folly if a person gurantees his good health only by visiting the doctor or eating supplements. Rather it has to be maintained by practicing good habits and changing our unhealthy patterns of eating and thinking in daily life. Thus, healthy life is only possible by following the recommendations prescribed on various food patterns in The Science of Healthy Diet—one of the time-tested disciplines of JKYog.

To sum up, JKYog is an elaborate discipline for the control and transcendence of the mind, senses, and inner faculties; it is associated with the unfoldment of intuition, the experience of Divine states, self-realization, and ultimately God-realization. JKYog enables aspirants to practice and apply these various aspects in daily lives.

This book is not intended to be a philosophical dissertation on "*Yog*." Rather, it is a practical guide for the application of *Yogic* sciences in our lives. The *asans*, *pranayam*, Subtle Body Relaxation, *dhyan*, *ṣhaṭkarmas*, *mudras*, and The Science of Healty Diet, documented here have been chosen to ensure maximum benefit, and also for the ease of practice for practitioners with varying degrees of physical and mental strength.

III. Warm-Up Exercises

Warm-up postures and Breathing exercises prepare the body for *Yogic* practices by warming-up your muscles, flexing stiff joints, and thus increasing suppleness of the joints. They also prepare your body for more strenuous activities. Warm-up exercises can prevent injuries by loosening up your joints and muscles. A proper warm-up increases the blood flow to the muscles, which results in decrease of muscle stiffness, less risk of injury, and improved performance. This section describes different warm-up exercises that can be included in the beginning of a *yogasan* session.

1. Twisting

Procedure

i. Stand up straight—in an upright position—with both feet joined together and arms by your sides, i.e. Saral Tadasan (See page 25).

ii. Keep a distance of about 2.5-3 feet between the two feet.

iii. As you inhale (Radhey), raise the hands sideways, keeping the arms parallel to the floor.

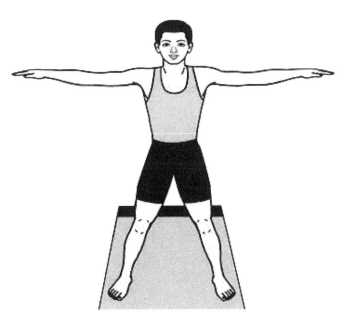

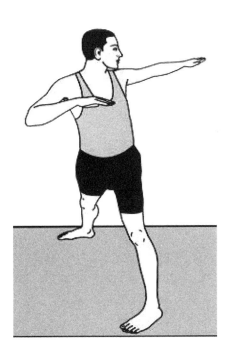

iv. Now standing firmly on the floor, exhale (Krishna) and twist to the right side without bending the right hand.

v. Simultaneously, bend the left hand to move it closer to the chest; then turn the head rightward and look at the right fingers.

vi. Now return to the centre while inhaling (Radhey) and repeat the same process leftward.

vii. Slowly, speed up to your comfort.

viii. Perform it for 25 rounds.

ix. Make sure twisting is done above the waist and the legs remain outstretched throughout.

x. Then, decrease the speed and and come to a standstill.

xi. Finally, come into Shithil Tadasan (See page 25) and relax.

2. Jumping Jacks

Procedure

i. Stand up straight—in an upright position—with both feet joined together and arms by your sides, i.e. Saral Tadasan (See page 25).

ii. With a vigorous jump, spread your feet about three feet apart—sideways—and simultaneously raise your arms to touch or clap the hands over your head.

iii. Now with another jump, come back to the initial position.

iv. Make sure your upper body reamains erect throughout the *asan*.

v. You should keep both arms straight while raising them over your head and lowering them down.

vi. As you jump to spread your feet, inhale (Radhey) and as you jump back to the initial position, exhale (Krishna).

vii. This completes one round; repeat these steps for 10-20 rounds.

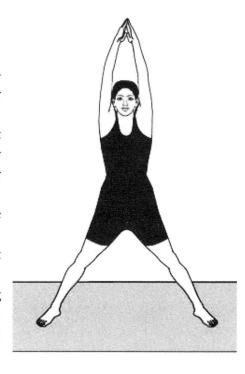

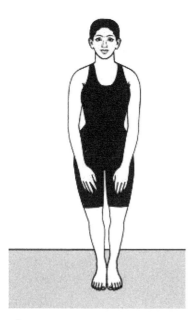

Variation - 1

Alternatively, instead of raising your hands sideways up, raise them vertically—from the front portion of your body.

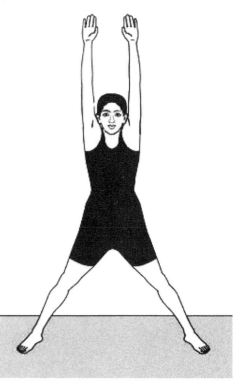

3. Forward and Backward Bending

Procedure

i.   Stand up straight—in an upright position—with both feet joined together and arms by your sides, i.e. Saral Tadasan (See page 25).

ii. Gradually, stretch out both arms straight above the head and keep the palms facing forward.

iii. As you inhale (Radhey), stretch the upper body backward as far as possible, making an arch-like shape with the upper body and arms.

iv. Make sure both the arms remain extended above your head.

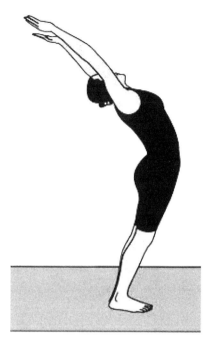

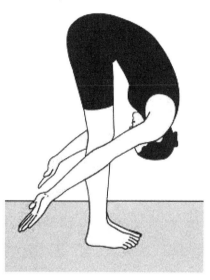
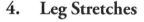

v.   As you exhale (Krishna), lean forward to your comfort.

vi.   Again while inhaling (Radhey), raise your upper body, stretch it backward and then without a pause, bend it forward with an exhalation (Krishna).

vii. Always bend only from the waist and try to make free and smooth movements.

viii. Practice the movements for 15-25 times.

ix.   Lastly, slow down your movement and come to a standstill.

4. Leg Stretches

Procedure

i.   Stand up straight—in an upright position—with both feet joined together and arms by your sides, i.e. Saral Tadasan (See page 25).

ii. Gradually, spread your feet about 2.5-3 feet apart and also gently swivel your left foot to the left.

iii. Then, gently raise your arms

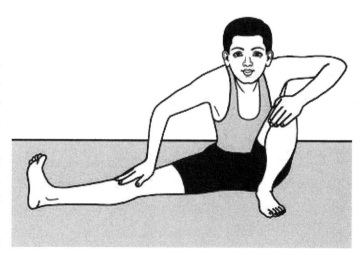

in front of you at shoulder level.

iv. Now, inhale (Radhey) in this position.

v. While exhaling (Krishna), slowly bend your right knee and lower your buttocks down to the floor in such a way that they almost touch your right ankle.

vi. When your left leg is fully outstretched, make sure your back remains erect as well.

vii. Maintain this position for 15-20 seconds, breathing normally.

viii. Come back to the standing position.

ix. Repeat the same method with the left leg.

Variation – 1

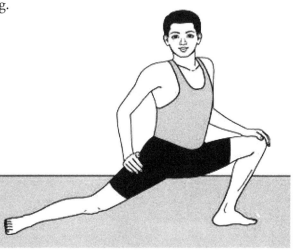

i. Stand up straight—in an upright position—with both feet joined together and arms by your sides, i.e. Saral Tadasan (See page 25).

ii. Comfortably, spread your feet about 2.5-3 feet apart.

iii. Gently swivel your left foot to the left completely and inhale (Radhey).

iv. While exhaling (Krishna), bend your left leg at the left knee and let your right leg outstretch fully.

v. Simultaneously, arch back your upper body—as much as you can.

vi. Place your left hand on your left knee and overlap the right hand on the left hand.

vii. Maintain this position for 15-20 seconds, breathing normally.

viii. Come back to the standing position.

ix. Repeat the same method with your right leg.

Variation – 2

i. Stand up straight—in an upright position—with both feet joined together and arms by your sides, i.e. Saral Tadasan (See page 25).

ii. Spread your feet about 2.5-3 feet apart.

iii. Gently sviwel both the feet to the right completely.

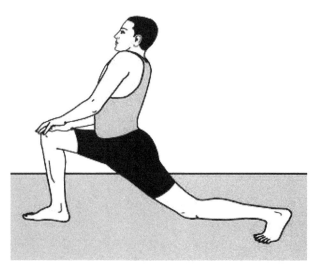

iv. Inhale (Radhey) in this state.

v. While exhaling (Krishna), slowly bend your right knee and let your left leg stretch fully.

vi. Simultaneously, arch your upper body slightly backward to your comfort.

vii. Place your right hand on your right knee and your left hand on your left waist.

viii. Maintain this position for 15-20 seconds, breathing normally.

ix. Return to the standing position.

x. Repeat the same method by turning both your feet leftward.

Variation - 3

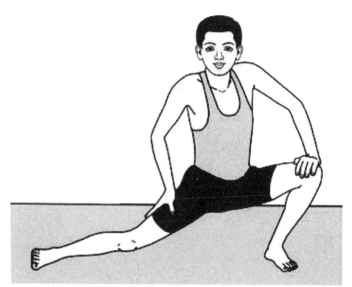

i. Stand up straight—in an upright position—with both feet joined together and arms by your sides, i.e. Saral Tadasan (See page 25).

ii. Now, spread your feet about 2.5-3 feet apart.

iii. Inhale (Radhey) in this state.

iv. While exhaling (Krishna), slowly bend your left knee and let your right leg stretch fully.

v. Simultaneously, arch your upper body backward to your comfort.

vi. Place your left hand on your left knee and your right hand on your right thigh.

vii. Maintain this position for 15-20 seconds, breathing normally.

viii. Come back to the standing position.

ix. Repeat the same method with your right leg.

5. On-Spot Jogging

Everyone is familiar with Jogging. Here, we will learn about "On-Spot Jogging." It is quite similar to the normal Jogging, except that it is done without actually moving your whole body back and forth, and thus it is called On-Spot Jogging. It is a very good way to warm up your joints and muscles prior to the start of *yogasans* and *pranayams*. On-Spot Jogging can be done without going outdoors; it can even be practiced in the balcony or veranda, near a window, etc.

Procedure

i. Stand up straight—in an upright position—with both feet joined together.

ii. Perform it by moving your arms back and forth customarily. For this, fold your arms at elbows, keeping the fists loose with the thumbs remaining outside. Now, start performing the following variations serially.

iii. Keep your shoulders relaxed.

Note: Do not speed up your jogging immediately on starting. Increase the speed gradually and comfortably.

The following variations form a single package of On-Spot Jogging. They are not individual exercises by themselves. So, the practitioner is advised not to come to a stand-still until all the four variations are performed.

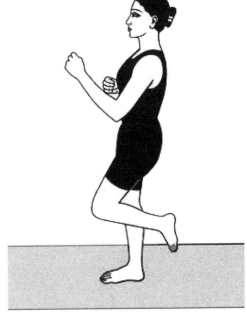

Variation - 1 (On-Spot Slow Jogging)

i. Gradually, start jogging on your toes.

ii. Jog for nearly 40-60 times, increasing your speed as much as you can.

iii. Now, slow down your speed; do not stop jogging.

iv. Reducing the speed gradually, prepare for the next variation, within next 15-20 on-spot strides.

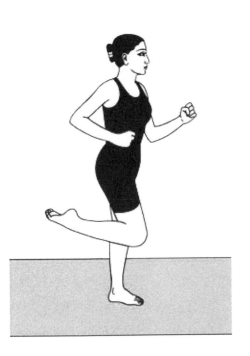

Variation - 2 (On-Spot Backward Jogging)

i. Lean slightly forward and slowly start jogging backward.

ii. While moving your foot backward, try to touch your buttocks with your heels lightly.

iii. Jog for 40-60 times, increasing your speed as much as you can.

iv. Now, slow down your speed but do not stop jogging.

v. Reducing the speed gradually, prepare for the next variation, within next 15-20 on-spot strides.

Variation - 3 (On-Spot Forward Jogging)

i. Lean backward a bit and start jogging.

ii. Try to lift your knees as high as possible.

iii. Slowly increase the speed.

iv. Jog for 40-60 times.

v. Now, slow down your speed; do not stop jogging.

vi. Reducing the speed gradually, prepare for the next variation, within 15-20 on-spot strides.

Variation - 4 (On-Spot Sideward Jogging)

i. Jog slowly while throwing your heels sideways—as if kicking sideways.

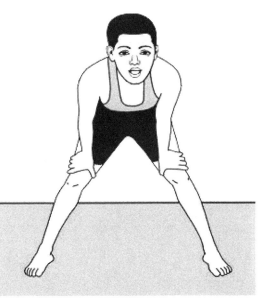

ii. As you speed up, try to lift your heels up, closer to the elbows.

iii. Jog for 30-40 times with speed.

iv. Now, slow down your speed and do slow jogging for 10-15 times, gradually coming to a stand-still.

v. Finally, come to a standstill.

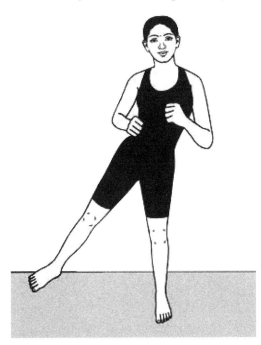
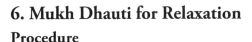

6. Mukh Dhauti for Relaxation

Procedure

i. Stand up straight—in an upright position—with both feet joined together and arms by your sides, i.e. Saral Tadasan (See page 25).

ii. Gradually, spread your feet about 1.5-2

19

feet apart.

iii. Gently lean forward, with both hands resting on the thighs slightly above your knees.

iv. Also, curl your upper body, creating a concave-like shape and look ahead.

v. Keeping your arms locked, inhale (Radhey) deeply through the nose.

vi. As you exhale (Krishna), blast out the air with maximum force through the mouth.

vii. Finally, come into Shithil Tadasan (See page 25) and relax.

Breathing Exercises

1. Arms In and Out Breathing

Procedure

i. Stand up straight—in an upright position—with both the feet joined together and arms by your sides, viz. Saral Tadasan (See page 25).

ii. Extend your arms in front of the chest, then bring them to your shoulder level and join your palms together.

iii. Breathing in (Radhey), gently spread both arms sideways.

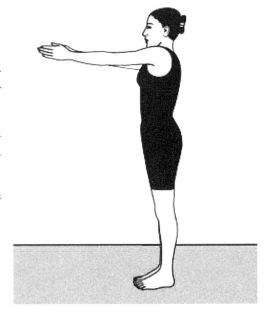

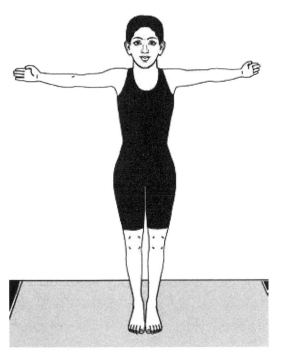

iv. Keep your arms parallel to the floor.

v. Breathing out (Krishna), smoothly move your arms forward, with both palms in contact with each other.

vi. Do it up to 10 times either slowly or dynamically.

vii. Make sure you do it non-stop by synchronizing with your breaths.

viii. Then, come into standing position with 6-12 inches' gap between your feet and relax.

ix. Be aware of your breathing rhythm.

2. Arms Stretch Breathing

Procedure

i. Stand up straight—in an upright position—with both feet joined together and arms by your sides, i.e. Saral Tadasan (See page 25).

ii. Maintain 4-6 inches' gap between the toes of your two feet forming "V" shape; join both heels together.

iii. Gently move your hands to the front of the chest.

iv. Interlock your fingers and rest them on the chest.

v. Then, move your elbows downward and relax.

Note: This is the initial position for all the variations.

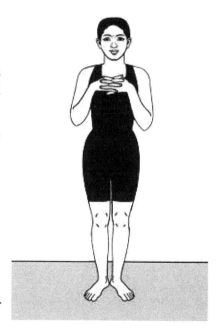

Variation - 1 (Horizontal Stretch at Shoulder Level)

i. Breathing in (Radhey), extend the arms in front of your chest by keeping your arms at shoulder level.

ii. Simultaneously, twist your hands in such a way that your palms turn outward.

iii. Breathing out (Krishna), reverse the process and draw your palms back to the chest.

iv. Lower your elbows downward and relax. This completes one cycle. Repeat it five times.

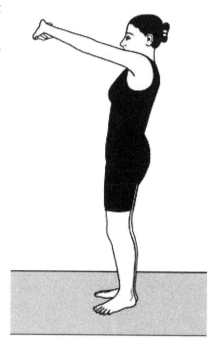

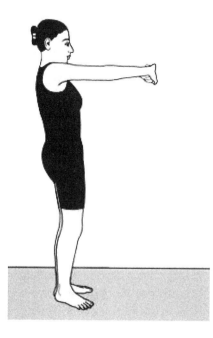

Variation - 2 (Forehead Level at 135 degrees)

i. Breathing in (Radhey), extend the arms in front— at the level of your forehead at 135 degrees.

ii. Simultaneously, twist your hands in such a way that your palms turn outward.

iii. Breathing out (Krishna), reverse the process and draw your palms back to the chest.

iv. Lower your elbows downward and relax.

v. This completes one cycle. Repeat it five times.

Variation - 3 (Vertical Stretch - Upward Level)

i. Breathing in (Radhey), stretch your arms upward, keeping them vertical; ensure your biceps stay on either side of your head.

ii. Simultaneously twist your hands—turning the palms upward.

iii. Breathing out (Krishna), reverse the process by taking your hands downward.

iv. Lower your elbows and relax.

v. This completes one cycle. Repeat it five times.

vi. Finally, return to normal, standing position by unlocking the fingers and dropping your hands.

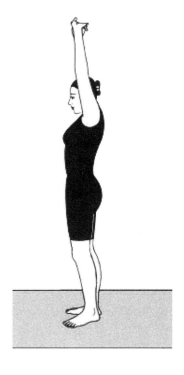

3. Ankles Stretch

Procedure

i. Stand up straight—in an upright position—with both the feet joined together and arms by your sides, i.e. Saral Tadasan (See page 25).

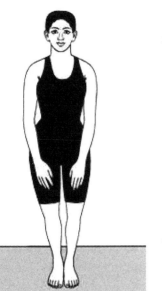

ii. Now, gaze at a point in front of you and keep your palms on the thighs.

iii. As you inhale (Radhey), raise your arms above the head and gradually lift the body on your toes.

iv. While exhaling (Krishna), lower both the arms and heels down.

v. Do it up to 10 times with the simultaneous movements of both—the arms and ankles.

vi. Ensure you do it non-stop and synchronizing with rhythmical breathing.

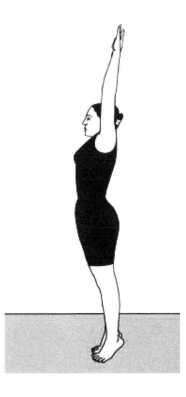

vii. Also, be aware of your breathing and on the stretched portion between the ankles and tiptoes.

viii. Eventually, come into Shithil Tadasan (See page 25) and relax.

4. Dog Breathing

Procedure

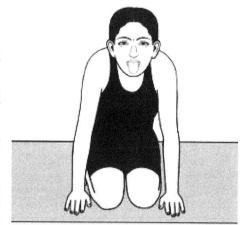

i. Sit down in Vajrasan (See page 113).

ii. Now, stretch your hands and keep your palms on the floor—beside the outer knees.

iii. Bending forward, arch your back slightly and look ahead.

iv. Open your mouth widely and stick out your tongue as much as you can.

v. Now, breathe in (Radhey) and breathe out (Krishna) through the mouth rapidly and forcibly; simultaneously expand and contract your abdomen dynamically—like a dog.

vi. Practice this process for around 20-40 seconds.

vii. Finally, get into Shashankasan (See page 117) and relax.

Contraindications

- Persons with epilepsy and high blood-pressure should not do it.

5. Rabbit Breathing

Procedure

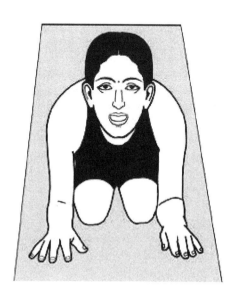

i. Come into Vajrasan (See page 113).

ii. Keeping your knees closer, lean forward and then place both the forearms flat on the ground so that the elbows lie on either side of your knees.

iii. Keep your chin about one foot above the ground; open your mouth and stick out your tongue partially—settling it between the lower lip and lower jaw.

iv. Fix both eyes on a point in front of you, look ahead.

v. Now, breathe like a rabbit by using the upper part of the chest.

vi. With the abdomen lying in-between your thighs, breathe rapidly through your mouth.

vii. Pant for 30-60 seconds in this state.

viii. Finally, regain the initial position and relax in Shashankasan (See page 117).

6. Raising Legs Straight

a. Alternate Legs Raising

Procedure

i. Lie flat on your back with both the feet joined together and touch the outer sides of the thighs with your hands, viz. Simple Supine Pose (See page 227).

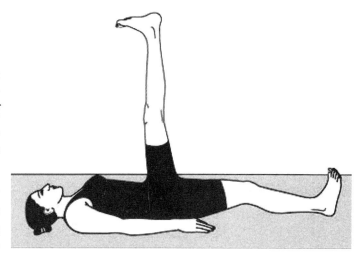

ii. As you inhale (Radhey), slowly lift your right leg upward as high as you can—keeping it stretched and perpendicular to the floor.

iii. As you exhale (Krishna), slowly lower the leg back to the ground.

iv. Repeat the above steps with your left leg.

v. This finishes one round; repeat these steps for 10-20 rounds.

b. Both Legs Raising

Procedure

i. Lie flat on your back with both the joined feet together and touch the outer sides of the thighs with your hands, viz. Simple Supine Pose (See page 227).

ii. As you inhale (Radhey), gradually lift both legs upward until they become perpendicular to the floor.

iii. As you exhale (Krishna), lower your legs down to the floor comfortably.

iv. This completes one round; repeat these steps for 10-20 rounds.

Contraindication

- Avoid this exercise if you suffer from lower back problems.

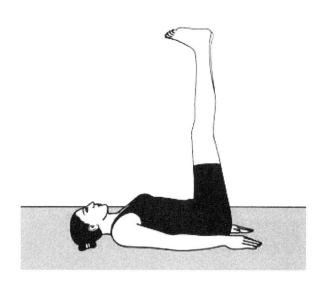

24

IV. Radhey Krishna Yogasans

A. Standing Asans

1. Saral Tadasan (Simple Palm Tree Pose)

Procedure

i. Come to a standing position.

ii. Now, keep both of your feet together.

iii. Then, distribute your body-weight equally on both feet.

iv. Keep your legs, spine, and head aligned.

v. Make sure your hands hang along the thighs, with the fingers outstretched.

vi. Breathe normally.

Note: This is the initial position for all standing *asans*.

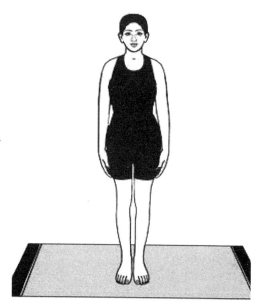

2. Shithil Tadasan (Relaxing Palm Tree Pose)

Procedure

i. Come to an upright position with the feet about 6-12 inches apart.

ii. Keep both hands hanging freely by the sides of your body, with the shoulders fully relaxed.

iii. Then, close your eyes; take some deep breaths and relax the whole body.

iv. Now, become aware of your breaths and feel the changes throughout the body.

Note: This is the relaxing pose after each standing *asan*.

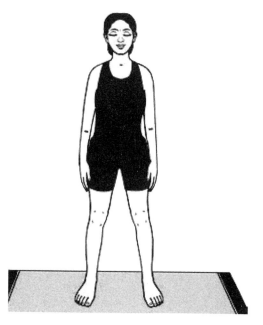

3. Hasta Utthanasan (Hand Raising Pose)

Procedure

i. Stand up straight—in an upright position—with both feet joined together and arms by your sides, i.e. Saral Tadasan (See page 25).

ii. Inhaling (Radhey), raise your arms sideways up to the shoulder level.

iii. When you exhale (Krishna), drop your head slightly backward and also move your arms above the head simultaneously.

iv. Cross the elbows above your face.

v. Keep your arms straight and gaze at the hands in this position.

vi. As you inhale (Radhey), lower your arms to the shoulder level and updrop the head to the initial position.

vii. Repeat the process for 5-10 times.

viii. Finally, come into Shithil Tadasan (See page 25) and relax.

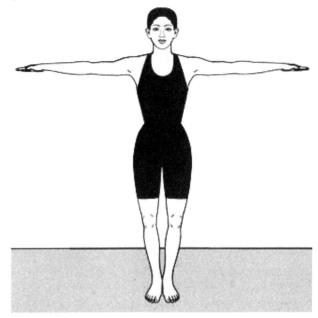

Awareness

✧ On the breaths synchronized with the physical movements

✧ On the extension of the arms, shoulders, and the expansion of the chest

✧ On mental uttering of the Divine Names "Radhey Krishna" along with your breaths

Benefits

✓ Hasta Utthanasan adds strength and suppleness to your arms and shoulders.

✓ When performed by synchronizing the breaths with the bodily movements, respiratory problems are naturally alleviated.

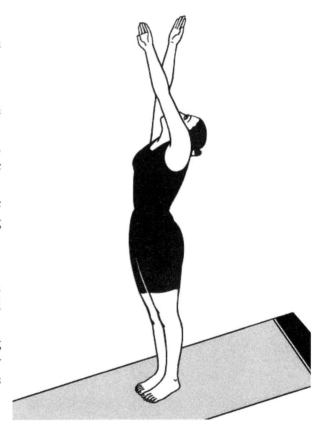

26

4. Akarna Dhanurasan (Bow and Arrow Pose)

Procedure

i. Stand up straight—in an upright position—with both feet joined together and arms by your sides, i.e. Saral Tadasan (See page 25).

ii. Now, spread your feet slightly apart and move the right leg with a short step forward.

iii. Then, clench your right fist and move your arm in front of the body—keeping it almost over the right foot and a bit above eye level.

iv. Now, slightly twist from your waist toward the left side.

v. Clench the left fist and take it slightly behind the right fist.

vi. Look at your right fist as if holding a bow and arrow, and then focus the eyes on an imaginary point.

vii. Inhaling (Radhey), gradually pull the left fist backward to the left ear—stretching both arms as though pulling the bow string.

viii. Move your head a bit backward with this motion, and keep the left elbow at the shoulder level.

ix. With an exhalation (Krishna), let the imaginary arrow go away and bring the left fist back behind the right fist.

x. Repeat the process for five more times.

xi. Then, repeat the same process on the other side.

xii. Ultimately, come to Shithil Tadasan (See page 25) and relax completely.

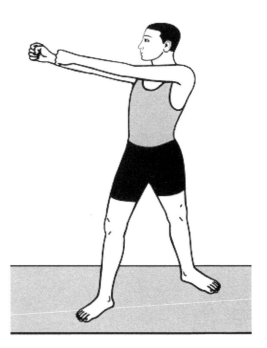

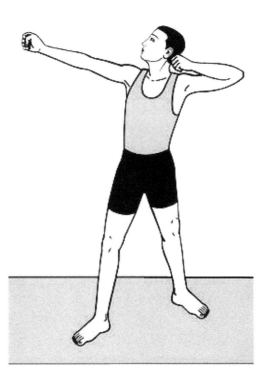

Awareness

✧ On the breaths synchronized with the movements of the arms

✧ On the extension in the arms and shoulders

✧ On becoming conscious of the presence of "Radhey Krishna" in your breaths

Benefits

✓ Akarna Dhanurasan is extremely beneficial for providing strength and suppleness to the shoulders and arms.

✓ It aids in removing stiffness from the neck and even helps in case of spondylitis.

✓ As in Vishwamitrasan (See page 86), it increases concentration ability too.

5. Kati Chakrasan (Waist Rotating Pose)

Procedure

i. Stand up straight—in an upright position— with both feet joined together and arms by your sides, i.e. Saral Tadasan (See page 25).

ii. Keep a distance of about 1.5-2 feet between your feet.

iii. Raise your arms in front and up to the level of your shoulders—with the palms facing each other.

iv. Let the distance between your arms be the same as the shoulder-width.

v. Inhale (Radhey) deeply in this position.

vi. Now exhale (Krishna) and twist your upper body to the right, as much as possible.

vii. Keep your arms locked at elbows throughout the process.

viii. Remain in this pose for 15-20 seconds with normal breathing.

ix. Inhale (Radhey) while returning to the centre.

x. Repeat each step three times on either side.

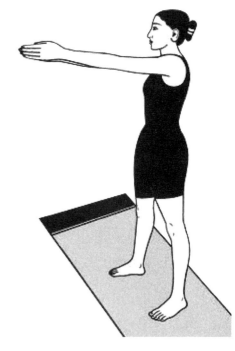

Note: Kati Chakrasan can also be done with fast movements—without maintaining the final position. Done this way, it can be practiced about 10-20 times.

Awareness

✦ On your bodily movements and breaths synchronized with them

✦ On the stretches and strains of the abdomen and spinal muscles

✦ On feeling the unbroken presence of "Radhey Krishna" along with your breathing

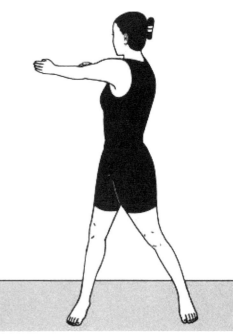

Benefits

- ✓ Kati Chakrasan tones up the abdomen, back, and buttocks.
- ✓ As this is a relaxing pose, it greatly benefits those who work the entire day at the office or home.

6. Monkey Stretch

Procedure

i. Stand up straight—in an upright position—with both feet joined together and arms by your sides, i.e. Saral Tadasan (See page 25).

ii. Spread your feet about 1.5 feet apart and loosen the fists, resting them on the upper thighs.

iii. Inhale (Radhey) deeply and with a slow exhalation (Krishna), bend your torso laterally rightward.

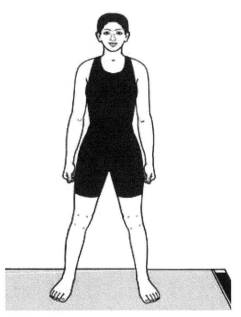

iv. Also, slide the left hand downward along the outer side of the left leg, and pull your right hand up into the armpit.

v. Make sure your hips and shoulders face forward and the spine is stretched laterally.

vi. Inhale (Radhey); then slowly return to the centre by moving both hands back to the thighs.

vii. Repeat the same process on the opposite side.

viii. This completes one round, practice for 5-10 rounds.

ix. Finally, come to Shithil Tadasan (See page 25) and relax.

Awareness

- ✧ On the breaths synchronized with the rightward and leftward movements
- ✧ On the stretched sides
- ✧ On spontaneously chanting Divine Names "Radhey Krishna" mentally, along with your breaths

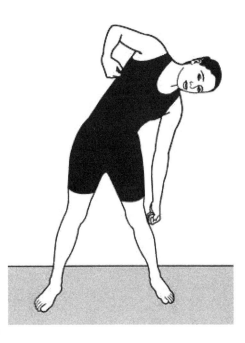

Benefits

- ✓ Monkey Stretch massages, loosens, and exercises the sides of the waist.
- ✓ It also balances the right and left groups of postural muscles.

7. Samakonasan (Right Angle Pose)

Procedure

i. Stand up straight—in an upright position —with both feet joined together and arms by your sides, i.e. Saral Tadasan (See page 25).

ii. Inhaling (Radhey), raise your arms straight above the head and bend the wrists to point the fingers forward—allowing your hands to go limp freely.

iii. Exhaling (Krishna), slowly bend forward from the hips by pushing the buttocks outward a bit until the upper body is parallel to the floor.

iv. Ensure your legs remain locked—forming a right angle with the trunk.

v. Align the head, neck, spine, and arms.

vi. Gaze continuously, at the fingers in the final state.

vii. With normal breathing, remain in this pose for 15-20 seconds.

viii. Inhaling (Radhey), slowly regain the base position.

ix. Repeat it twice.

x. Lastly, come into Shithil Tadasan (See page 25) and relax.

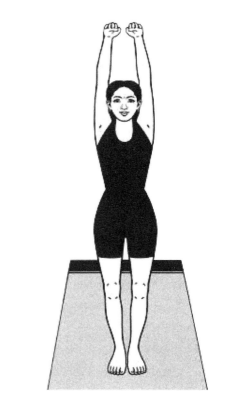

Awareness

✧ On the forward bends and upward movements synchronized with the breaths

✧ On the balance

✧ On uttering the Sacred Names "Radhey Krishna" flowing with your breaths

Benefits

✓ Particularly, Samakonasan is considered to be effective for the upper back and the spinal curvature.

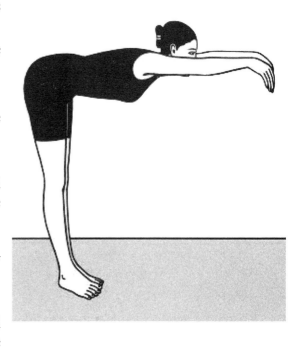

✓ It also reduces tension and anxiety as one remains longer in the forward bending position.

Contraindication

- People with severe sciatica should avoid it.

8. Ardh Kati Chakrasan (Lateral Arc Pose)

Procedure

i. Stand up straight—in an upright position—with both feet joined together and arms by your sides, i.e. Saral Tadasan (See page 25).

ii. With an inhalation (Radhey), slowly raise your right arm above the head with the biceps touching the right ear.

iii. Make sure your arms, head, and legs remain straight in this position.

iv. Now, stretch the right arm upward and while exhaling (Krishna), slowly bend the trunk to the left—as low as possible.

v. Let the left palm slide down slowly along the left thigh.

vi. Do not bend your right elbow or the knees.

vii. Hold the pose for 15-20 seconds with normal breathing.

viii. Inhaling (Radhey), come back to the centre and lower the right arm.

ix. Similarly, perform the above process with your left arm.

x. Repeat it up to three times on either side.

xi. Finally, come into Shithil Tadasan (See page 25) and relax.

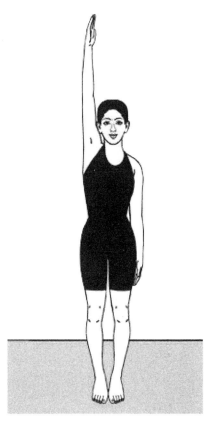

Awareness

✧ On the inhalations and exhalations along with the movements synchronized with them

✧ On the stretch in the arms, legs, hips, and the neck

✧ On feeling the Holy Names "Radhey Krishna" in your breaths

Benefits

✓ Ardh Kati Chakrasan helps decrease fat in the waist girlde and strengthens the spine.

✓ Additionally, it improves the functioning of the liver.

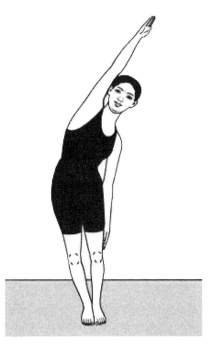

9. Meru Prishthasan (Spinal Back Pose)

Procedure

i. Stand up straight—in an upright position—with both feet joined together and arms by your sides, i.e. Saral Tadasan (See page 25).

ii. Keep a distance of about 1.5-2 feet between both the feet and spin both the toes slightly outward.

iii. Inhaling (Radhey), raise the arms sideways up in line with the shoulders, and then turn the palms upward.

iv. Now, fold your arms at the elbows and place the finger-tips on the shoulders.

v. Make sure that the elbows point sideways in the stretched position.

vi. With an exhalation (Krishna), slowly twist to the right side as much as possible.

vii. Remain in this position for 15-20 seconds with normal breathing.

viii. With an inhalation (Radhey), return back to the centre.

ix. Similarly, practice on the left side.

x. Practice for three times on either side.

xi. Finally, come back to the initial position, and relax in Shithil Tadasan (See page 25).

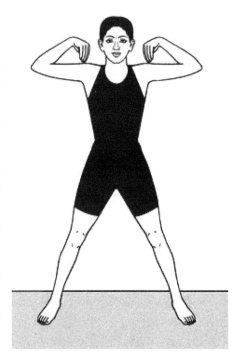

Note: Meru Prishthasan can be done dynamically too—without stopping on either side.

Awareness

✧ On the breaths and the movements synchronized with them

✧ On the stretch of upper back muscles

✧ On realizing the presence of "Radhey Krishna" in your breaths

Benefits

✓ Meru Prishthasan gives a perfect stretch to the spine.

✓ It strengthens the back muscles.

✓ It also removes stiffness from your shoulders and upper back.

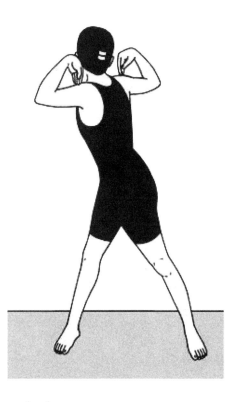

Contraindications

- People suffering from the back problems should not practice it.

10. Dolasan (Pendulum Pose)

Procedure

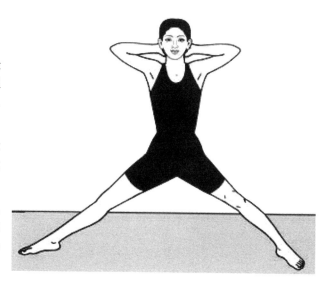

i. Stand up straight—in an upright position—with both feet joined together and arms by your sides, i.e. Saral Tadasan (See page 25).

ii. Spread your feet about 3-4 feet apart, and turn the right foot completely to the right.

iii. Inhaling (Radhey), raise your arms, and interlock the fingers at the back of the neck, pointing the elbows sideways.

iv. Exhaling (Krishna), slowly twist to the right and bend forward gradually, bringing your head as close to the right knee as possible.

v. Make sure the legs remains locked throughout the process.

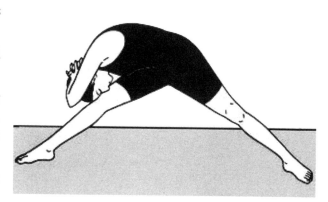

vi. Breathing normally, move your head and the torso to the left knee, and then from left knee to the right knee.

vii. Repeat the method around 5-10 times.

viii. Carefully, regain the upright position.

ix. Lastly, come into Shithil Tadasan (See page 25) and relax.

Awareness

✧ On the bodily movements synchronized with the breaths
✧ On the stretch of the back and knees
✧ On mentally chanting the Divine Names "Radhey Krishna" with your each breaths
✧ On the balance in the final position

Benefits

✓ Dolasan energizes tendons at the back of the knees and gives suppleness to the back.
✓ It tones up the spinal nerves.

Contraindications

- Dolasan should not be practiced by people suffering from backache, high blood pressure, and hiatus hernia.

11. Tadasan (Palm Tree Pose)

Procedure

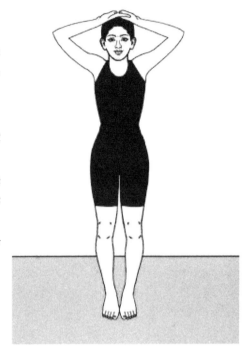

i. Stand up straight—in an upright position—with both feet joined together and arms by your sides, i.e. Saral Tadasan (See page 25).

ii. Spread your feet about 4-6 inches apart.

iii. Hold your body steady and distribute the weight equally on both feet.

iv. Raise your arms above the head; interlock the fingers with your palms facing upward, and place them on top of the head.

v. Fix your eyes on any point in front of you, slightly above the level of the head.

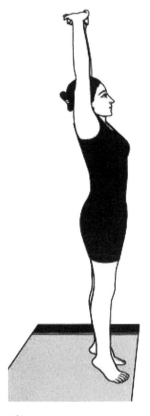

vi. With an inhalation (Radhey); stretch the arms, shoulders, and thighs as much as you can, and then expand the chest to your ability.

vii. Simultaneously, raise your heels and try to stand on the toes.

viii. Try and outstretch the body thoroughly.

ix. Continue to fix the eyes on the point to maintain the balance.

x. Maintain this position for 15-20 seconds with normal breathing.

xi. Initially, it is difficult to hold the balance but with practice, it becomes easier.

xii. Then, with an exhalation (Krishna), gradually lower the heels; bring down the hands and keep them on top of the head.

xiii. This is one round; practice this twice.

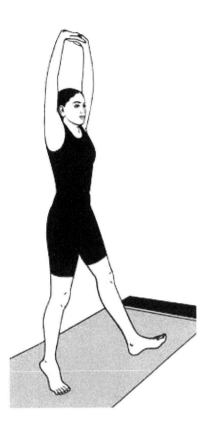

xiv. Finally, come to Shithil Tadasan (See page 25) and relax with deep breathing.

Variation - 1

i. Come to the final position of Tadasan (steps vi-ix).

ii. Then, lift one leg and extend it either forward or backward.

iii. Repeat the same process with the other leg.

iv. Practice it twice.

Variation - 2

i. Come to the final position of Tadasan (steps vi-ix).

ii. Gaze the eyes at your interlocked fingers, by stetching your neck slightly backward.

iii. This will require a longer period of practice to maintain the balance.

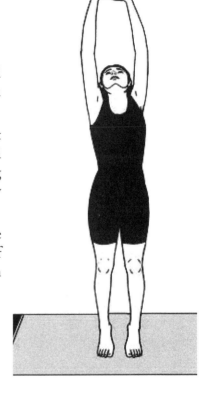

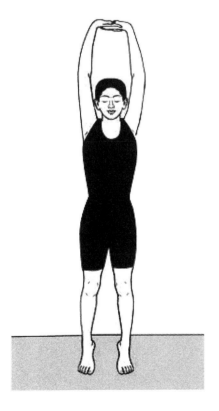

Variation - 3

i. Come to the final position of Tadasan (steps vi-ix).

ii. Close both the eyes.

iii. It is difficult to maintain the balance at first.

iv. After continuous practice, you can master this *asan* with eyes closed.

Note: You can do this variation only after mastering the main procedure of Tadasan with the eyes open.

Awareness

✧ On the breaths synchronized with the bodily movements

✧ On the balance

✧ On the stretches and strain caused by it

✧ On always feeling the omnipresence of "Radhey Krishna" in your breaths

Benefits

✓ Tadasan brings about exceptional stretching and loosening of the spine, which help clear the congestion of the spinal nerves.

✓ It is helps develop physical and mental balance.

✓ The stretching of the intestinal and digestive systems makes them healthier.

✓ It is also useful during the first six months of pregnancy to keep the abdominal muscles and nerves toned up well.

12. Tiryak Tadasan (Swaying Palm Tree Pose)

Procedure

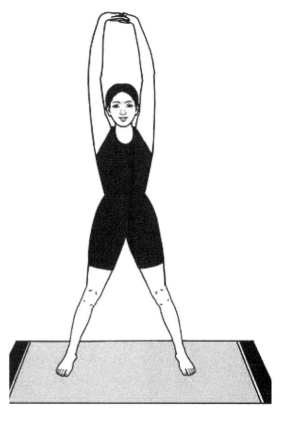

i. Stand up straight—in an upright position—with both feet joined together and arms by your sides, i.e. Saral Tadasan (See page 25).

ii. Now, spread out your feet, keeping a distance of about 1.5-2 feet between each other.

iii. Breathing in (Radhey), raise your arms above your head.

iv. Interlock your fingers and twists the wrists so that the palms face the sky.

v. Make sure your arms remain straight.

vi. Breathing out (Krishna), comfortably bend rightwards from the waist.

vii. Ensure you always bend laterally, keeping the spinal cord erect.

viii. Also, do not twist the head; it must be aligned with the arms.

ix. Maintain the final position to your comfort.

x. Breathing in (Radhey), come to an upright position.

xi. Practice on the other side.

xii. Finally exhaling (Radhey), lower the arms by the thighs and relax.

Awareness

✧ On the breaths synchronized with the bodily movements

✧ On the stretch of the sides of the waist

✧ On feeling the presence of "Radhey Krishna" in your each breath

✧ On the balance in the last state

Benefits

✓ Its benefits are the same as that of Tadasan (See page 34).

✓ Besides, it mainly gives a good massage to the waist, resulting in removing excessive fats from the waist girdle.

✓ It also gives a lateral stretch to the spine, making it extremely flexible.

13. Trikonasan (Triangle Pose)

Procedure

i. Stand up straight—in an upright position—with both feet joined together and arms by your sides, i.e. Saral Tadasan (See page 25).

ii. Now, spread your feet about 3-4 feet apart, with the toes pointing forward.

iii. Breathe in (Radhey) and raise your arms sideways to the shoulder level, with the palms facing downward.

iv. While breathing out (Krishna), gently bend down rightward from your waist, and try to touch your right foot with right hand.

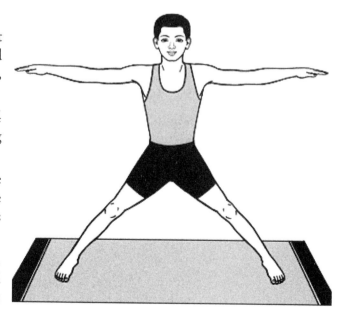

v. Do not bend either forward or backward; also make sure the hips, back of the legs, and the backbone stay in aligned.

vi. Keep your knees and the elbows locked.

vii. Straightening your left arm, align it with the right hand; ensure the right palm faces forward.

viii. Slightly twist your head to look at the left palm.

ix. Remain in this position for 15-20 seconds with normal breathing.

x. With a slow inhalation (Radhey), return to the central position; now outstretch both arms horizontally.

xi. Practice on the left side in the similar manner.

xii. This finishes one round; complete two more rounds.

xiii. Lastly, come into Shithil Tadasan (See page 25) and relax.

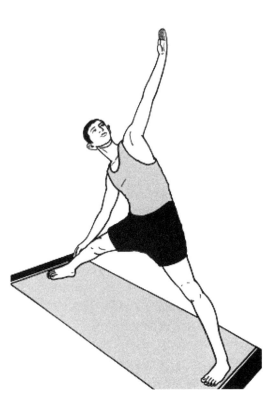

Variation - 1

i. Come to the final position of Trikonasan (steps vii-viii).

ii. Now, instead of keeping the left arm straight in line with the right arm, lower it over the ear until it is parallel to the floor, with the palm facing downward.

iii. Try to keep your body in one vertical level by not letting it lean forward or backward.

iv. Stretching the neck a little upward, try to look at the left palm.

v. Maintain the pose for 15-20 seconds with normal breathing.

vi. With an inhalation (Radhey), come to the central position with both hands stretched out horizontally.

vii. Perform the exercise on the left side in the same manner.

viii. This is one round; perform two more rounds.

ix. Lastly, come into Shithil Tadasan (See page 25) and relax.

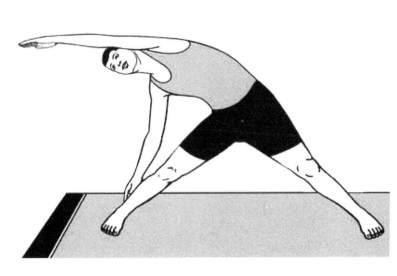

Variation – 2

i. Stand up straight—in an upright position—with both feet joined together and arms by your sides, i.e. Saral Tadasan (See page 25).

ii. Spread your feet about 3-4 feet apart from each other, with the toes pointing forward and both hands hanging along the sides of the body.

iii. Inhale (Radhey) in this position.

iv. While exhaling (Krishna), slowly bend down rightward from the waist.

v. Simultaneously, slide the right hand down along the outer side of the right leg as low as possible.

vi. Try to touch the right foot with the right hand, keeping the left arm loose along the left side of the body.

vii. Ensure neither to strain nor to bend forward or backward.

viii. Maintain the pose for 15-20 seconds with normal breathing.

ix. Breathing in (Radhey), come back to the upright position.

x. Repeat the same process on the left side.

xi. This is one round; perform for two more rounds.

xii. Finally, come to Shithil Tadasan (See page 25) and relax.

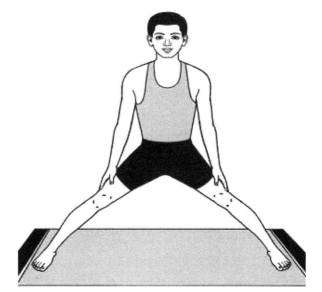

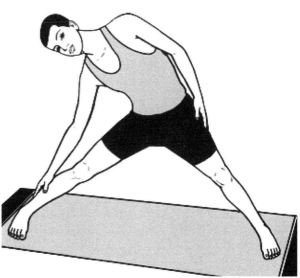

Note: All the above mentioned variations can also be done with the right foot swiveling to the right while bending to the right, and the left foot swiveling to the left while bending to the left.

Awareness

✧ On mentally chanting "Radhey Krishna" with your each breath and the movements synchronized with them

✧ On the balance

✧ On the stretches and strains of the side portions of the body in the final state

Benefits

✓ Trikonasan tones the nervous system and alleviates nervous depression.

✓ It alleviates constipation and improves digestion as there is induction of *jaṭharāgni* (digestive fire) and activates intestinal peristalsis.

✓ This pose not only prevents from flat foot, but it also helps correct the curvatures of the back and makes the spine extremely flexible.

✓ While stretching the sides of the body, the waist becomes very flexible and if regularly practiced, the waistline's fat is reduced considerably.

✓ It is also effective in strengthening both—the calf and the thigh—muscles.

Contraindications

- People with poor back conditions, and/or those who have undergone a recent abdominal surgery should avoid this *asan*.

14. Konasan (Angle Pose)

Procedure

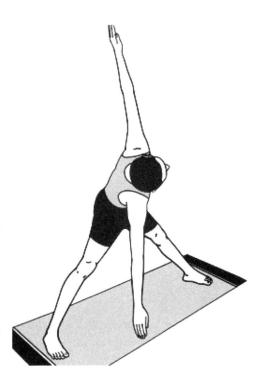

i. Stand up straight—in an upright position—with both feet joined together and arms by your sides, i.e. Saral Tadasan (See page 25).

ii. Spread your feet about 3-4 feet apart.

iii. Raise both arms sideways to the shoulder level, with the palms facing downward.

iv. Inhale (Radhey) in this position.

v. While exhaling (Krishna), twist your upper body and bend diagonally leftward from your waist.

vi. Touch the left foot with the right hand—whereas the left arm will slowly move into a slanted position above the shoulder—leveling both the arms in a single line.

vii. Turn your head to the left and look up toward the raised left hand.

viii. Stay in this posture for 15-20 seconds with normal breathing.

ix. Inhaling (Radhey) slowly and evenly, come back to the standing position.

x. Make sure your arms remain outstretched to the sides.

xi. Repeat the same process on the left side.

xii. This finishes one round; do two more rounds.

xiii. Lastly, come into Shithil Tadasan (See page 25) and relax.

Variation - 1 (Dynamic Konasan)

i. Practice the *asan* in the same way but unlike maintaining the final position (vii step of Konasan), return to the upright position—without any pause, and repeat on the other side.

ii. Practice this for at least ten rounds.

iii. Then come to Shithil Tadasan (See page 25) and relax.

Awareness

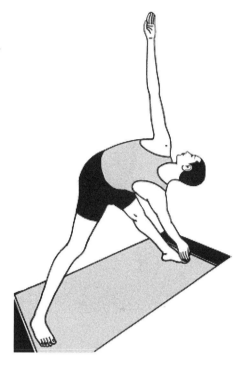

✦ On the twisting and bending movements and the breaths synchronized with them

✦ On the balance

✦ On the Divine Names "Radhey Krishna" in your each breath

✦ On the stretches of the sides of the body at the final state

Benefits

✓ Konasan gives rotational movements to your spine.

✓ It improves the functioning of the kidneys.

✓ *Yog* therapists also believe it as a suitable posture for strengthening the thigh muscles and toning the entire body.

✓ Exercises the leg and waist muscles, improves digestion, stimulates appetite, and thus alleviates constipation.

✓ It is very useful for women as it tones the reproductive organs.

✓ Further, it assists in reducing unnecessary fat from the abdominal area.

Contraindications

- People with severe back conditions, recent abdominal operations, heart problems, and severe hypertension should not do this *asan*.

15. Natarajasan (Lord Shiv's Dance)

Procedure

i. Stand up straight—in an upright position—with both feet joined together and arms by your sides, i.e. Saral Tadasan (See page 25).

ii. Spread your feet slightly apart; now gently bend and raise the left knee so that the left thigh is horizontal to the floor and the left foot is pointing away from the body and also slightly to the right side.

iii. Flex your right knee a bit, take your left arm across the body—almost paralleling the left thig with the palm facing downward.

iv. Now, bend your right elbow, right palm facing forward and forearm vertical.

v. Make sure that your right elbow lies exactly behind the left wrist.

vi. Perform Gyan Mudra with the right hand and look at the horizon at the same time.

vii. Try to remain in this stance as long as comfortable with normal breathing.

viii. Come back to the starting position by lowering your hands and legs carefully.

ix. Repeat on the other side in the same way.

x. Finally, come into Shithil Tadasan (See page 25) and relax.

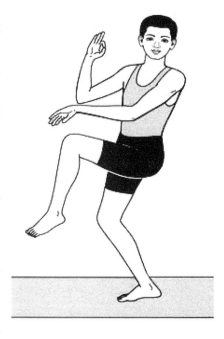

Awareness

✧ On always feeling the omnipresence of "Radhey Krishna"

✧ On the balance while maintaining the final position

Benefits

✓ As in Natavarasan, Natarajasan develops concentration and gives control over your body.

✓ Plus, your nervous system is balanced well, and legs are given extra suppleness.

16. Dhruvasan (Dhruv's Pose)

Procedure

i. Stand up straight—in an upright position—with both feet joined together and arms by your sides, i.e. Saral Tadasan (See page 25).

ii. Bending the right knee gently, place the right sole on the left thigh.

iii. Set the right heel at the root of the left thigh, with the toes pointing downward.

iv. To maintain balance, firmly hold your left foot on the ground.

v. Join your hands in Namaskar Mudra.

vi. With normal breathing, be in this position for as long as you are comfortable.

vii. Then, slowly release your hands and bring the right

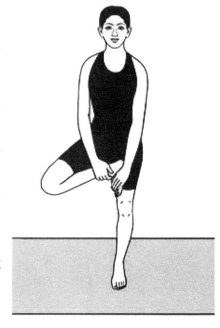

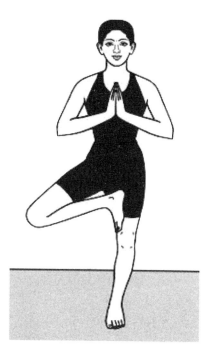

leg down to the ground.

viii. Repeat with the other leg similarly.

ix. Lastly, come to Shithil Tadasan (See page 25) and relax.

Variation – 1

In the final position—as explained above in step iv—raise your arms above your head and join the palms.

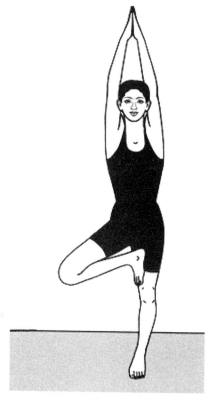

Awareness

✧ On the Divine Names "Radhey Krishna" flowing with your breaths
✧ On the raised foot and the rooted foot on the ground
✧ On the balance in the final position

Benefits

✓ Dhruvasan improves both—physical and mental balance.
✓ The nervous system develops well.
✓ The leg muscles are toned excellently.

17. Utthit Lolasan (Swinging while Standing)

Procedure

i. Stand up straight—in an upright position—with both feet joined together and arms by your sides, viz. Saral Tadasan (See page 25).

ii. Spread the feet 3-4 feet apart.

iii. Now inhale (Radhey); raise the arms up above the head; keep them straight.

iv. Next, bend the wrists to let the hands hang freely, with the palms facing downward.

v. Exhaling (Krishna), lean the upper body from the waist, letting it move freely downward; simultaneously allow your head and the arms to pass through the legs.

vi. Move your head and hands as far behind the feet as possible.

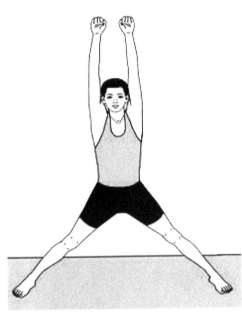

vii. Ensure that the knees and the elbows remain locked.

viii. Your trunk should move freely—without any jerks.

ix. Inhaling (Radhey), return slowly to the upright position with the hands above the head.

x. Repeat it for 5-10 times.

xi. Eventually, come into Shithil Tadasan (See page 25) and relax.

Awareness

◇ On the movements and breaths synchronized with them
◇ On becoming conscious of the omnipresence of "Radhey Krishna"
◇ On loosening your body

Benefits

✓ Utthit Lolasan keeps us very vigorous because it helps eliminate fatigue by improving blood-circulation and toning up the spinal nerves.

✓ It provides adequate exercise to the back muscles, loosens the hips, and massages the

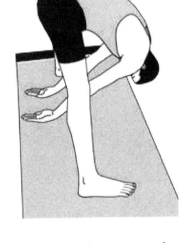

internal organs.

✓ It is a blessing for those who have been suffering from respiratory problems like asthma, as it stimulates the lungs by opening up the alveoli.

✓ It also eases tension and various psychiatric cases.

Contraindications

- People affected with high blood-pressure and back problems should avoid this *asan*.

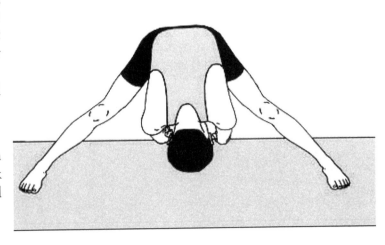

18. Natavarasan (Lord Krishna's Pose)

Procedure

i. Stand up straight—in an upright position—with both feet joined together and arms by your sides, i.e. Saral Tadasan (See page 25).

ii. Focus on a fixed point at the eye level.

iii. Move your right foot to the outer side of the left calf so that outer side of your left foot touches the right toes; rest your right toes on the floor.

iv. Ensure the sole of the right foot remains almost vertical.

v. Fold both arms at the elblows to the right side as if playing a flute like Lord Krishna.

vi. Make sure your right palm faces forward and the left palm backward.

vii. The index and the little fingers of your hands should be straight, while the remaining fingers should be folded.

viii. Turning the head a little bit to the left side, look at a point, slightly on the right side and downward.

ix. Remain in this stance for as long as possible with normal breathing.

x. While regaining the Saral Tadasan, lower your arms to the sides, and right foot to the floor.

xi. Repeat the above procedure with the other set of hands and feet.

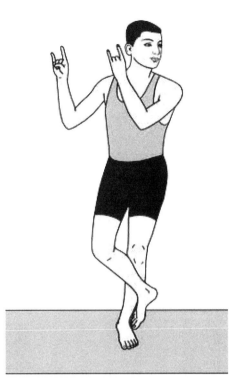

Awareness

✧ On mentally chanting "Radhey Krishna" with your breaths
✧ On the balance in the final position

Benefits

✓ Natavarasan particularly develops concentration.
✓ It helps in controlling the nerves.

19. Dwikonasan (Double Angle Pose)

Procedure

i. Stand up straight—in an upright position—with both feet joined together and arms by your sides, i.e. Saral Tadasan (See page 25).

ii. Now, spread your feet about 1-1.5 foot apart.

iii. Gradually, bring your arms behind the back and interlock the fingers tightly, resting them on your coccyx (tailbone).

iv. Breathe in (Radhey).

v. While breathing out (Krishna), start leaning your body downward in front from the hips; and simultaneously lift up your arms behind the back as higher as possible.

vi. Keep your legs and arms stretched.

vii. Raise your head a bit and look forward.

viii. Be in this pose for 15-20 seconds with deep and even breathing.

ix. Return to the upright position by lowering your arms smoothly.

x. Repeat it around three times.

xi. Finally, come into Shithil Tadasan (See page 25) and relax.

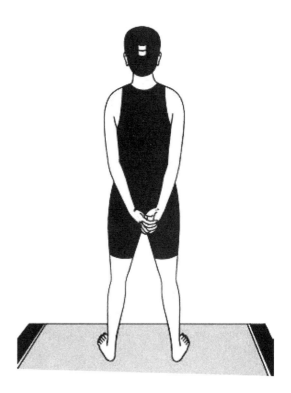

Awareness

✧ On mentally chanting "Radhey Krishna" along with breaths and the bodily movements synchronized with them

✧ On the stretch of the arms, shoulders, upper back, and the buttocks

✧ On spontaneously feeling the omnipresence of "Radhey Krishna"

Benefits

✓ The whole body gains superb flexibility.

✓ The chest is flattened and the neck becomes shapely.

✓ Dwikonasan is considerably helpful for the internal muscles of the upper back and the shoulders.

Contraindications

- People having problems in the shoulder joints should not include this *asan* in their *Yog* package.

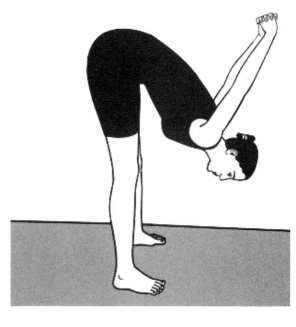

46

20. Tiryak Kati Chakrasan (Swaying Waist Rotating Pose)

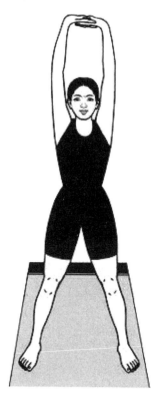

Procedure

i. Stand up straight—in an upright position— with both feet joined together and arms by your sides, viz. Saral Tadasan (See page 25).

ii. Keep a distance of about 1.5-2 feet between your feet.

iii. Interlock your fingers comfortably; then inhaling (Radhey), raise your arms above the head and turn the palms upward.

iv. With an exhalation (Krishna), bend forward from the hips, keeping your trunk, head, and arms parallel to the floor.

v. Fixing your eyes on the back of hands, try to keep your back horizontally straight.

vi. With normal breathing, slowly move the arms and trunk to the left as far as possible and then to the right.

vii. Keep moving the arms and trunk to either side for 5-10 times, breathing normally.

viii. Inhaling (Radhey), come back to the centre and return to Saral Tadasan.

ix. Finally, come into Shithil Tadasan (See page 25) and relax.

Awareness

✧ On breathing in and out along with the movements

✧ On the balance while moving on either side

✧ On the stretch of the abdomen and spinal muscles

✧ On the Sacred Names "Radhey Krishna" with your breaths

Benefits

✓ By Tiryak Kati Chakrasan, the abdomen, back, and buttocks are toned up superbly.

✓ As in Kati Chakrasan, it relaxes your whole body after a long day's work.

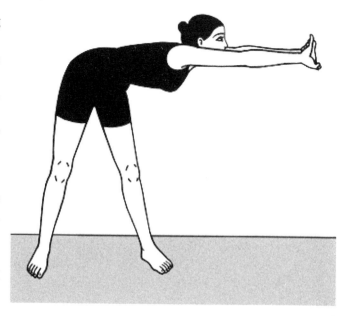

21. Utthit Janu Shirasan (Standing Head between Knees Pose)

Procedure

i. Stand up straight—in an upright position—with both feet joined together and arms by your sides, i.e. Saral Tadasan (See page 25).

ii. Spread your feet about 2-3 feet apart.

iii. Raise your arms slowly above the head while inhaling (Radhey), and then turn the palms forward.

iv. With an exhalation (Krishna), bend forward from the hips, and try to wrap your legs with the arms through the calves.

v. Either grasp the other wrist or anchor both hands behind the calves.

vi. Bring your head toward the knees by bending the elbows a bit and tightening the grip.

vii. Make sure your legs stay locked without any strain.

viii. Rest the body against the thighs while holding the wrist and elbows behind calves at this stage.

ix. Try to stay in this position for 15-20 seconds with normal breathing.

x. Now while inhaling (Radhey), return gently to Saral Tadasan.

xi. This is one round; practice for up to three rounds.

xii. Finally, come to Shithil Tadasan (See page 25) and relax.

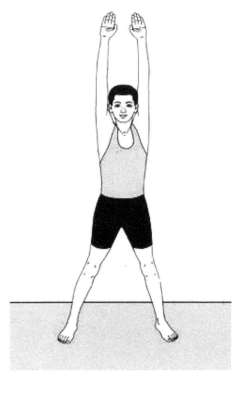

Variation – 1

i. Stand up straight—in an upright position—with both feet joined together and arms by your sides, i.e. Saral Tadasan (See page 25).

ii. Spread your feet about 2-3 feet apart.

iii. With an inhalation (Radhey), raise your arms slowly above the head; turn the palms forward.

iv. While exhaling (Krishna), bend forward from the hips to touch the knee with the forehead, and wrap your arms around the tendons, bending the legs a little.

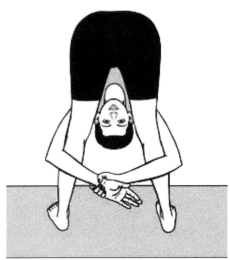

v. Ensure your arms stays horizontal with the elbows pointing out to the sides.

vi. Now, try to bring the hands forward in between the legs; pushing your head backward, interlock the fingers firmly behind the back of the neck.

vii. Slowly straighten your legs without letting the fingers slip from behind the neck; do not strain.

viii. Hold this position as long as you are comfortable with normal breathing.

ix. With an inhalation (Radhey), gently release the hands by bending the knees, and return to the standing position.

x. This is one round; practice for up to three rounds.

xi. Finally, drop the arms and relax fully in Shithil Tadasan (See page 25).

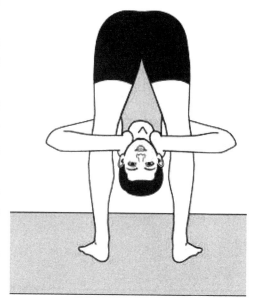

Note: This variation can be practiced by those who have perfected the first one.

Awareness
✧ On breathing in and out along with the various movements of your body
✧ On the straightened legs, the stretch of the back muscles, and the neck
✧ On spontaneous chanting (mental) of Holy Names "Radhey Krishna" with your breaths

Benefits
✓ Utthit Janu Shirasan activates the pancreas, gives massage to the spinal nerves, and enhances the blood flow to the head region, resulting in revitalizing the brain to a large extent.
✓ This pose not only relaxes the hip joints and hamstring muscles, but also strengthens the knees tremendously.

Contraindications
- People affected with severe back conditions, heart disease, and hypertension should omit this *asan* from their exercise package.

22. Shirsha Angushth Yogasan (Head to Toe Pose)
Procedure
i. Stand up straight—in an upright position—with both feet joined together and arms by your sides, i.e. Saral Tadasan (See page 25).

ii. Spread the feet about 3-4 feet apart; bring the hands back and interlock the fingers with the palms facing inward.

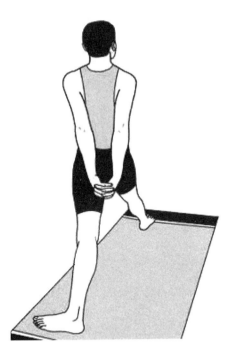

iii. Keeping your arms straight, twist the body to the right and turn the right foot slightly to the right.

iv. Inhale (Radhey) in this position.

v. With an exhalation (Krishna), bend forward, stretching your arms as high as possible.

vi. Slightly bend your right knee and bring the head to the inner side of the right foot; try to touch the big toe with the head.

vii. Keeping the arms locked, relax the shoulders and allow the arms to fall forward to the limit of your comfort.

viii. Stay in this position for 15-20 seconds, breathing normally.

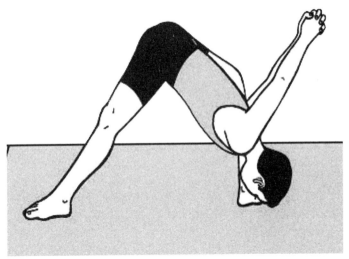

ix. Inhaling (Radhey), return to the standing position.

x. Repeat the whole process on the other side in the same manner.

xi. This completes one round; practice for two more rounds.

xii. Lastly, come into Shithil Tadasan (See page 25) and relax.

Awareness

✧ On the breaths synchronized with the various movements
✧ On feeling the presence of "Radhey Krishna" in your breaths
✧ On the stretches and strains caused by them
✧ On the balance

Benefits

✓ As lateral stretch is given to the spine, Shirsha Angushth Yogasan activates the nervous system.
✓ It improves the digestive organs, alleviates constipation, and thus induces good appetite.
✓ In this pose, the hamstring muscles are also stretched.
✓ Besides, it makes the waist flexible and reduces unwanted fat.

Contraindications

- People suffering from heart disease, high blood-pressure, and poor back conditions like slipped-disc, sciatica, and sacral infection, etc. should not include it in their *Yog* package.

23. Utthit Ek Pada Janu Shirasan (Standing Separate Leg Head to Knee Pose)

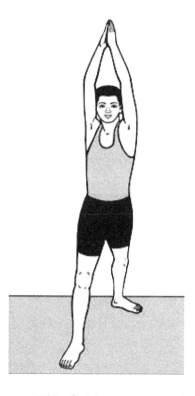

Procedure

i. Stand up straight—in an upright position—with both feet joined together and arms by your sides, i.e. Saral Tadasan (See page 25).

ii. Spread your feet about 2-3 feet apart and turn the right foot rightward.

iii. Also, turn your hips, torso, and face directly to the right.

iv. Inhaling (Radhey), slowly raise your arms above the head and join the palms together.

v. Exhaling (Krishna), slowly lean forward from the hips, move the forehead downward and touch the right knee; then place the joined hands over the toes.

vi. You should stretch the hands forward until the elbows are straight.

vii. Stay in this pose for 15-20 seconds, breathing normally.

viii. Slowly, regain the central position.

ix. Perform the process with the left leg too.

x. This finishes one round; practice for two more rounds.

xi. Then, lower the arms slowly.

xii. Lastly, come into Shithil Tadasan (See page 25) and relax.

Awareness

✧ On the breaths synchronized with the forward and upward movements

✧ On the stretches and strains in the arms, legs, hips, and neck

✧ On feeling the presence of "Radhey Krishna" along with your each breath

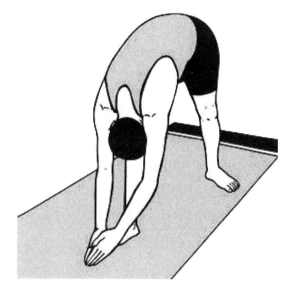

Benefits

✓ Utthit Ek Pada Janu Shirasan tones up the various digestive organs and removes gastric, constipation, indigestion, and menstrual problems.

✓ Not only making the spine flexible, but it also activates and tones up all the spinal nerves.

✓ It increases the blood flow to the brain, helping circulation to the pituitary and thyroid glands.

✓ Utthit Ek Pada Janu Shirasan removes nasal and throat diseases; strengthens the thighs, and slims the abdomen, waistline, hips, and buttocks.

✓ Additionally, it also gives mental benefits like improving concentration, memory power, etc.

Contraindications

- People who have severe hypertension, vertigo (dizziness), cenical spondylitis, serious back problems, sciatica, heart disease, hernia, and disc prolapses should avoid this *asan*.

24. Ek Pada Bakasan (One Legged Crane Pose)

Procedure

i. Stand up straight—in an upright position—with both feet joined together and arms by your sides, i.e. Saral Tadasan (See page 25).

ii. Now, gaze at a fixed point in front of you.

iii. Lift your right leg off the floor until the thigh becomes parallel with the floor.

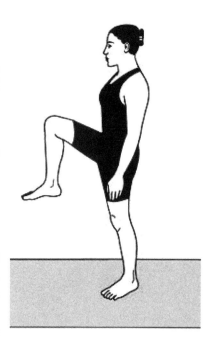

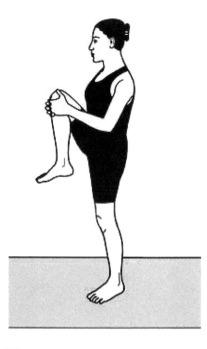

iv. Ensure that the left leg stays firm and stretched so that the whole body-weight can be transferred onto it.

v. Slowly raise the hands and interlock the fingers and place them on the outer side of the right knee and hold it firmly.

vi. Inhale (Radhey) and while exhaling (Krishna) draw the right knee toward the chest and at the same time keep the head erect and arch the spine slightly.

vii. Stay in this posture for 15-20 seconds, breathing normally.

viii. Inhaling (Radhey), lower the right foot to the floor; return to the starting position.

ix. Likewise, repeat it with the other set of arms and legs.

x. This ends one round; do up to three rounds.

xi. Finally, come to Shithil Tadasan (See page 25) and relax.

Awareness
- ✧ On the balance
- ✧ On always feeling the presence of "Radhey Krishna" with your breaths

Benefits
- ✓ Ek Pada Bakasan superbly tones up the leg muscles.
- ✓ It helps increase the flexibility of the hip portion.
- ✓ It naturally brings one's body and mind into balance.

25. Utthanasan (Squat and Rise Pose)

Procedure

i. Stand up straight—in an upright position—with both feet joined together and arms by your sides, i.e. Saral Tadasan (See page 25).

ii. Keep a distance of one foot between your feet.

iii. Outstretch the hands to the front at the shoulder level and inhale (Radhey).

iv. Exhaling (Krishna), slowly bend your knees until the thighs become parallel to the floor (as if you are sitting on an imaginary chair).

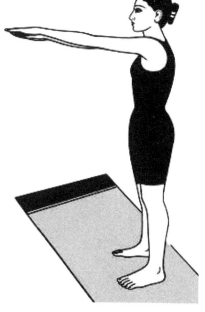

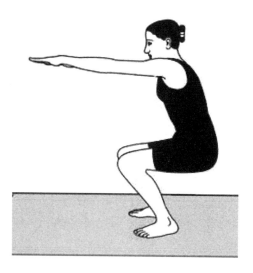

v. Maintaining your balance, keep the spine and head as much straight as possible.

vi. Be in this position for 15-20 seconds with normal breathing.

vii. Inhale (Radhey) while coming up to the standing position.

viii. Repeat it up to three times.

ix. Lastly, come into Shithil Tadasan (See page no. 25) and relax.

Variation – 1

i. Keep a distance of one foot between your feet.

ii. Bring the hands to the front at shoulder level and then inhale (Radhey).

iii. Now, exhale (Krishna); next slowly go downward to a squatting position, and also simultaneously raise the heels so that you can stand on the toes.

iv. Keep the spine and head erect; then bend the legs, making sure they do not touch the floor.

v. Try to remain in this pose for 15-20 seconds with normal breathing.

vi. Inhale (Radhey) while returning to the standing position.

vii. Do it up to three times.

viii. Lastly, come into Shithil Tadasan (See page 25) and relax.

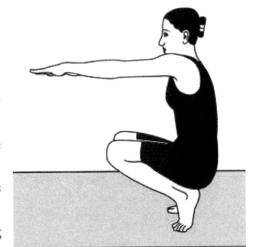

Awareness

✧ On the downward and upward movements of your legs and the breaths synchronized with them

✧ On the balance in the final state

✧ On mental chanting of the Holy Names "Radhey Krishna" in your breaths

Benefits

✓ Its regular and diligent practice helps strengthen the knees and leg muscles.

✓ Utthanasan also strengthens the muscles in the middle of the back, pelvis, and uterus.

✓ It tones up both—the thighs and ankles.

Contraindications

- Women with prolapse of the uterus should avoid it. It should not be practiced after the first pregnancy trimester.

26. Utthit Pashchimottanasan (Standing Separate Leg Stretching Pose)

Procedure

i. Stand up straight—in an upright position—with both feet joined together and arms by your sides, i.e. Saral Tadasan (See page 25).

ii. Spread your feet about 3-4 feet apart, and simultaneously raise your arms to the sides—aligning with the shoulders.

iii. Inhale (Radhey) in this position.

iv. As you exhale (Krishna), gradually bend forward from the lower back, and move your hands down to the outer sides of the feet and ankles.

v. Grasp the middle part of the feet near the heels.

vi. Pulling on the feet and keeping the legs locked, take your forehead downward as far as possible, trying to touch the floor; look ahead.

vii. With normal breathing, stay in this pose for 15-20 seconds.

viii. Now release your hands, and with an inhalation (Radhey), gradually return to Saral Tadasan.

ix. Also, bring the arms to the level of the shoulders simultaneously.

x. This ends one round; repeat for two more rounds.

xi. Ultimately, come to Shithil Tadasan (See page 25) and relax.

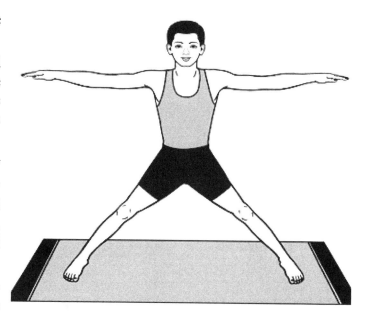

Awareness

✧ On the forward and upward movements along with breaths synchronized with them

✧ On the stretch in the arms, legs, shoulders, and the lower back

✧ On mental uttering of "Radhey Krishna" spontaneously with your breaths

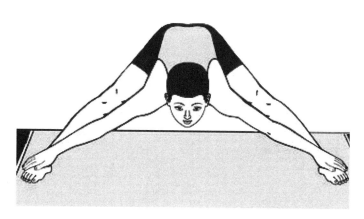

Benefits

✓ Utthit Pashchimottanasan helps prevent sciatica; it gives flexibility to the thighs, calves, pelvis, ankles, hip joints, and the lower part of the spine.

✓ It also stimulates the function of the internal abdominal

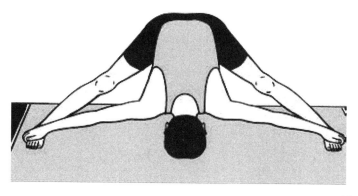

organs, along with strengthening of the stomach muscles.

Contraindications

- People who have sever hypertension, vertigo (dizziness), spondylitis, serious back problems, sciatica, heart disease, hernia, and disc prolapses should not practice this *asan*.

27. Veerbhadrasan (Warrior's Pose)

Procedure

i. Stand up straight—in an upright position—with both feet joined together and arms by your sides, i.e. Saral Tadasan (See page 25).

ii. Spread your feet about three feet apart; turn the right foot to the right and twist the whole body to the right side.

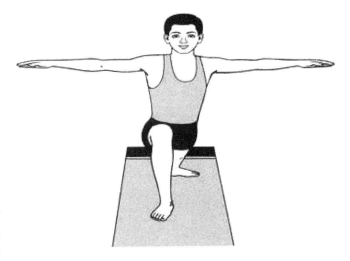

iii. Now inhale (Radhey); while exhaling (Krishna), fold your right knee in such a way that your right thigh becomes parallel to the floor.

iv. Simultaneously, slide the left foot backward to form a strong base for the posture.

v. Ensure that the right shin remains perpendicular to the floor.

vi. Also, push your left heel back to stretch the left leg.

vii. With an inhalation (Radhey), raise your arms out to the sides and then overhead and form Namaste Mudra.

viii. Exhaling (Krishna), try to fix your eyes on the joined hands with Namaste Mudra.

ix. Now with an inhalation (Radhey), try to stretch your spine and head as much backward as possible.

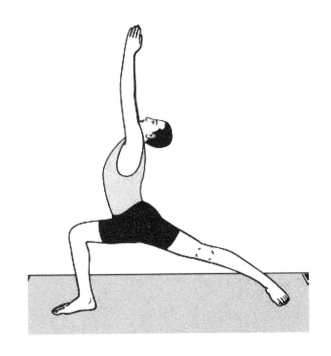

x. Stretch out your arms backward with a gaze at the joined hands with Namaste Mudra for the balance of the whole body.

xi. Stay in this position at your ease with normal breathing.

xii. To come back to the base pose, follow the reverse order of the whole process.

xiii. Repeat the same process with the other leg.

xiv. Lastly, come to Shithil Tadasan (See page 25) and relax.

Variation - 1

i. Stand up straight—in an upright position—with both feet joined together and arms by your sides, i.e. Saral Tadasan (See page 25).

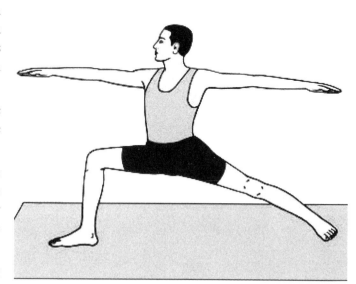

ii. Spread your feet about three feet apart, and then swivel the right foot to the right.

iii. Now inhale (Radhey); while exhaling (Krishna), fold the right knee in such a way that the right thigh becomes parallel to the floor.

iv. Simultaneously, slide the left foot backward to form a strong base for the posture.

v. With a slow inhalation (Radhey), stretch out your arms to the sides at the shoulder level, with both palms facing downward.

vi. The arms should be stretched and parallel to the floor.

vii. Now, turning your face to the right, gaze at the finger-tips of the right hand to maintain the balance.

viii. Stay in this position to your comfort with normal breathing.

ix. Now following the reverse order of the steps to return back to the starting position.

x. Repeat the same process with the other leg.

xi. Lastly, come into Shithil Tadasan (See page 25) and relax.

Awareness

✧ On the breaths synchronized along with the physical movements
✧ On pressing the hips and knees
✧ On the unbroken remembering the Holy Names "Radhey Krishna" with your breaths
✧ On the balance in the final position

Benefits

✓ Veerbhadrasan is a great boon for all (especially women) as it exercises the lower abdomen, spinal column, and reproductive organs.

✓ Particularly, it relieves rheumatic pain, stiffness in the neck and shoulders, strengthens the legs, and makes the waist slimmer.

✓ It stimulates the heart and generates heat.

✓ The pain from standing or sitting all day while working is easily removed by practicing it systematically.

28. Ardh Chakrasan (Half Wheel Pose)

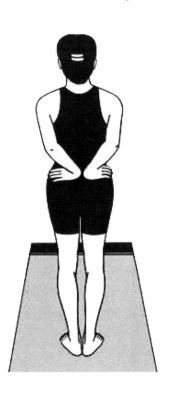

Procedure

i. Stand up straight—in an upright position—with both feet joined together and arms by your sides, i.e. Saral Tadasan (See page no 25).

ii. Place your palms and fingers at the back of the waist to support your back.

iii. All the fingers (including the thumb) will point forward.

iv. Inhale (Radhey), and simultaneously recline backward slowly and carefully from the lower back, letting your head fall backward.

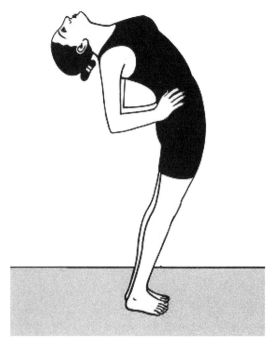

v. Keep the legs locked with a regular forward push at the hips.

vi. Attempt to stay for 15-20 seconds in this pose with normal breathing.

vii. Exhaling (Krishna), comfortably regain the upright position.

viii. Perform two more times in the same manner.

ix. Then, lower hands down gradually.

   x. Lastly, come into Shithil Tadasan (See page 25) and relax.

Awareness
✧ On the breaths synchronized with the different bodily movements
✧ On the stretch of the legs, hips, lower back, and neck
✧ On becoming conscious of the omnipresence of "Radhey Krishna" while breathing in and out

Benefits
✓ Ardh Chakrasan has several benefits such as removing back pain, relocating the spine, and even activizing the spinal nerves.
✓ It improves blood circulation to the head.
✓ It strengthens the neck muscles and shoulders; also shapes the body by widening the chest.

Contraindications
- People who have undergone a recent abdominal surgical operation and those with giddiness should not perform it.

29. Pada Hastasan (Standing Head to Knee Pose)

Procedure

   i. Stand up straight—in an upright position—with both feet joined together and arms by your sides, i.e. Saral Tadasan (See page 25).

   ii. Inhale (Radhey) slowly, and simultaneously raise both hands above the head with the palms facing forward.

  iii. Keeping your hands straight, stretch the body upward from the waist.

  iv. As you exhale (Krishna), bend forward from your hips till your hands touch the floor; then slowly letting the trunk go down, place both the hands down on either side of the feet, and try to touch the knees with the chin.

   v. Try not to bend the trunk at the middle; keep it straight from the waist to the neck.

  vi. Also, keep both knees locked in this condition.

 vii. With normal breathing, hold the position for 15-20 seconds.

viii. Keep the whole body relaxed in this state.

  ix. With an inhalation (Radhey), return to Saral Tadasan.

   x. This is one round; do it for two more rounds.

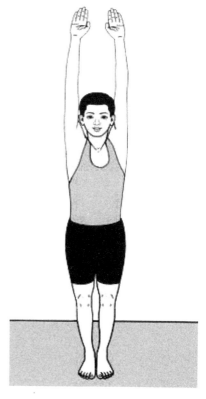

xi. Lastly, come to Shithil Tadasan (See page 25) and relax.

Note: Pada Hastasan can also be done with fast movements—without maintaining the final position. In the beginning, it can be practiced 5-10 rounds and with a regular practice, it can be done for about 20-30 rounds.

Variation - 1

i. Stand up straight—in an upright position—with both feet joined together and arms by your sides, i.e. Saral Tadasan (See page 25).

ii. Slowly inhale (Radhey).

iii. Now with an exhalation (Krishna), slowly lean forward, letting your arms go limp.

iv. Next, place your fingers underneath the toes, and pull the feet upward while trying to touch the knees with the forehead.

v. Remain in this position for 15-20 seconds with normal breathing.

vi. Then, return to Saral Tadasan with an inhalation (Radhey).

vii. This ends one round; repeat for two more rounds.

viii. Finally, come to Shithil Tadasan (See page 25) and relax.

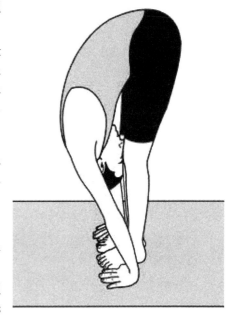

Awareness

✧ On the breaths synchronized with the movements
✧ On the mental chanting of the Holy Names "Radhey Krishna" through your breaths
✧ On the relaxation of the back muscles and hamstrings in the final position

Benefits

✓ The movements in Pada Hastasan massage and tone the digestive organs; it rectifies flatulence, constipation, indigestion, and strengthens the thighs.

✓ Besides all these, the hamstrings and spinal nerves are strengthened and the spine is made extremely flexible.

✓ Pada Hastasan is great boon for women as it helps in preventing menstrual problems.

✓ Many *Yog* practitioners do it mostly for enhancing the blood flow to the head region.

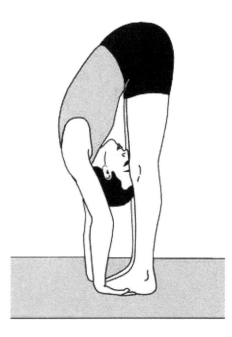

✓ It even eliminates problems related to the thyroid and pituitary glands.

Contraindications

- People who have sever hypertension (high blood pressure), vertigo (dizziness), serious back problems, sciatica, heart disease, hernia, and disc prolapses should avoid this *asan*.

30. Utthit Ardh Chandrasan (Standing Half Moon Pose)

Procedure

i. Stand up straight—in an upright position—with both feet joined together and arms by your sides, i.e. Saral Tadasan (See page 25).

ii. Inhaling (Radhey), raise your arms above the head, then interlock your fingers tightly, and point the index fingers upward.

iii. As you exhale (Krishna), slowly bend laterally from the waist to the right, letting the trunk go down as low as possible.

iv. Then, stretch your legs and the arms with the biceps touching the ears.

v. Push the hips forward to maintain proper balance.

vi. With normal breathing, try to hold this pose for 15-20 seconds.

vii. While inhaling (Radhey), gradually return back to the centre, and then bend gradually to the left side in the same way.

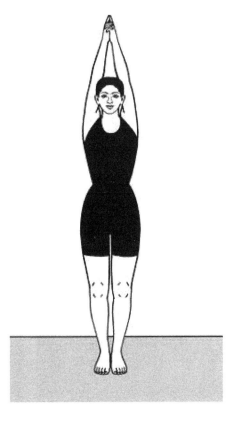
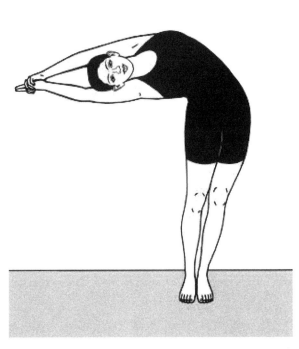

viii. This is one round; practice up to three rounds.

ix. Now lowering the arms, return to Saral Tadasan.

x. Finally, come into Shithil Tadasan (See page 25) and relax.

Awareness
- ✧ On the breaths synchronized with the sideward bends
- ✧ On becoming conscious of the omnipresence of "Radhey Krishna"
- ✧ On the stretch of the shoulder blades, hips, and the arms
- ✧ On the balance

Benefits
- ✓ Utthit Ardh Chandrasan rejuvenates the body by supplying instant energy and vitality, developing and strengthening every muscle in the central part of the body (particularly in the abdomen), and increasing the suppleness of the body.
- ✓ It perfects the kidney function.
- ✓ It cures enlargement of the liver and spleen, dyspepsia (indigestion), and even constipation.

Contraindications
- - People with back conditions and those who have undergone recent abdominal surgery should omit this practice.

31. Moordhasan (Crown-Based Pose)

Procedure

i. Stand up straight—in an upright position—with both feet joined together and arms by your sides, i.e. Saral Tadasan (See page 25).

ii. Spread your feet about 3-4 feet apart.

iii. Inhale (Radhey); while exhaling (Krishna), bend forward from the hips, and place the hands on the floor.

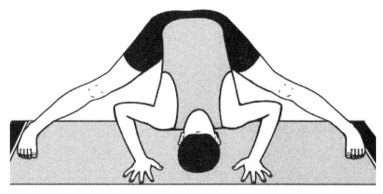

iv. Distribute the body-weight equally on the limbs.

v. Place the crown of the head on the floor between the hands.

vi. Balancing on your head and legs, raise the arms; bring them over the back and catch hold of one of the wrists.

vii. Now, raise your heels, and maintain balance on your head and toes.

viii. Remain in this position for 15-20 seconds with normal breathing.

ix. With an inhalation (Radhey), regain the central position after replacing the hands on the floor.

x. This finishes one round; practice for up to three rounds.

xi. Eventually, come to Shithil Tadasan (See page 25) and relax.

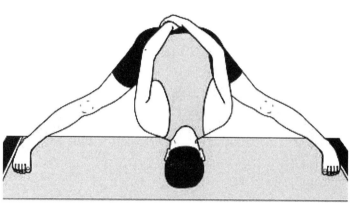

Awareness

✧ On the breaths synchronized with the various movements
✧ On the stretches and strains caused by them
✧ On the balance in the final position
✧ On mental chanting of the Sacred Names "Radhey Krishna" along with inhalations and exhalations

Benefits

✓ Moordhasan is extremely good for people suffering from low blood pressure.
✓ This *asan* also acts as a boon as it helps increase the balance of the nervous system.
✓ As other standing poses, it makes the neck and head muscles stronger.
✓ It supplies sufficient blood to the brain, and thus rejuvenates the practitioners.
✓ Many *Yog* therapists also take it as a supportive pose for Shirshasan.

Contraindications

- People suffering from high blood pressure, heart problems, ear problems, eye problems, organically defective pituitary or thyroid glands, arteriosclerosis, cerebral or other thrombosis, asthma, tuberculosis, slipped-disc, cold or sinusitis, impure blood, and weak spine should omit it.

32. Drut Utkatasan (Dynamic Energy Pose)

Procedure

i. Stand up straight—in an upright position—with both feet joined together and arms by your sides, i.e. Saral Tadasan (See page 25).

ii. Inhaling (Radhey), raise your arms up above the head and join the palms together.

iii. As you exhale (Krishna), slowly lower your body and bend the knees until the buttocks rest on the floor.

iv. Hold this pose for 15-20 seconds with normal breathing.

v. Keep your knees and feet together throughout the process.

vi. Also, straighten both—the arms and trunk—at all times.

vii. Inhaling (Radhey), gradually raise your body to the upright position, with both hands above the head.

viii. This is one round; practice two more rounds.

ix. Finally, come to Shithil Tadasan (See page 25) and relax.

Awareness

✧ On the breaths synchronized along with the different physical movements

✧ On the stretch of the thighs, buttocks, trunk, and the arms

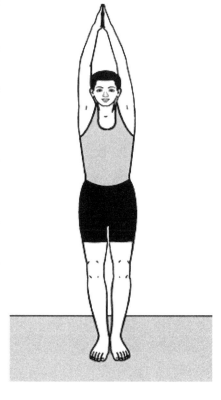

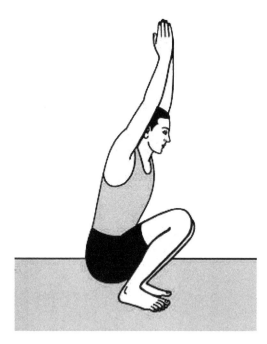

✧ On becoming conscious of the presence of "Radhey Krishna" in your breaths

Benefits

✓ Drut Utkatasan helps prevent the risk of sciatica and slipped-disc.

✓ It alleviates back pains.

✓ It strengthens the muscles of the back and legs.

Contraindications

- Women with prolapse of the uterus should avoid it. It should not be performed after three months of pregnancy.

33. Hasta Utthan Ardh Chakrasan (Hands Stretched Half Wheel Pose)

Procedure

i. Stand up straight—in an upright position—with both feet joined together and arms by your sides, i.e. Saral Tadasan (See page 25).

ii. Inhaling (Radhey), raise your arms above the head, interlock the fingers tightly, with the index fingers pointing upward.

iii. Inhaling (Radhey), slowly and carefully recline backward from the lower back.

iv. Make sure your legs remain locked throughout the process.

v. Now smoothly push your hips forward to stretch further.

vi. Attempt to stay for 15-20 seconds in this pose with normal breathing.

vii. Exhaling (Krishna), return to the upright position gently.

viii. Practice two more times likewise.

ix. Finally, lower the arms down and return back to Shithil Tadasan (See page 25) and relax.

For Other Details: See Ardh Chakrasan (Page 58)

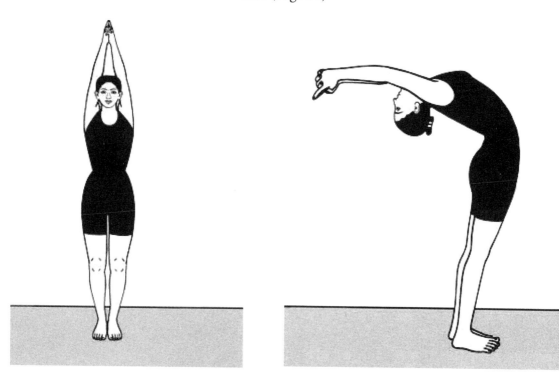

34. Parshwa Konasan (Lateral Angle Pose)
Procedure

i. Stand up straight—in an upright position—with both feet joined together and arms by your sides, i.e. Saral Tadasan (See page 25).

ii. As in Konasan (See page 40), spread both feet about 3-4 feet apart.

iii. Swivel your right foot 90 degrees to the right side of the body and your left leg slightly to the right, keeping it stretched out and locked at the knee.

iv. Without any force, push the hips and stomach forward.

v. Now, lean your upper body backward with the face, trunk, and the left leg facing forward.

vi. With an inhalation (Radhey), raise your hands up to the level of the shoulder.

vii. Then, bend down your right knee directly to the right, lowering the right thigh until it becomes parallel to the floor.

viii. Keep your arms straight at all times.

ix. With an exhalation (Krishna), bend the upper body rightward—slowly and consciously, placing the right elbow in front of the right knee and the fingertips touching the toes, with the right palm facing the front.

x. Ensure you raise your left arm vertically up and that you do not shift weight on the fingers; instead try to bear the whole weight on the bent leg.

xi. When both hands are in a straight line, turn the head to the left and look up toward the raised left hand.

xii. Hold the posture for 15-20 seconds with normal breathing.

xiii. Then inhaling (Radhey), slowly come back to the central position, with the hands stretched out.

xiv. Repeat the process on the left side.

xv. This ends one round; practice for two more rounds.

xvi. Finally, come to Shithil Tadasan (See page 25) and relax.

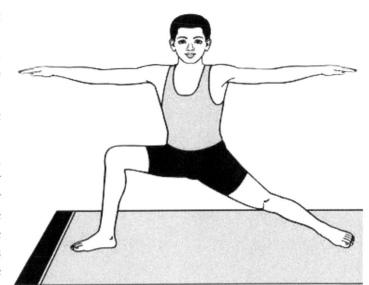

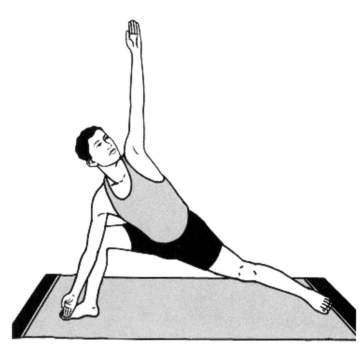

Awareness

✧ On breathing in and out along with the bending movements

✧ On always feeling the presence of "Radhey Krishna" in your every breath

✧ On the balance

Benefits

✓ This sideward bending exercise, Parshwa Konasan, expands the thorax (the part of the body between the neck and the stomach) along with strengthening the shoulder joints, hip joints, thighs, tendons, calf muscles, and the ankles.

✓ It helps reduce fat from your waist and the hip region.

✓ It helps cure lumbago (backache).

✓ It improves the spinal condition, and relieves arthritic and sciatic pains.

✓ Additionally, intestinal peristalsis is stimulated wonderfully by its regular practice.

Contraindications

- People with cardiac problems and recent abdominal surgeries should avoid this posture.

35. Parivritt Parshwa Konasan (Turned Back Lateral Angle Pose)

Procedure

i. Stand up straight—in an upright position—with both feet joined together and arms by your sides, i.e. Saral Tadasan (See page 25).

ii. Spread the feet about 3-4 feet apart.

iii. Turn the right foot 90 degrees to the right side of the body, and the left foot slightly to the right, keeping it outstretched and tight at the knee.

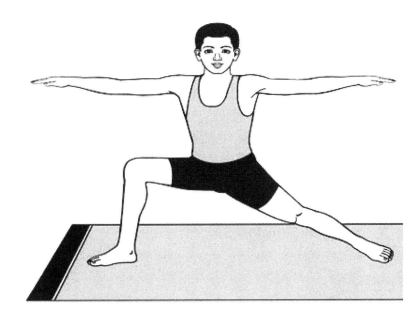

iv. Push your hips and stomach forward and lean the upper body backward with the face, trunk, and left leg facing the front.

v. With an inhalation (Radhey), raise hands up to the shoulder level.

vi. Bend the right knee directly to the right, lowering the right thigh until it is parallel to the floor.

vii. While exhaling (Krishna), twist and bend diagonally right from waist.

viii. Touch the right foot with the left fingers; your right hand will slowly move into a vertical position, above the shoulder.

ix. Use the fingers only to touch the right leg; do not put any pressure on the fingers.

x. Outstretch the left arm vertically to align both the arms in a single line.

xi. Turn your head to the right and look up toward the right hand.

xii. Remain in this position for 15-20 seconds with normal breathing.

xiii. Inhaling (Radhey), slowly come back to the central position in the reverse manner of the steps above.

xiv. Repeat the process on the left side.

xv. This completes one round; practice for two more rounds.

xvi. Come to Shithil Tadasan (See page 25) and relax.

Awareness

✧ On breathing in and out along with the twisting and bending movements
✧ On mentally chanting "Radhey Krishna" with your breaths
✧ On the balance in the final position

Benefits

✓ This effectual *asan* tones up the digestive organs, stimulates intestinal peristalsis, and helps in removing constipation.
✓ Parivritt Parshwa Konasan reduces unnecessary fat around the waist girdle—slimming the body down.
✓ Your spine is rejuvenated wholly.
✓ The the shoulders and hips are strengthened in extreme as well.
✓ The function of the kidneys improves greatly.

Contraindications

- People with spinal problems, recent abdominal surgeries, heart problems, and severe hypertension should avoid this posture.

36. Garudasan

Procedure

i. Stand up straight—in an upright position—with both feet joined together and arms by your sides, i.e. Saral Tadasan (See page 25).

ii. Fix your eyes at a fixed point in front of you—slightly below the eye level.

iii. Raise your right foot and intertwine the lower left leg with the right leg (especially left calf as shown in the figure) from the outer side.

iv. Make sure that your right thigh rests on the left thigh; the top of the right foot lies on the left calf, and the right big toe lies just above the inner side of the left ankle.

v. As you inhale (Radhey), fold your arms and bring them in front of the chest; then place the right elbow crossing the left elbow.

vi. Now, intertwine the forearms around each other, and join the palms to resemble an eagle's beak, or form Namaste Mudra.

vii. As you exhale (Krishna), slowly bend the left knee and lower your body until the right big toe touches the ground.

viii. Stretch your spine more; then turn the hips to the left, and force both knees on either side.

ix. Fixing eyes on a point, hold this final position to your capacity with normal breathing.

x. Return to the initial position as you inhale (Radhey); then slowly raise the body and eventually release the legs and hands.

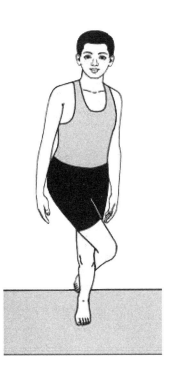
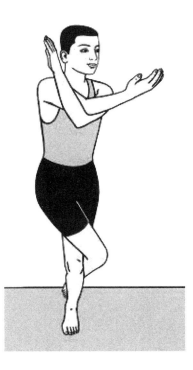
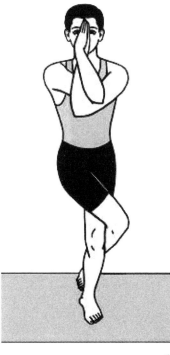

xi.   Practice the same process with the alternate set of legs and arms.

xii. Lastly, come into Shithil Tadasan (See page 25) and relax.

Awareness
- ✧ On the balance and the focus at a fixed point
- ✧ On the presence of "Radhey Krishna" in your each breath

Benefits
- ✓ Garudasan is extremely good for sciatica, rheumatism, and hydrocele.
- ✓ The nervous system gets toned very well.
- ✓ The joints of the legs and the arms are made more flexible along with the rise of strength in the muscles.
- ✓ It also removes stiffness in the shoulder.
- ✓ It offers a great relief in urinal problems.
- ✓ It is even recommended in case of cramps in the calf muscles for healing naturally.
- ✓ Females are also benefited because reproductive organs are toned well, and the kidneys get activated with adequately oxygenated blood.
- ✓ Most *Yog* experts even consider this *asan* helpful in controlling sexual passion.

Contraindication
- People with weak knees may avoid this practice.

37. Prishthasan (Back Pose)

Procedure

i.   Stand up straight—in an upright position—with both feet joined together and arms by your sides, i.e. Saral Tadasan (See page 25).

ii.   Spread your feet about one foot apart, with the toes slightly out to the sides.

iii. Inhaling (Radhey), bend your knees, taking them close to the floor as much as possible.

iv.   Meanwhile, also bend the trunk backward from the waist, and by moving your arms back, slowly reach down to hold your ankles.

v.   Now maintain balance, drop your head backward, trying to lower both—the head and the back—as closer to the floor as possible.

vi.   Hold this position from 15-20 seconds with normal breathing.

vii. Exhaling (Krishna), come back to the initial pose with both the feet apart.

viii. Repeat this for up to two times.

ix.   Finally, come into Shithil Tadasan (See page 25) and relax.

Variation – 1

As an alternative process, the hands could be placed on the waist to give support to the backward movement of the backbone, and then the hands be taken down stepwise to the thighs and legs.

70

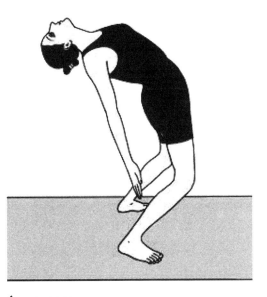 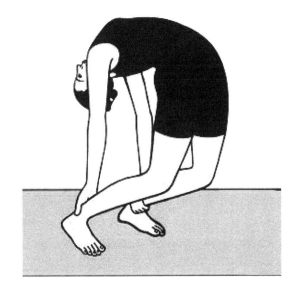

Awareness

✧ On your breaths synchronized with the different bodily movements
✧ On the stretches and strains caused by them
✧ On becoming conscious of the presence of "Radhey Krishna" in your each breath
✧ On the balance in the final position

Benefits

✓ Prishthasan strengthens the abdominal muscles and organs by stretching them fully.
✓ The blood circulation in the back is improved well, which stimulates and tones the nerves of the backbone.
✓ It makes the legs stronger and moresupple.

Contraindications

- People suffering from stomach ulcers, high blood pressure, coronary thrombosis, or back ailments should not practice it.

38. Parshwavottanasan (Standing Runner's Pose)

Procedure

i. Stand up straight, in an upright position, with both feet joined together and arms by your sides, i.e. Saral Tadasan (See page 25).

ii. Spread the feet about three feet apart.

iii. Bring your hands together behind the back to form Namaste Mudra.

iv. Inhaling (Radhey), turn your right foot to the right and twist the whole body to the right side.

v. With an exhalation (Krishna), bend forward from the hips with a straight spine until your nose touches the right knee.

vi. Stay in this pose at your ease with normal breathing.

vii. Come back to the starting position in the reverse order.

viii. Repeat the process on the next side in the similar manner.

ix. Lastly, come into Shithil Tadasan (See page 25) and relax.

Awareness

✧ On the bodily movements synchronized with the breaths

✧ On the stretch in the hamstrings

✧ On the pressure in the arms

✧ On mental uttering of "Radhey Krishna" with your breaths

Benefits

✓ Parshwavottanasan trims the waist by eliminating unnecessary fat.

✓ It also loosens the limbs of the body, removes rheumatic or joint pain, and thus helps the body to become very light and agile.

Contraindications:

- Those who are weak, ill, or with defective hands should not do it without proper guidance of a *Yog* expert.

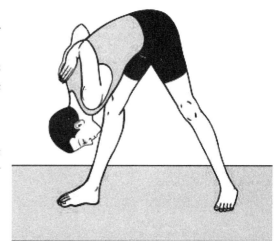

39. Utthit Hasta Padangushthasan

Procedure

i. Stand up straight—in an upright position—with both feet joined together and arms by your sides, i.e. Saral Tadasan (See page 25).

ii. Focus your eyes at a point in front of you at eye level.

iii. Inhaling (Radhey), bend your right knee and bring the right thigh as close to the chest as possible.

iv. Lock the left knee by stretching the left leg a bit backward.

v. Placing the right arm around the outside of the right thigh, catch hold of the big toe.

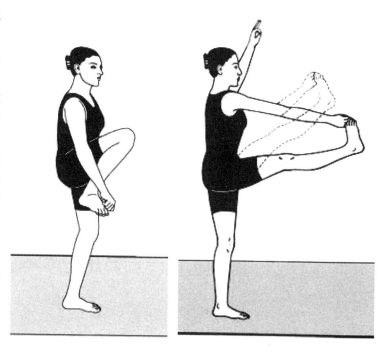

vi. Now, raise the left hand to the side for balance.

vii. As you exhale (Krishna), straighten the right leg; and slowly pull the big toe backward, as far as possible.

viii. Without bending the knees, maintain this posture for as long as comfortable with normal breathing.

ix. While coming back to the Saral Tadasan, inhale (Radhey); then exhaling (Krishna), release your right big toe from the grasp; bend the right leg slowly and unhurriedly; finally lower it to the floor.

x. Repeat these steps with alternate set of legs and arms.

xi. Eventually, come into Shithil Tadasan (See page 25) and relax.

Variation - 1

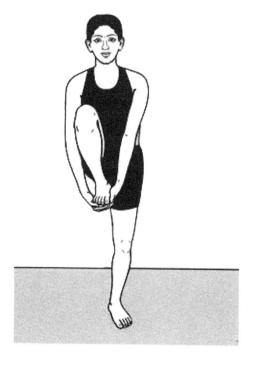

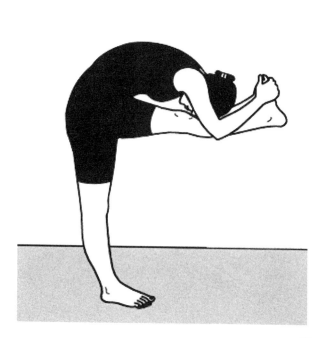

i. Stand up straight—in an upright position—with both feet joined together and arms by your sides, i.e. Saral Tadasan (See page 25).

ii. Fix the eyes at a point in front of you at eye level.

iii. Inhaling (Radhey), flex the right knee and bring the right thigh as close to the chest as possible.

iv. Lock your left knee, stretching the left leg a bit backward; then interlock your fingers and place them under the heel.

v. With an exhalation (Krishna), straighten the right leg and while using the arms as a lever, pull the right leg toward the head.

vi. Bending forward as necessary, try to touch your raised leg with the chin.

vii. Remain in this position for as long as is comfortable with normal breathing.

viii. To return to the base pose, first inhale (Radhey); then exhaling (Krishna), bend your right knee; release your heel unhurriedly from the interlocked fingers and finally lower it to the floor.

ix. Repeat the process with the other leg.

x. Lastly, come into Shithil Tadasan (See page 25) and relax.

Variation – 2

i. Stand up straight—in an upright position—with both feet joined together and arms by your sides, i.e. Saral Tadasan (See page 25).

ii. Then, focus the eyes in front of you at eye level.

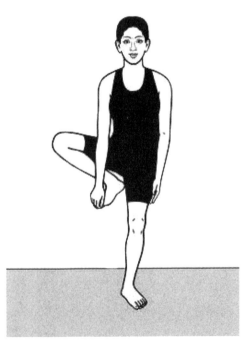
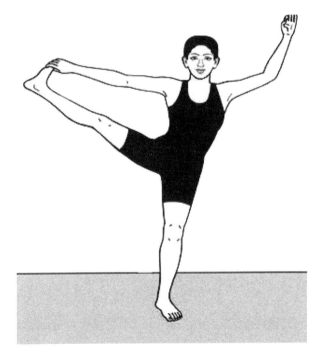

iii. Now inhaling (Radhey), bend the right knee and gradually bring the right thigh as close to the chest as possible.

iv. Place the right arm along the inside of the right leg and catch hold of the big toe.

v. With an exhalation (Krishna), turn the right knee to the right and slowly stretch it sideways.

vi. For balance, lift the left hand to the left side and form Gyan or Chin Mudra with it.

vii. Then, raise the right leg slowly, keeping it locked, as high as possible and pull it closer to the body.

viii. With normal breathing, stay in this final position to your comfort.

ix. To return back to Saral Tadasan, first inhale (Radhey); then exhaling (Krishna), release your right big toe unhurriedly from the right hand and finally lower it to the floor.

x. Repeat on the opposite side.

xi. Ultimately, come into Shithil Tadasan (See page 25) and relax.

Awareness
✧ On a point for balance
✧ On breaths synchronized with the bodily movements
✧ On continuous mental chanting of the Divinely Names "Radhey Krishna" with your breaths
✧ On the balance in the final positions

Benefits
✓ Generally, it grows concentration of the mind and strengthens the hip and leg muscles.
✓ The coordination of the muscular and nervous balance in this posture gives steadiness and poise perfectly.

Contraindications:
- Utthit Hasta Padangushthasan should be performed very carefully without giving any strain to the legs. People with knee problems, hip problems, and sciatica should not practice it.

40. Padangushthasan (Standing on the Toes)

Procedure
i. Stand up straight—in an upright position—with both feet joined together and arms by your sides, i.e. Saral Tadasan (See page 25).

ii. Now, focus at a point in front of you.

iii. Shift the body-weight onto the left leg; lift the right foot and keep it on top of the left thigh, turning the right sole upward.

iv. If it slips, lock the left knee without any worry.

v. Inhaling (Radhey), join the palms in front of the chest to form Namaste Mudra.

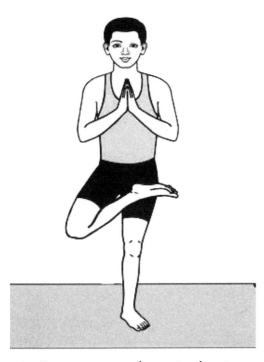

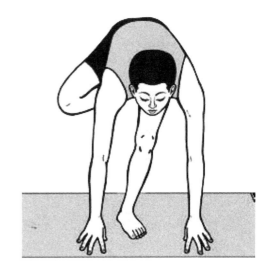

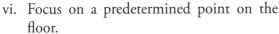

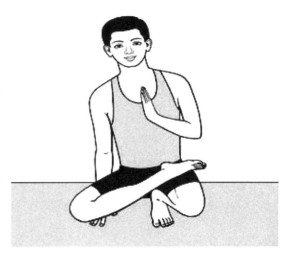

vi. Focus on a predetermined point on the floor.

vii. Now exhaling (Krishna), slowly bend your left leg at the knee.

viii. Keep on lowering the body with the hands in the praying pose as long as possible.

ix. Then while bending forward, place both the hands on the floor for support.

x. Now with the support of the fingers, slowly lower your whole body, and rest the right buttock on the left heel.

xi. Shift the body-weight to the left toes on the ground.

xii. Supported with both hands, try to balance properly.

xiii. Then, one by one, bring the palms close to the chest and join them together in a Namaskar Mudra.

xiv. With normal breathing, stay in this position for as long as your are comfortable.

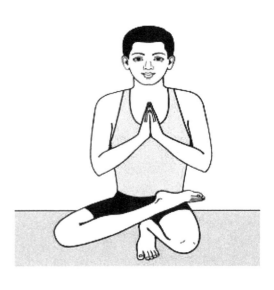

xv. Return to the upright position reversing the steps in which you had gone down, and then lower your right foot carefully.

xvi. Repeat the same steps on the other side.

xvii. Lastly, return to Shithil Tadasan (See page 25) and relax.

Awareness
✧ On a point on the floor
✧ On the balance
✧ On the bodily movements synchronized with your breaths
✧ On the mental chanting of the Holy Names "Radhey Krishna" with your breaths

Benefits
✓ It generates patience and thus helps develop both—physical and mental balance.
✓ It helps in curing gout and rheumatism of the knees, ankles, and feet.
✓ It also assists in healing hemorrhoid (piles) problems.
✓ If done regularly, it vitalizes the body, and even contributes to the maintenance of celibacy.

Contraindications
- People with severe knee or foot problems may avoid this practice. Besides, those who are overweight should do this only if they feel comfortable.

41. Tul Dandasan / Ek Padasan (Balancing Stick Pose)

Procedure
i. Stand up straight—in an upright position—with both feet joined together and arms by your sides, i.e. Saral Tadasan (See page 25).

ii. Inhaling (Radhey), raise your arms above the head; interlock the fingers tightly; you may also point the index fingers upward.

iii. With an exhalation (Krishna), bend forward slowly from your hips with the trunk, head, and arms in a straight line.

iv. Raise your left leg straight back simultaneously, and also keep it aligned with your trunk, and focus the eyes at the hands to maintain

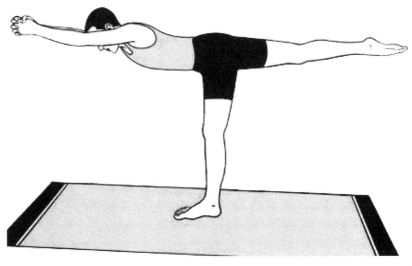

balance.

v. Ensure the right hip joint remains the pivotal point for your whole body.

vi. The left leg, the trunk, the head, and the arms should stay aligned when the right leg remains perpendicular to the floor.

vii. Be in this pose for as long as possible with normal breathing.

viii. Inhaling (Radhey), smoothly return to Saral Tadasan.

ix. Repeat the same process by raising the right leg back.

x. Eventually, return to Shithil Tadasan (See page 25) and relax.

Awareness

✧ On mentally uttering the Sacred Names "Radhey Krishna" with your breaths

✧ On the balance in the final position

Benefits

✓ Tul Dandasan / Ek Padasan strengthens your arms, wrists, hips, and leg-muscles.

✓ It relaxes the lower back.

✓ It also helps develop the nervous system and increases concentration ability wonderfully.

Contraindications

- People suffering from high blood pressure and heart ailments should omit it from their *Yogic* package.

42. Natarajasan - 1 (Lord Shiv's Dance - 1)

Procedure

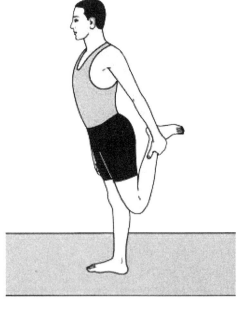

i. Stand up straight, in an upright position, with both feet joined together and arms by your sides, i.e. Saral Tadasan (See page 25).

ii. Focus at a fixed point at eye level.

iii. Inhaling (Radhey), fold your right leg so that you can hold its ankle with your right hand behind the body.

iv. Keeping the inner thighs together, maintain your balance.

v. With an exhalation (Krishna), slowly raise and outstretch your right leg backward, as high as possible.

vi. Without twisting the right hip, try to raise right leg directly behind your body.

vii. Move the left arm upward and forward so as to maintain the balance.

viii. Try to hold the position as long as possible with normal breathing.

ix. To regain the base position, inhale (Radhey) and lower both, the left arm and the right leg slowly by bringing the knees together.

x. Then, release your right ankle, simultaneously lower the foot down to the floor, and also lower the right arm to the side.

xi. Perform the same process with the left leg.

xii. Ultimately, come into Shithil Tadasan (See page 25) and relax.

Note: One should not do it unless the body is flexible enough.

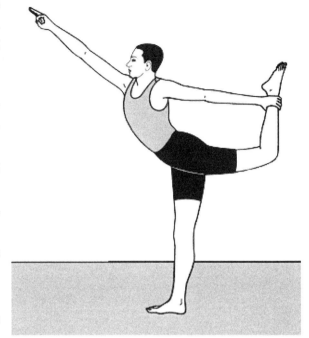

Awareness

✧ On spontaneously feeling the omnipresence of "Radhey Krishna"

✧ On the balance in the final position

Benefits

✓ Natarajasan develops concentration and gives control over your body.

✓ Plus, your nervous system is balanced well.

✓ Legs are given extra suppleness.

43. Vatayanasan (Flying Horse Pose)

Procedure

i. Stand up straight—in an upright position—with both feet joined together and arms by your sides, i.e. Saral Tadasan (See page 25).

ii. Look at a fixed point at eyes level.

iii. Bending your left knee, place the outer left foot on the right thigh in Half Lotus Position (See page 111).

iv. Now, grasp the left ankle until your body is steady.

v. Do Namaste Mudra and inhale (Radhey).

vi. With an exhalation (Krishna),

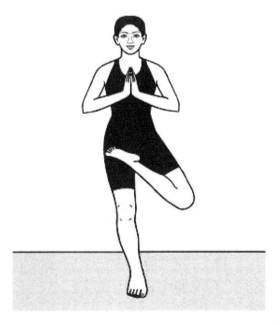

maintain the balance and then bend the right knee and lower the body until the left knee rests completely on the floor.

vii. Try to keep your trunk and the head erect in the final pose.

viii. Hold this position to your capacity with normal breathing.

ix. With an inhalation (Radhey), raise the body gradually, straightening the left knee.

x. Now, release your left leg smoothly, and bring it down to the floor.

xi. Practice the same process with the alternate legs.

xii. Ultimately, come to Shithil Tadasan (See page 25) and relax.

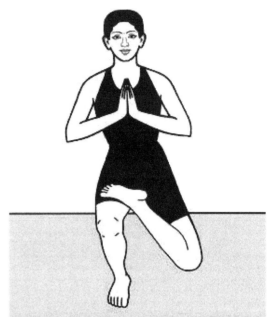

Awareness

✧ On your breaths synchronized with the different body movements

✧ On becoming conscious of the presence of "Radhey Krishna" in your each breath

✧ On the balance in the final position

Benefits

✓ Vatayanasan chiefly strengthens the leg muscles and knee joints.

✓ It also reduces hyperactivity of the kidneys and diuresis.

✓ Most significantly, it is a blessing for celibates as it plays a great role in retaining seminal fluid for celibacy.

Contraindications

- People affected with severe knee pain, weak legs, and slipped-disc should avoid this *asan*.

44. Ardh Baddh Padmottanasan (Half Lotus Forward Bending)

Procedure

i. Stand up straight—in an upright position—with both feet joined together and arms by your sides, i.e. Saral Tadasan (See page 25).

ii. Look at a fixed point at eye level.

iii. Shift the body-weight on the left leg; then bend the left knee and place the foot as high as possible on the right thigh, near the perineum, as in Half Lotus Position (See page 111).

iv. Raise your arms above the head, and while inhaling (Radhey), join your palms together.

v. Ensure your elbows and right knee remain locked.

vi. Relax the whole body in this position.

vii. Now while exhaling (Krishna); slowly lean forward, keeping the arms straight.

viii. Place both palms flat on either side of the right foot; balance the body on the hands and the right foot and also try to touch the knee with your forehead.

ix. Try to be in this position at your ease with normal breathing.

x. With an inhalation (Radhey), slowly come back to the standing position, lower the arms carefully, and then release the left leg.

xi. Repeat with the next leg similarly.

xii. Finally, come to Shithil Tadasan (See page 25) and relax.

Awareness

✧ On the breaths synchronized with your bodily movements

✧ On the balance

✧ On becoming conscious of the presence of "Radhey Krishna" in your each breath

Benefits

✓ Ardh Baddh Padmottanasan has several effects such as improving digestion, eliminating constipation, maintaining normal blood circulation, and strengthening the legs.

✓ It expands the chest and helps in breathing freely and deeply.

Contraindications

- People with the problems like sciatica, slipped-disc, hernia, weak legs, and high blood pressure should not perform this *asan*.

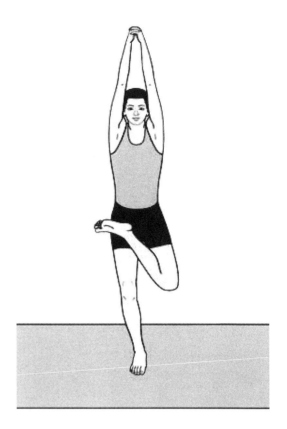

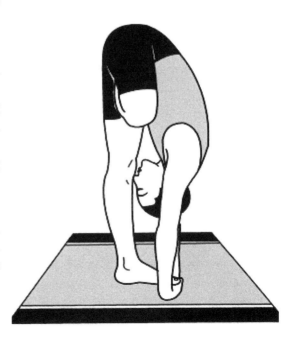

45. Ashtavakrasan (Eight-Twist Pose)

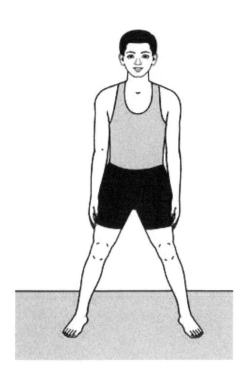

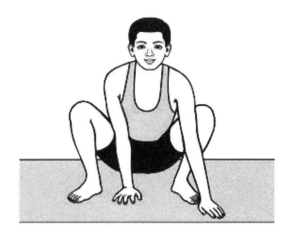

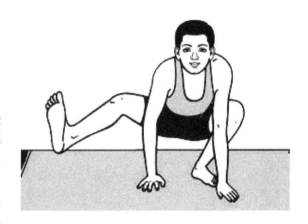

Procedure

i. Stand up straight—in an upright position —with both feet joined together and arms by your sides, i.e. Saral Tadasan (See page 25).

ii. Spread your feet about 1.5-2 feet apart.

iii. Inhale (Radhey); while exhaling (Krishna), slowly go down to a squatting position.

iv. Place the right palm on the floor between the feet and the left palm slightly in front of the left foot.

v. Now stretching the right leg gently, place it above the right arm, keeping the thigh on the back of the upper right arm, exactly above the elbow.

vi. Inhale (Radhey); move the left foot forward, between the arms; while

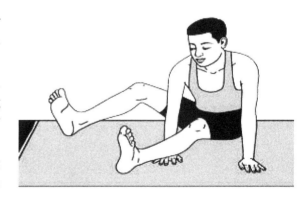

exhaling (Krishna), slowly raise both legs from the floor.

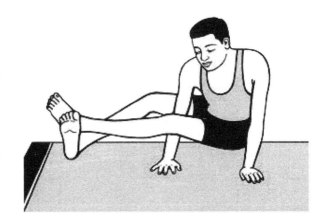

vii. Now inhaling (Radhey), interlock the two legs by keeping the left foot on the right ankle and extend both legs to the right side slowly.

viii. You may bend the right elbow a bit below the thighs to give support and balance on the arms.

ix. With an exhalation (Krishna), gradually bend your elbows and lower the trunk and the head until they become horizontal to the floor.

x. With normal breathing, try to stay in this *asan* for as long as possible.

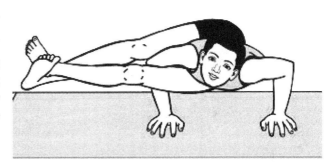

xi. Inhale (Radhey) and exhaling (Krishna), make your arms straight; then raise your trunk comfortably and release the legs without any strain.

xii. Again, regain the squatting pose.

xiii. Perform it wither the alternate pattern of arms and legs.

xiv. Lastly, come up to the base position and relax in Shithil Tadasan (See page 25).

Awareness

✧ On breathing in and out along with the movements
✧ On the Sacred Names "Radhey Krishna" with your breaths
✧ On the balance in the final position

Benefits

✓ Ashtavakrasan provides sterling coordination between the mind and body.
✓ It is very helpful for celibates to maintain celibacy.
✓ It slims-down the body along with strengthening the wrists, arms, and leg muscles; it gives a wholesome exercise to the abdomen as well.

Contraindications

- Persons with weak or defective hands may exclude it from their daily *Yog* exercise.

46. Saral Konasan (Straight Angle Pose)

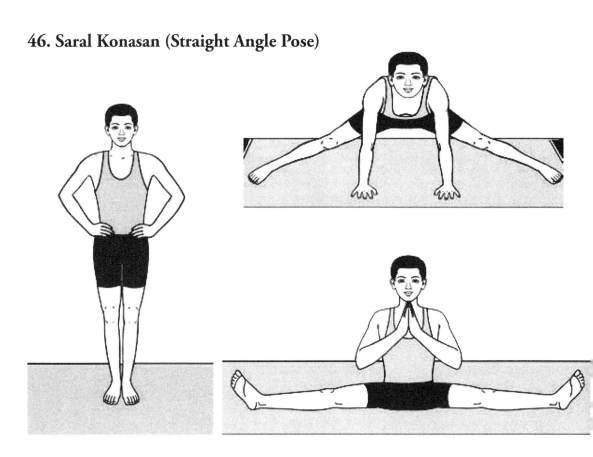

Procedure

i. Stand up straight—in an upright position—with both feet joined together and arms by your sides, i.e. Saral Tadasan (See page 25).

ii. Now, place your hands on the waist.

iii. Slowly and gently, move your feet sideways apart.

iv. Rest your palms on the floor and inhale (Radhey).

v. With an exhalation (Krishna), extend the feet further until your buttocks touch the floor with both legs in a straight line.

vi. Try to make your spine, neck, and head completely erect.

vii. Also, join the palms together in front of the chest.

viii. Maintain the posture for as long as is comfortable with normal breathing.

ix. Gradually, with the support of the hands, come back to the standing position.

x. Finally, come into Shithil Tadasan (See page 25) and relax.

Awareness

✧ On the stretch of your legs

✧ On feeling the presence of "Radhey Krishna" in front of you, watching you with a smile

Benefits

✓ This *asan* helps prevent hernia, gives relief from sciatic cases, and helps cure defects in the lower part of the spine.

✓ It also keeps the pelvic region and the genital organs healthy by proper blood-circulation through them.

✓ Along with strengthening the leg muscles, it also exercises the hip joints and helps develop extra suppleness in the legs.

Contraindications

- Persons affected with physical problems like slipped-disc, sciatica, hernia, and dislocation of the hip joints should not attempt this pose.

47. Bakasan (Crane Pose)

Procedure

i. Stand up straight—in an upright position—with both feet joined together and arms by your sides, i.e. Saral Tadasan (See page 25).

ii. With an inhalation (Radhey), raise your arms above the head; then join the palms.

iii. Exhaling (Krishna), bend forward from the hips and hold the toes of the right foot with both the hands.

iv. Continuing to exhale, stretch the left leg backward as high as possible, and simultaneously bring your head towards the knees, as much close as possible.

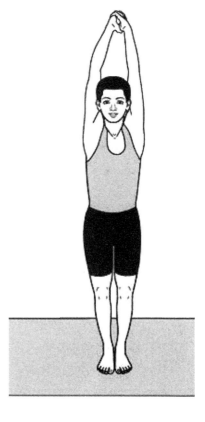

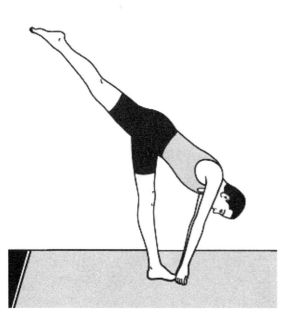

v. In the final position, make sure your legs stay straight at the knees and your left leg and the trunk stay aligned.

vi. With normal breathing, remain in this posture to your comfort.

vii. Now, lower the left leg and regain the base position.

viii. Perform the same steps with the right leg too.

ix. This completes one round; repeat for two more rounds.

x. Lastly, come into Shithil Tadasan (See page 25) and relax.

Awareness

✧ On the breaths synchronized with the movements of your legs and arms

✧ On the balance

✧ On the mental chanting of "Radhey Krishna" with your inhalations and exhalations

Benefits

✓ Bakasan is a very invigorating pose as it strengthens hip and leg muscles.

✓ As it helps in circulating sufficient blood to the brain, it is supportive in improving concentration power and nervous coordination.

Contraindications

- People suffering from high blood pressure and heart problems should omit it.

48. Vishwamitrasan (Sage Vishwamitra's Pose)

Procedure

i. Stand up straight—in an upright position—with both feet joined together and arms by your sides, i.e. Saral Tadasan (See page 25).

ii. Now, inhale (Radhey); with an exhalation (Krishna), lean forward and place your arms on the floor, as in Parvatasan (See page 285).

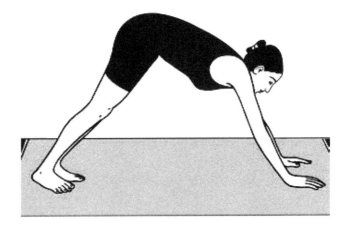

iii. Now, move your right leg forward and place it just in front of the right hand.

iv. Keeping your arms fixed; inhale (Radhey) and separate both the feet backward about 3.5-5 feet.

v. Exhale (Krishna); then rest the head on the floor, raising the buttocks.

vi. As you inhale (Radhey), gradually raise your head.

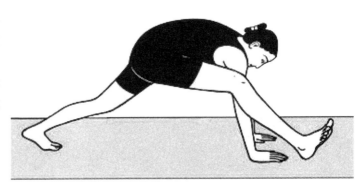

vii. Then exhaling (Krishna), bring your right leg over the right hand and place the back of the right thigh on the right triceps.

viii. Do not touch the floor with the right foot.

ix. Without delay, slowly flip your body to the left and keep the left arm along the left thigh; maintain the balance.

x. Twist your left foot sideways and push the left heel on the floor.

xi. Also, keep your right leg straight.

xii. While inhaling (Radhey), pull the left arm up vertically.

xiii. Try to gaze at the extended left hand in this state.

xiv. Be in this pose for as long as possible with normal breathing.

xv. As you come back to the central position, let go of your right leg slowly.

xvi. Try the pose on the other side.

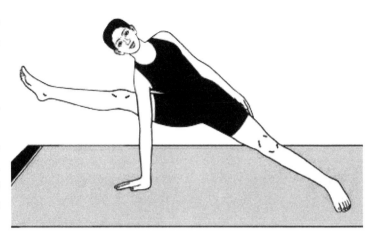

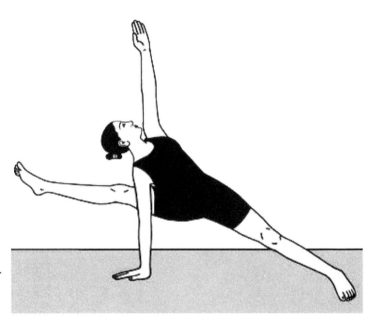

xvii. Lastly, come into Shithil Tadasan (See page 25) and relax.

Awareness

✧ On breathing in and out along with the various movements

✧ On the balance

✧ On the mental chanting of "Radhey Krishna" with each breath and feeling Their presence at all times

Benefits

✓ Vishwamitrasan nicely exercises the muscles of your arms and the legs, as well as the

sciatic nerves.
- ✓ By massaging the internal organs, it improves the digestive system tremendously.
- ✓ It also aids in developing the concentration power and sense of balance.

Contraindication

- People without enough flexibility in their body should not attempt it.

B. *Sūkṣhma Vyāyāms* (Subtle Exercises)

Introduction

Subtle Exercises (*Sūkṣhma Vyāyāms*) are ancient techniques that integrate subtle *Yogic* warm-ups with gentle stretching, breathing, and relaxation. They promote overall well-being and increase fitness level. These simple exercises, done with awareness, help develop concentration and induce relaxation.

In Subtle Exercises, there are exercises for every part of the body—the head, neck, ears, eyes, etc.—from top to toe. These exercises exercise each organ, each joint, and each muscle, either through a particular exercise or set of exercises, combined with a particular breathing system.

1. Padanguli Naman (Tow Bending)

Procedure

i. Sit down with your legs outstretched in front and keeping the back erect, place your palms on the floor behind the buttocks, with the fingers pointing backward, i.e. Dandasan (See page 117).

ii. Spread your feet slightly apart and rest your hands behind the buttocks.

iii. With the support of the arms, rested on either side of the buttocks, lean a little bit backward.

iv. Make your spine erect in this state.

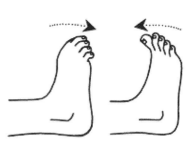

v. While inhaling (Radhey), slowly stretch your toes of both feet forward; while exhaling (Krishna), slowly pull them backward; don't move your feet.

vi. Practice this exercise about 15-20 times.

Awareness

◇ On the stretch of the toes and their movements
◇ On recalling "Radhey Krishna" with inhalations and exhalations

Benefits

✓ Padanguli Naman assists in rejuvenating a motionless lymph and venous blood, which results in relieving tiredness, relieving cramps, and also preventing venous thrombosis.

2. Gulf Naman (Ankle Bending)

Procedure

i. Sit down with your legs outstretched in front and keeping the back erect, place your palms on the floor behind the buttocks, with the fingers pointing backward, i.e. Dandasan (See page 117).

ii. Spread your feet slightly apart and rest your hands behind the buttocks.

iii. With the help of your arms, recline slightly backward.

iv. Ensure your spine stays erect in this position.

v. Now slowly move both feet backward and forward, bending them from the ankle joints.

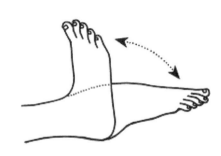

vi. While bending the feet forward, inhale (Radhey); while bending them backward, exhale (Krishna).

vii. Stretching as much as comfortable, attempt to touch the floor with your toes, and then pull them backward.

viii. Practice this exercise for 10-20 times.

Awareness
- ✧ On the stretch of the foot, ankle, calf, and leg joints, and their movements
- ✧ On mentally uttering the Divine Names "Radhey Krishna" along with the breaths flowing in and out through your nose

Benefits
- ✓ Gulf Naman *asan* helps rejuvenate a motionless lymph and venous blood, which results in relieving tiredness, relieving cramps, and also preventing venous thrombosis.

3. Gulf Chakra (Ankle Rotation)

Procedure

i. Sit down with your legs outstretched in front and keeping the back erect, place your palms on the floor behind the buttocks, with the fingers pointing backward, i.e. Dandasan (See page 117).

ii. Now, place your feet together touching each other.

iii. Make sure that your spine remains vertical, with the heels on the ground, at all times.

iv. Now, slowly start rotating both feet together clockwise.

v. While bending your feet forward, inhale (Radhey); while bending them backward, exhale (Krishna).

vi. While rotating your feet, do not let the feet separate from each other; and fix your knees well to the ground.

vii. Practice for about 10-20 times, both—clockwise and counterclockwise.

Variation - 1

i. Sit down with your legs outstretched in front and keeping the back erect, place your palms on the floor behind the buttocks, with the fingers pointing backward, i.e. Dandasan (See page 117).

ii. Keep a slight distance between the two feet.

iii. Make sure that your spine remains erect, with the heels on the ground, at all times.

iv. Slowly, rotate both feet from the ankles simultaneously in opposite directions.

v. While bending the feet forward, inhale (Radhey); while bending them backward, exhale (Krishna).

vi. Practice about 10-20 rotations in either direction.

Awareness

✧ On the rotations of your feet
✧ On remembering "Radhey Krishna" while performing inhalations and exhalations

Benefits

✓ Like Padanguli Naman, this *asan* helps rejuvenate a motionless lymph and venous blood, which results in relieving tiredness, relieving cramps, and also preventing venous thrombosis.

4. Padanguli Ghurnan (Toes Rotation)

Procedure

i. Sit down with your legs outstretched in front and keeping the back erect, place your palms on the floor behind the buttocks, with the fingers pointing backward, i.e. Dandasan (See page 117).

ii. Fold your right leg at the knee, then rest the right foot on top of the left thigh in such a way that the sole faces upward and the knee touches the floor.

iii. Grasp your right foot with your right hand and make it stable.

iv. Grasp the toes of the right foot with the left hand.

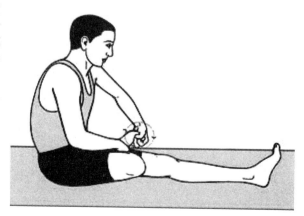

v. Now, start rotating the toes 10-20 times, clockwise and counterclockwise.

vi. While rotating the toes forward, inhale (Radhey); while rotating them backward, exhale (Krishna).

vii. Repeat the same process with the left foot.

Awareness

✧ On the rotations

✧ On spontaneous remembering "Radhey Krishna" while performing inhalations and exhalations

Benefits

✓ Like Padanguli Naman, this *asan* helps rejuvenate a motionless lymph and venous blood, which results in relieving tiredness, relieving cramps, and also preventing venous thrombosis.

5. Gulf Ghurnan (Ankle rotation)

Procedure

i. Sit down with your legs outstretched in front and keeping the back erect, place your palms on the floor behind the buttocks, with the fingers pointing backward, i.e. Dandasan (See page 117).

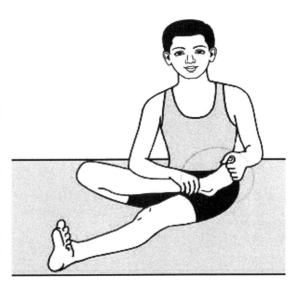

ii. Bend your right leg at the right knee, and then rest the foot on top of the left thigh so that the sole faces upward and the knee touches the floor.

iii. Grasp your right leg firmly just above the ankle with the right hand, and also grasp the right toes with the left hand.

iv. Now using the left hand, comfortably rotate the right foot 10-20 times, clockwise and counterclockwise.

v. While bending your foot forward, inhale (Radhey); while bending it backward, exhale (Krishna).

vi. Also, practice with the left foot.

Awareness

✧ On the rotations

✧ On remembering "Radhey Krishna" while performing inhalations and exhalations

Benefits

✓ Like Padanguli Naman (See page 89), this *asan* helps rejuvenate a motionless lymph and venous blood, which results in relieving tiredness, relieving cramps, and also preventing venous thrombosis.

6. Janu Naman (Knee Bending)

Procedure

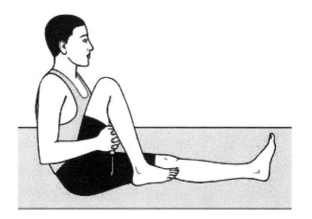

i. Sit down with your legs outstretched in front and keeping the back erect, place your palms on the floor behind the buttocks, with the fingers pointing backward, i.e. Dandasan (See page 117).

ii. Comfortably folding your right leg, catch hold of your right thigh with the interlocked fingers of either of the hands, and move it closer to your chest.

iii. You may also cross both arms instead of interlocking the fingers of either of the hands, and catch the elbows.

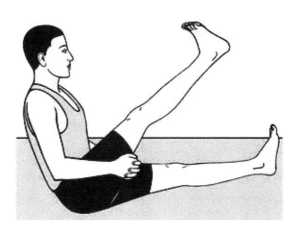

iv. Make sure the spine and head stay erect.

v. While inhaling (Radhey), straighten your right leg; make sure your right thigh remains unmoved.

vi. While exhaling (Krishna), slowly drop your right feet to the floor.

vii. This completes one round.

viii. Repeat the process for 10-20 rounds with the right leg.

ix. Perform the same number of rounds with the left leg.

Awareness

✧ On the stretches in the thigh muscles
✧ On unbroken rememberance of "Radhey Krishna" while performing inhalations and exhalations

Benefits

✓ The effects of this pose are same as those of Padanguli Naman (See page 89).

7. Janu Chakra (Knee Crank)

Procedure

i. Sit down with your legs outstretched in front and keeping the back erect, place your palms on the floor behind the buttocks, with the fingers pointing backward, i.e. Dandasan (See page 117).

ii. Comfortably fold your right leg, move your hands underneath the right thigh and either interlock the fingers, or cross both arms and catch the elbows.

iii. Make sure your trunk and head remain erect.

iv. Keep your arms straight so that the heels or toes do not touch the floor.

v. Slowly lift your right foot upward, and start rotating the leg from the knee in a big circle.

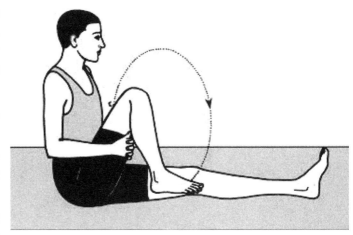

vi. Inhale (Radhey) during the upper half rotation, and exhale (Krishna) during the lower half rotation.

vii. Keep your upper part of the leg and the body entirely motionless throughout the practice.

viii. Rotate around 10-20 times—clockwise and counterclockwise.

ix. Perform the same process with the other leg.

Awareness
✧ On the circular movements
✧ On mentally chanting the Divine Names "Radhey Krishna" during inhalations and exhalations

Benefits
✓ Janu Chakra provides perfect exercise to the knee joints, strengthens the quadriceps muscle and ligaments, and thus relieves knee injuries, sprains, osteoarthritis, etc.

8. Shroni Chakra (Hip Rotation)

Procedure

i. Sit down with your legs outstretched in front and keeping the back erect, place your palms on the floor behind the buttocks, with the fingers pointing backward, i.e. Dandasan (See page 117).

ii. Place your right foot on the left thigh close to the root of the leg (groin area); hold it properly with your left hand.

iii. Hold your right knee with the right hand.

iv. Now rotate your right knee in a circle with the help of the right hand, making a circle as big as possible.

v.   Inhale (Radhey) when your knee goes toward the ground and exhale (Krishna) when the knee comes toward the chest.

vi. Repeat 10 times—clockwise and counterclockwise.

vii. Practice with the other leg likewise.

viii. Finally, come into Shithil Dandasan (See page 117) and relax.

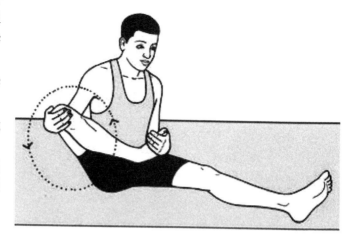

Awareness

✧ On the breaths synchronized with the various movements

✧ On the rotation of the hips

✧ On mentally recalling "Radhey Krishna" along with your breathing

Benefits

✓ It loosens the back muscles and tones the spinal nerves.

✓ As both hips are rotated wonderfully, this pose makes the hip joints supple and helps increase blood circulation. Thus, it releases pain of the legs, knees, hips, and the buttocks.

9. Ardh Titali Asan (Half Butterfly Pose)

Procedure

i.   Sit down with your legs outstretched in front and keeping the back erect, place your palms on the floor behind the buttocks, with the fingers pointing backward, i.e. Dandasan (See page 117).

ii. Slowly flex your right leg and place your right foot on top of the left thigh, close to the root of the leg (groin area).

iii. Now rest your right hand on right knee and grasp the right toes firmly with the left hand.

iv. While inhaling (Radhey), gently pull the right knee upward to touch the chest, and while exhaling (Krishna) slowly push the knee downward to the floor.

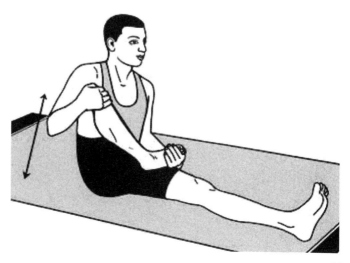

v. Make sure your spine and head remain erect and that the leg muscles remain relaxed as the movement should be done only by the force of the right arm.

vi. Repeat it as many times as possible.

vii. Repeat the same process on the other side.

Awareness

✧ On the movements of your legs and breaths synchronized with them
✧ On the movement of the hip joints
✧ On the relaxation of the thigh muscles
✧ On always feeling the presence of "Radhey Krishna" in your breaths

Benefits

✓ Ardh Titali Asan makes the knees and hip joints very supple by loosening them with the dynamic flapping of the legs.
✓ It is chiefly effective for those who cannot sit in any crossed legged poses such as Padmasan or Siddhasan.

10. Purna Titali Asan (Butterfly Pose)

Procedure

i. Sit down with your legs outstretched in front and keeping the back erect, place your palms on the floor behind the buttocks, with the fingers pointing backward, i.e. Dandasan (See page 117).

ii. Gently bend your legs and place the soles of the feet against each other, with the heels touching the perineum.

iii. Now, interlock your fingers and hold the toes.

iv. Raise your knees and lower them in a flapping motion—similar to the movement of a

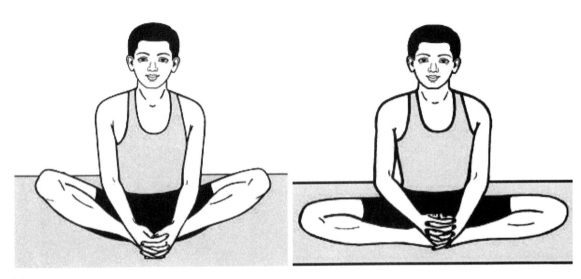

butterfly's wings.

v. As this completes one round; do it about 50-60 rounds.

vi. Eventually, come into Shithil Dandasan (See page 117) and relax.

Awareness

✧ On the movements and the relaxation of the thighs and the pelvic joints

✧ On always feeling the presence of "Radhey Krishna" in your breaths

Benefits

✓ The effects of this pose are the same as those of Shroni Chakra (See page 94).

Contraindication

- Those who are suffering from either sciatica or sacral conditions should omit it.

11. Mushtik Bandh (Hand Clenching)

Procedure

i. Sit in either Sukhasan (see page 111) or Vajrasan (See page 113), with your spine erect.

ii. Now, raise both arms straight in front of the chest at shoulder level; then open the hands completely and with the palms downward, extend the fingers widely.

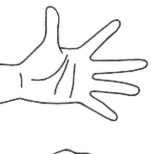

iii. While inhaling (Radhey), form tight fists, placing the thumbs inside.

iv. Then while exhaling (Krishna), open the hands again and outstretch the fingers as wide as possible.

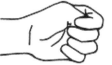

v. Ensure your arms and wrists remain locked throughout the process.

vi. Likewise, repeat the method 15-20 times.

Awareness

✧ On the stretch of the finger-joints

✧ On always realizing the presence of "Radhey Krishna" in your breath

Benefits

✓ This exercise of the fingers, Mushtik Bandh, alleviates the stress due to excessive writing, typing, etc.

✓ It is also effective in relieving arthritis of the related joints.

12. Manibandh Chakra (Wrist Joint Rotation)

Procedure

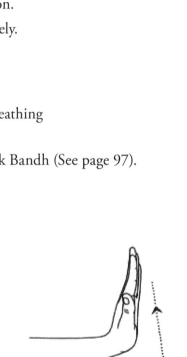

i. Sit in either Sukhasan or Vajrasan, keeping your spine erect.

ii. Now stretch both arms in front of the body—at shoulder level; form tight fists, with the thumbs inside.

iii. Then, slowly rotate both the fists by rotating the wrist joints simultaneously in the same direction.

iv. Try to form extended circles for enhanced effect on the wrists.

v. While making the circle, inhale (Radhey) in the lower half and exhale (Krishna) in the upper half.

vi. Ensure that the arms and elbows remain straight and still while rotating the wrists.

vii. Practice for more than 20 rounds in one direction.

viii. Repeat equal number of rounds in the opposite direction.

ix. Ultimately, lower both the arms and rest them completely.

Awareness

✧ On the movements synchronized with the breath
✧ On the pressure in the wrist joints
✧ On spontaneously recalling "Radhey Krishna" while breathing

Benefits

✓ The effects of this pose are the same as those of Mushtik Bandh (See page 97).

13. Manibandh Naman (Wrist Bending)

Procedure

i. Sit in either Sukhasan or Vajrasan, keeping your spine erect.

ii. Stretch both arms in front of your body at the shoulder level, with both palms open and the fingers extended.

iii. While inhaling (Radhey), fold the arms at the wrists in such a way that the fingers point toward the ceiling.

iv. While exhaling (Krishna), fold them forward in such a way that the fingers point toward the floor.

v. Make sure that your elbows remain locked and the fingers stretched at all times.

vi. Practice nearly 20-30 rounds.

Awareness

✧ On the movement of the wrist joints and the breaths synchronized with them
✧ On the stretch of the forearm muscles
✧ On the mental chanting of the Holy Names "Radhey Krishna" while breathing

Benefits

✓ The effects of Manibandh Naman are same as that of Mushtik Bandh (See page 97) and Shroni Chakra (See page 94).

14. Kehuni Naman (Elbow Bending)

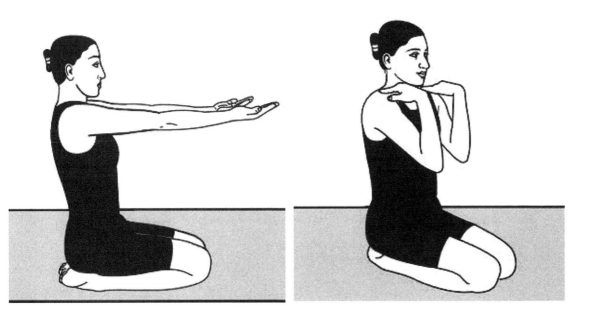

Procedure

i. Sit in either Sukhasan or Vajrasan, with your spine erect.

ii. With an inhalation (Radhey), stretch both arms in front of the body at the shoulder level; ensure both hands reamain open and the palms face upward.

iii. Now, while exhaling (Krishna), slowly fold your arms at the elbows and take the fingers up to the shoulders.

iv. Again inhale (Radhey), and straighten your arms.

v. Perform 20-30 rounds with normal breathing.

Variation – 1

Alternatively, it can also be practiced by stretching the arms sideways at the shoulder level, in the same manner.

Awareness

- ⬥ On the movement of the wrist joints and the breaths synchronized with them
- ⬥ On the stretch of the forearm muscles
- ⬥ On the mental chanting of the Holy Names "Radhey Krishna" in your breaths

Benefits

- ✓ The effects of Kehuni Naman are same as that of Mushtik Bandh (See page 97).

15. Skandh Chakra (Shoulder Socket Rotation)

Procedure

i. Sit in either Sukhasan or Vajrasan, keeping your spine erect throughout.

ii. Stretch out both arms sideways at the shoulder level, with both hands open and the palms facing up.

iii. Fold both the arms at the elbows and rest the fingers of the right hand on the right shoulder and the fingers of the left hand on the left shoulder.

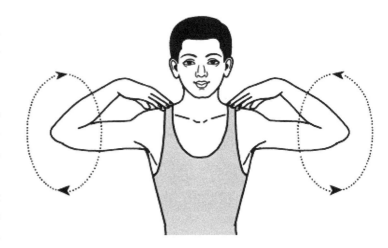

iv. Now rotate both elbows simultaneously in a big circle, trying to touch with each other at elbows in front of the chest while moving forward and touch the ears while going up.

v. Inhale (Radhey) during the backward half of the rotation, and exhale (Krishna) during the forward half of the rotation.

vi. Stretch the arms while moving backward, and also touch the sides of the trunk while moving downward.

vii. Perform clockwise and counterclockwise—10 times each.

Awareness

- ⬥ On the breaths synchronized with the movements of the arms and shoulders
- ⬥ On the stretch and pressure on the shoulder joints
- ⬥ On realizing the presence of "Radhey Krishna" along with your breathing

Benefits

- ✓ Skandh Chakra is also like a relaxing exercise because it relieves fatigue generated from routine office work and activities like driving, cycling, etc.
- ✓ It is quite helpful in relieving cervical spondylitis and frozen shoulders.
- ✓ It trims your whole body so well by shaping the shoulders and chest beautifully.

16. Kati Ghurnan (Waist Rotation)

Procedure

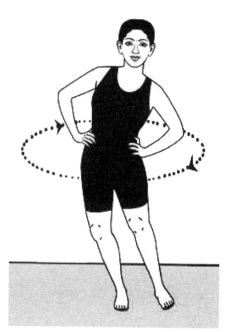

i. Stand up straight, in an upright position, with both feet joined together and arms by your sides, i.e. Saral Tadasan (See page 25).

ii. Spread your feet about 6-12 inches apart.

iii. Hold your waist and rotate it 10 times, both—clockwise and counterclockwise.

iv. Inhale (Radhey) when your waist comes forward and exhale (Krishna) when your waist goes backward.

v. Attempt to make big and perfect horizontal circles with your waist while rotating it.

vi. Keep your knees locked while rotating your waist.

vii. Finally, bring your hands down, and then come into Saral Tadasan.

Awareness

✧ On the breaths synchronized with the movements
✧ On rotating and the pressure around the waist
✧ On always recalling "Radhey Krishna" with each breath

Benefits

✓ Kati Ghurnan makes your waist flexible and activates the liver and kidneys.
✓ It trims your body by reducing the unnecessary fat from waist girdle.

17. Greeva Sanchalan (Neck Movement)

Procedure

i. Sit in either Sukhasan or Vajrasan, keeping your head and spine erect.

ii. While inhaling (Radhey), turn your face to the right (as if looking at an object or a person), so that your chin comes above the right shoulder.

iii. Ensure you twist your neck as much as possible but slowly and without strain.

iv. While exhaling (Krishna), bring your face to the centre.

v. Repeat it on the other side.

vi. Practice about five times in either direction.

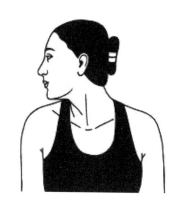

Variation - 1

i.   Sit in either Sukhasan or Vajrasan, keeping your head and spine erect.

ii. While inhaling (Radhey), tilt your head to the right so that the right ear touches the right shoulder, and while exhaling (Krishna), bring your head to the centre.

iii. Repeat it on the other side.

iv. Practice about five times in either direction.

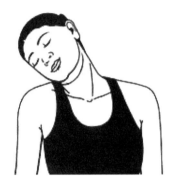

Variation - 2

i.   Sit in either Sukhasan or Vajrasan, keeping your head and spine erect.

ii. While inhaling (Radhey), tilt your head backward; while exhaling (Krishna), bring your head to the centre.

iii. While inhaling (Radhey), tilt your head forward and try to touch the chest with the chin; while exhaling (Krishna), bring your head to the centre; do it gently.

iv. Repeat the exercise for five times.

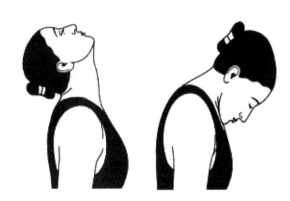

Variation - 3

i.   Sit in either Sukhasan or Vajrasan, keeping your head and spine erect.

ii. Start rotating your neck rightward (so that your chin comes above the right shoulder), then downward (so that your chin touches the pit below the throat), then leftward (so that your chin comes above the left shoulder) and finally again to the centre.

iii. Try to create a (vertical) circular motion in this rotational act.

iv. Inhale (Radhey) during the upper half of the rotation, and exhale (Krishna) during the lower half of the rotation.

v.   Repeat the exercise for five times.

Awareness

✧ On the breaths synchronized with the movements
✧ On the stretching and strain of the muscles on the sides of the neck
✧ On the unbroken remembrance of "Radhey Krishna" while breathing

Benefits

- ✓ Greeva Sanchalasan relieves tension from the neck and shoulders.
- ✓ It removes *prāṇic* energy blockages from the neck region.
- ✓ It also helps in curing a stiff neck.

Contraindications

- Greeva Sanchalanasan should not be performed by elderly people with low or high blood pressure, and also by those who are suffering from cervical spondylitis.

18. Blinking

Procedure

i. Sit with your eyes open in any comfortable meditative position.

ii. Now, quickly start blinking your eyes 10 times, and then close them.

iii. Relax both eyes for 20 seconds in this position.

iv. Repeat this for five times.

Awareness

✦ On blinking your eyes, and simultaneously remembering "Radhey Krishna"

Benefits

- ✓ This subtle exercise removes irregular blinking resulting from habitual tension in the eyes.

19. Palming

Procedure

i. Sit in any meditative *asan* such as Sukhasan or Vajrasan (See page 113).

ii. Stay peacefully and close both the eyes.

iii. Now, rub your palms together until they turn warm.

iv. Then, without any force, comfortably place them over the eyes, and feel the warmth and Divine Energy emanating through the hands into the eyes.

v. Keep the palms over the eyes for as long as you are comfortable.

vi. Finally, lower your hands without opening the eyes, and then, slowly open them with a few gentle blinks.

vii. Practice this process at least two more times.

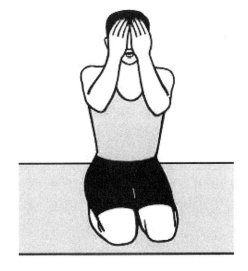

Awareness

✧ On the Divine Energy coming through your hands into the eyes

✧ On remembering "Radhey Krishna" with your normal breathing

Benefits

✓ By this Palming process, the eye muscles are relaxed and energized well.

✓ It also contributes in correcting any type of visionary defects by activating the circulation of the aqueous humor.

20. Sideways Viewing

Procedure

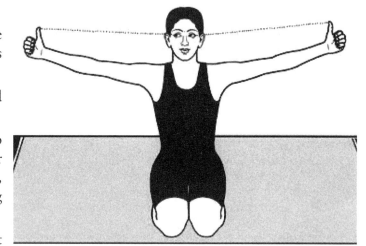

i. Sit in any comfortable meditative *asan* such as Sukhasan or Vajrasan.

ii. Ensure your spine and head remain erect throughout.

iii. Slowly lift both arms up sideways at the shoulder level and straighten them, with both thumbs pointing upward.

iv. Bring your thumbs a bit forward in case they are not visible to the eyes.

v. Now, gaze at a certain point in front which is at eye level, and level the head accordingly.

vi. Keeping your head fixed, focus your eyes on the left thumb, then slowly bring them between the eyebrow centre and then to the right thumb.

vii. In the same way, move them to the left thumb.

viii. This is one cycle; repeat 5-10 cycles likewise.

ix. Lastly, close your eyes and relax them fully with the Palming method (See page 103).

Awareness

✧ On the movement of the eyes

✧ On keeping your head stable—in the centre

✧ On mental remembrance of "Radhey Krishna," and feeling the gratitude for the graces showered

Benefits

- By practicing Sideways Viewing, the eyes are relieved of the strain of the muscle pain caused either by close work or long hours' reading.

21. Front and Sideways Viewing

Procedure

i. Sit down with your legs outstretched in front and keeping the back erect, place your palms on the floor behind the buttocks, with the fingers pointing backward, i.e. Dandasan (See page 117).

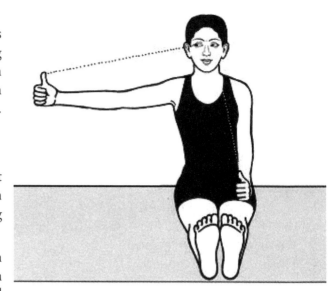

ii. Keep the head and spine erect.

iii. Slowly lift both arms sideways at the shoulder level and straighten them, with both thumbs pointing upward.

iv. Slowly bring the left hand down and to the front—in line with the left leg, with the thumb still pointing upward.

v. Now, keep your head fixed; focus the eyes on the left thumb; then move them diagonally up to the right thumb, and then back to the left thumb.

vi. Repeat this cycle about 5-10 times.

vii. Likewise, perform for 5-10 times with the alternate hands position.

viii. Lastly, close your eyes and relax them fully with the Palming method (See page 103).

Awareness

✧ On the movement of the eyes
✧ On keeping your head stable—in the centre
✧ On mentally remembering "Radhey Krishna," and feeling the gratitude for the graces showered upon you

Benefits

✓ Front and Sideways Viewing wonderfully coordinates the medial and lateral muscles.
✓ Additionally, the eyes are released from the tension of muscle pain caused either by close work or continuous reading.

22. Rotational Viewing

Procedure

i. Sit in any comfortable meditative *asan*, such as Sukhasan or Vajrasan, keeping your spine and head erect.

ii. Moving your eyeballs slowly, move them to the right side as far as possible without strain, then slowly upward, then to the left, then downward, and lastly to the right side again—

to complete one circle.

iii. In the same way, rotate the eyes for 5-10 times, both—clockwise and counterclockwise.

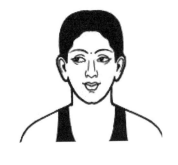
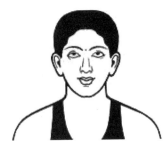

iv. Keep the head and spine erect throughout.

v. At last, close the eyes and relax the eyes for some time with Palming method (See page 103).

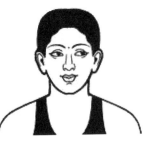
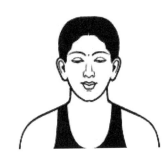

Awareness

✧ On the rotation of the eyes
✧ On keeping your head stable —in the centre
✧ On mentally recalling "Radhey Krishna," and feeling Their presence while breathing

Benefits

✓ Rotational Viewing recovers the proper balance in the eye muscles, and thus helps improve the various functions of the eyeballs.
✓ Additionally, the eyes are relieved from the strain of muscle pain caused either by close work or extended reading session.

23. Up and Down Viewing

Procedure

i. Sit down with your legs outstretched in front and keeping the back erect, place your palms on the floor behind the buttocks, with the fingers pointing backward, i.e. Dandasan (See page 117).

ii. Gently lift both arms up in front at the shoulder level and straighten them.

iii. Form fists with both the hands with the thumbs pointing upward and lower them to the knees.

iv. Slowly raise your right arm and simultaneously follow the movement

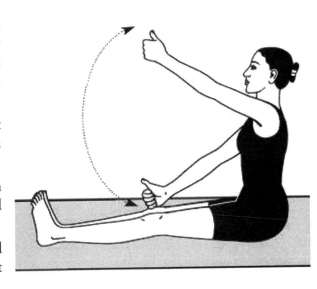

106

of the right thumb with the eyes.

v. As the thumb reaches the optimum point, gradually take it back to the base position.

vi. Make sure your eyes remain fixed on the thumb throughout the process, with the head remaining stable.

vii. Perform the same process with your left thumb too.

viii. Repeat 5-10 times with each thumb, keeping your spine erect at all times.

ix. Lastly, relax your eyes by first closing and then Palming (See page 103) them for some time.

Awareness
✧ On the movement of the eyes
✧ On keeping your head stable—in the centre
✧ On mental recalling of "Radhey Krishna," and feeling grateful for the graces showered

Benefits
✓ It keeps the upper and the lower portion of the eyeballs in an excellent balance.
✓ As in other exercises, the eyes are relieved of the strain of the muscle pain caused either by close work or an extended reading session.

24. Scattered Viewing (Defocusing)
Procedure
i. Sit in any meditative *asan* such as Sukhasan or Vajrasan.

ii. Keep your spine and neck erect throughout.

iii. Raise your arms in front at the shoulder level, keeping them locked.

iv. Form fists of either of the hands, with both the palm-bases touching each other and the thumbs pointing upward.

v. Then, focus your eyes at the thumbs.

vi. Now, slowly separate the fists and move them away sideways, while viewing both the thumbs at the same time as far as possible.

vii. Then, again viewing the thumbs, bring your hands back to the previous position.

viii. Repeat this 5-10 times.

ix. Finally, close your eyes and relax them for some time with the Palming method (See page 103).

Awareness

✧ On the movement of the eyes
✧ On keeping your head stable—in the centre
✧ On mental recalling of "Radhey Krishna," and feeling grateful for the graces showered

Benefits

✓ Scattered viewing is a very invigorating exercise for the eyes as it relaxes the eye muscles and improves eyesight.

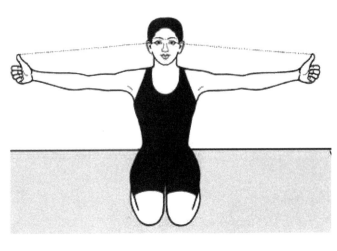

25. Prarambhik Nasikagra Drishti (Preliminary Nose Tip Gazing)

Procedure

i. Sit down with your legs outstretched in front and keeping the back erect, place your palms on the floor behind the buttocks, with the fingers pointing backward, i.e. Dandasan (See page 117).

ii. While inhaling (Radhey), bring your right arm exactly in front of the nose; lock it; then form a fist in such a way that the thumb points upward.

iii. Focusing your eyes on the tip of the thumb, slowly exhale (Krishna).

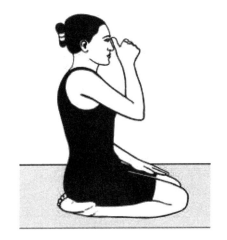

iv. Next, fold your arm and comfortably move the thumb to the nose tip.

v. Keeps your eyes fixed continuously on the tip of the thumb.

vi. Gently straighten the arm, and keep the eyes fixed on the tip of the thumb.

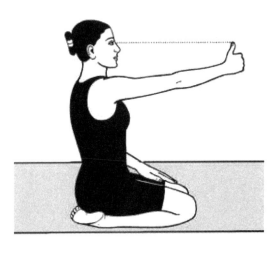

vii. This completes one round; do it up to three more rounds.

Awareness

✧ On the breaths flowing in and out along with mentally chanting the Divine Names "Radhey Krishna"

✧ On feeling Their omnipresence at all times

Benefits

✓ Prarambhik Nasikagra Drishti improves both—sight of the eyes and concentration of the brain.

26. Jhulanasan (Baby's Cradle Pose)

Procedure

i. Sit down with your legs outstretched in front and keeping the back erect, place your palms on the floor behind the buttocks, with the fingers pointing backward, i.e. Dandasan (See page 117).

ii. Place your right foot on the left thigh—closer to the root of the leg (the groin area), and hold it tightly with your left hand.

iii. Placing your right knee on right elbow and right foot on left elbow, interlock both the hands.

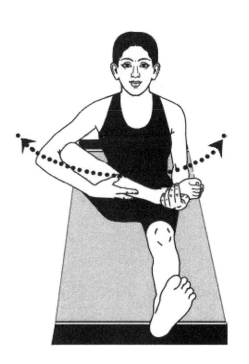

iv. Now swing your right leg with the help of your interlocked hands—both leftward and rightward.

v. Inhale (Radhey) when the knee goes rightward, and exhale (Krishna), when the knee goes leftward.

vi. Ensure your spine stays erect throughout.

vii. Continue the process for about 10-20 times in the same manner.

viii. Repeat the above method with the other leg for 10-20 times.

ix. Lastly, come into Shithil Dandasan (See page 117) and relax.

Awareness

✧ On the breaths synchronized with the rightward and leftward movements

✧ On spontaneous recalling of "Radhey Krishna" along with your breaths

Benefits

- ✓ Like Shroni Chakra (See page 94), Jhulanasan loosens the back muscles and firm the spinal nerves.
- ✓ Due to sideward movement of hips, the hip joints become supple and blood circulation is also increased copiously. Resultantly, tension is released from your legs, knees, hips, and buttocks.

C. *Dhyānātmak Asans* (Meditative Poses)

1. Sukhasan (Comfortable Pose)

Procedure

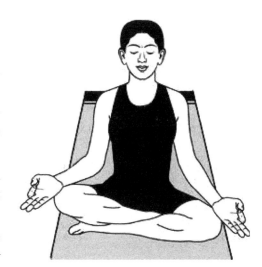

i. Sit down with your legs outstretched in front and keeping the back erect, place your palms on the floor behind the buttocks, with the fingers pointing backward, i.e. Dandasan (See page 117).

ii. Gradually, flex your legs one by one in such a way that the right foot comes just under the left thigh and the left foot under the right thigh.

iii. Sit comfortably with your spine vertical to the floor and rest the hands on the knees in any *mudra*.

iv. Make sure you do not feel strain while keeping the spine, head, and neck erect.

v. Close your eyes and relax the whole body.

vi. Stay in this pose for as long as comfortable, with slow and even breathing.

Awareness

✧ On the breaths flowing in and out of your nostrils
✧ On the Holy Names "Radhey Krishna" in your each breath
✧ On the erect spine in the final position

Benefits

✓ As the name suggests, Sukhasan is a "Comfortable Pose," the easiest meditative pose among all. Even beginners can practice it.
✓ It also stretches the spine wonderfully.
✓ It increases concentration ability by developing stability of the mind.

2. Ardh Padmasan (Half Lotus Pose)

Procedure

i. Sit down with your legs outstretched in front and keeping the back erect, place your palms on the floor behind the buttocks, with the fingers pointing backward, i.e. Dandasan (See page 117).

ii. Slowly pull the right leg along the floor, folding at the right knee and place the foot on the inner side of left thigh.

iii. Also, fold the left leg and bring the left foot under the right thigh.

iv. Adjusting the position comfortably, place the hands on the knees in any *mudra*.

v. In the final position, keep the back, neck, and the head erect.

vi. As in Sukhasan, close your eyes and relax the whole body.

vii. Be in this pose for a while with slow and even breathing.

viii. Repeat the above process by exchanging the legs.

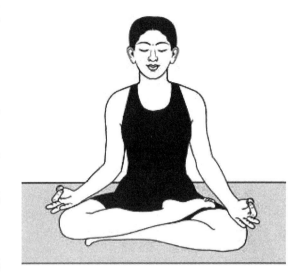

Awareness

✧ On recalling "Radhey Krishna" along with your breaths

✧ On the breaths in the final position

Benefits

✓ If performed for a long period of time, it helps to straighten the spine, which helps reduece depression and tension as the lower spine also becomes erect.

✓ It also develops the nervous system to a large extent and stimulates digestion as blood circulation gets concentrated in the abdominal area instead of the legs.

✓ Lastly, it trims the extra fat from the waist.

Contraindications

- People with sciatica or weak knees should not practice it.

3. Swastikasan (Propitious Pose)

Procedure

i. Sit down with your legs outstretched in front and keeping the back erect, place your palms on the floor behind the buttocks, with the fingers pointing backward, i.e. Dandasan (See page 117).

ii. Flex your right leg at the knee and keep the right sole of your foot against the left inner thigh and the right heel near the perineum.

iii. Flex your left leg and rest the foot in between the right inner thigh and the right calf muscle; left heel

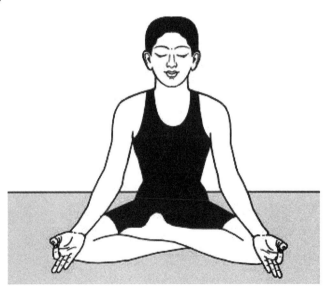

should rest near the pubis.

iv. Make sure that both the knees rest on the floor and both the heels remain away from each other.

v. Make your trunk, neck, and head stay erect in this position.

vi. Also, rest your hands on the knees in any *mudra* and relax the whole body.

vii. Maintain the posture for as long as possible with slow and even breathing.

viii. Perform the *asan* again with the legs crossed the other way.

Awareness

✧ On feeling the presence of "Radhey Krishna" in your breaths
✧ On the breaths flowing in and out in the final position

Benefits

✓ Swastikasan is useful to those who are afflicted with leg problems such as varicose veins, fluid retention, and tired and aching muscles.

Contraindications

- People with sacral infection and sciatica should omit this *asan* from their *Yogic* practice.

4. Vajrasan (Thunderbolt Pose)

Procedure

i. Sit down with your legs outstretched in front and keeping the back erect, place your palms on the floor behind the buttocks, with the fingers pointing backward, i.e. Dandasan (See page 117).

ii. Flex your right leg, and gradually bring your right heel under the right buttock, with the shin and knee resting on the floor.

iii. Bending your left leg similarly, move the left heel under the left buttock.

iv. Ensure your heels remain slightly apart and the big toes touch each other.

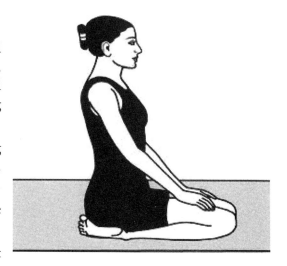

v. Sit comfortably in between heels, and rest the hands on the knees in any *mudra*.

vi. Make sure your back and head remain erect throughout.

vii. As you relax the whole body, close the eyes.

viii. Maintain the position at your ease, with slow and even breathing.

Awareness

✧ On the breaths flowing in and out

◆ On mentally chanting the Divine Names "Radhey Krishna" with your breaths

Benefits

✓ One of the relaxing *asans*, it relieves one from severe ailments such as acidity, gas, constipation, and indigestion.
✓ It also helps cure peptic ulcer, piles, menstrual disorder, and hydrocele.
✓ This is the only the *asan* which can be done for 10-15 minutes even immediately after a meal.

5. Dhyan Veerasan (Hero's Meditative Pose)

Procedure

i. Sit down with your legs outstretched in front and keeping the back erect, place your palms on the floor behind the buttocks, with the fingers pointing backward, i.e. Dandasan (See page 117).

ii. Now, fold your left leg underneath the right leg and touch the right buttock with your left heel.

iii. Folding the right leg and placing it over the bent left leg, touch the left buttock with the right heel.

iv. Make sure your right knee comes exactly on top of the left knee.

v. Keep your head, neck, and spine erect and aligned.

vi. Place your right palm on the right knee and the left palm on top of the right hand.

vii. Lastly, close your eyes and relax the whole body with slow and even breathing.

viii. Repeat the *asan* with the alternate arrangement of hands and legs.

Awareness

◆ On the breaths flowing in and out
◆ On the Divine Names "Radhey Krishna" in your breaths

Benefits

✓ This meditative posture, Dhyan Veerasan, has a marvelous effect on the pelvic structure.
✓ The outer muscles of the thighs are stretched well.
✓ It massages and strengthens the pelvic and reproductive organs.

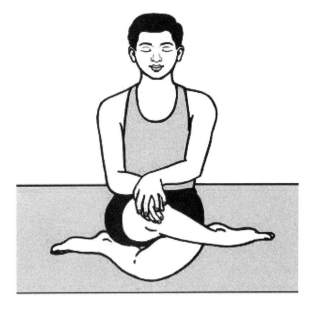

✓ It cures rheumatic pain in the knees and gout, and also shows improvment on the problem of flat feet.

6. Siddhasan (Accomplished Pose)

Procedure

i. Sit down with your legs outstretched in front and keeping the back erect, place your palms on the floor behind the buttocks, with the fingers pointing backward, i.e. Dandasan (See page 117).

ii. Now, fold your left leg and place the left sole beside the right inner thigh with the heel touching the perineum (the area between the genital and the anus).

iii. Then, fold the right leg and place the right heel above the left heel in such a way that the right heel touches the pelvic floor.

iv. Now, insert the right toes between the left thigh and calf; pull up the left toes to place them between the right thigh and the calf.

v. Keep your hands on the knees in any *mudra*.

vi. Make sure that the knees lie on the floor and the heels on top of each other in the final position.

vii. Make the head, neck, and spine erect in a single line.

viii. Close the eyes and relax the whole body with slow and even breathing.

ix. Repeat the *asan* with alternate set of the hands and legs.

Awareness

✧ On breathing in and out
✧ On the Sacred Names "Radhey Krishna" with your each breath

Benefits

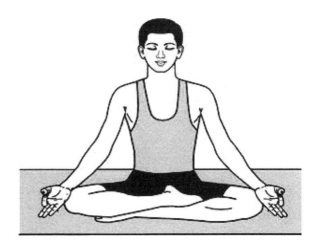

✓ Siddhasan helps direct sexual energy upward to the brain.
✓ It helps in building excellent memory power.
✓ It stimulates and strengthens the digestion system as blood circulation gets concentrated in the abdominal area instead of the legs.
✓ It also activizes your nervous system wonderfully.

Contraindications

- Persons suffering from sciatica or sacral infection should not do this *asan*.

7. Padmasan (Lotus Pose)

Procedure

i. Sit down with your legs outstretched in front and keeping the back erect, place your palms on the floor behind the buttocks, with the fingers pointing backward, i.e. Dandasan (See page 117).

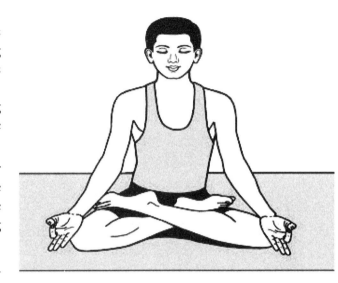

ii. Slowly and carefully, fold your right leg at the knee and place your right foot on top of the left thigh, with the sole facing upward.

iii. Similarly, fold the left leg and place the left foot on top of the right thigh with comfort.

iv. The heels should be close to the pubic bones and both knees should be touching the ground.

v. Make sure your head and the spine remain erect; also there is no tension in the shoulders.

vi. Now, place your hands on the knees in any *mudra*.

vii. Finally, close your eyes and relax your body with slow and even breathing.

viii. Repeat the *asan* by placing the left foot on top of the right thigh.

Awareness

✧ On breathing in and out
✧ On always recalling "Radhey Krishna" along with breathing in and out

Benefits

✓ If performed for a long period of time, Padmasan helps to straighten the spine automatically, which supports to relieve one from depression and tension as the lower spine becomes perfectly erect.
✓ It also develops the nervous system to a large extent.
✓ It stimulates digestion as blood circulation gets concentrated in the abdominal area instead of the legs.
✓ Lastly, it trims the extra fat from the waist.

Contraindications

- People with sciatica, sacral infections, and weak or injured knees should not do it.

D. Sitting Poses

1. Dandasan (Simple Sitting Pose)

Procedure

i. Slowly, sit with your legs outstretched in the front, and the heels together.

ii. Keep your palms on the floor behind the buttocks.

iii. Make sure your fingers remain pointing backward.

iv. Recline your torso slightly, resting it lightly on your arms.

v. Breathe normally.

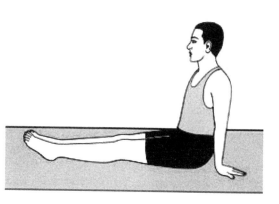

Note: This will be the starting or base position for all the sitting *asans*.

2. Shithil Dandasan (Relaxing Sitting Pose)

Procedure

i. Sit on the floor with your legs outstretched, keeping a distance of about 1-2 feet between them.

ii. Lean your body little bit backward, supporting it by placing your hands behind.

iii. Make sure your fingers remain pointing backward.

iv. Let your head go backward freely, or rest on either side of your shoulder.

v. Lastly, close your eyes and relax with deep breathing.

Note: This will be the final position for all the sitting *asans*.

3. Shashankasan (The Moon Pose)

Procedure

i. Sit down with your legs outstretched and joined together in front; keeping the back erect, place your palms on the floor behind the buttocks, with the fingers pointing backward, i.e. Dandasan (See page 117).

ii. Slowly come into Vajrasan (See page 113) and rest your palms on the thighs.

iii. Inhale (Radhey); raise your arms up above the head; straighten the trunk, head, and arms;

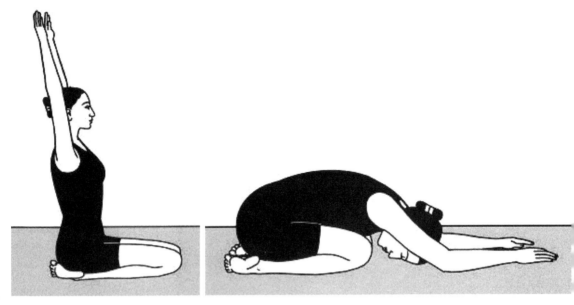

turn the palms forward.

iv. Now, while exhaling (Krishna), gently lean forward from the hips until the hands and forehead reach the floor.

v. Slightly flex your elbows and let them rest on the floor so that the whole body rests completely.

vi. Be in this posture for as long as possible with slow and even breathing.

vii. Ultimately, come back to the base position.

Awareness
✧ On the movements and the breaths synchronized with them
✧ On feeling relaxation on the stretched and contracted parts of your body
✧ On always remembering "Radhey Krishna" along with breaths

Benefits
✓ This tension relieving *asan*, Shashankasan, helps maintain a healthy body and sound mind by toning the spinal nerves, sciatic nerves, and the pelvic muscles.
✓ It corrects the position of the vertebral disc.
✓ Besides, it superbly assists in the functioning of the adrenal glands.
✓ It helps eliminate the disorder of the reproductive organs.
✓ If practiced continually, constipation is eradicated within a short duration.
✓ If one performs Ujjayi Pranayam in the final position, it yields an excellent soothing effect to the brain.

Contraindications
- People with high blood pressure and slipped-disc should not do this *asan*.

4. Veerasan (Hero's Pose)

Procedure

i. Come into Vajrasan progressively (See page 113).

ii. Slightly unfold your left leg and rest the left foot on the floor near the inner side of the right knee.

iii. Gently raise your left hand, put the left elbow on the left knee and rest the chin on the left palm.

iv. Make sure your trunk and head stay well erect.

v. Rest your right hand on your right knee, and then close your eyes.

vi. Hold the pose for as long as you are comfortable, with slow and even breathing.

vii. Gently return to Vajrasan and repeat the *asan* on the other side.

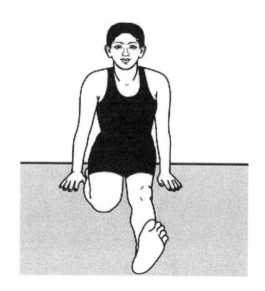

Awareness

✧ On the breaths flowing in and out
✧ On keeping the spine and head erect
✧ On spontaneously remembering "Radhey Krishna" along with the exhalations and inhalations

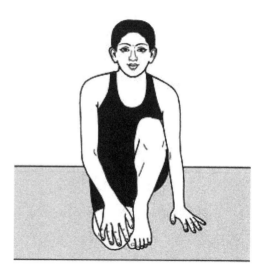

Benefits

✓ The aim of Veerasan is to improve the functions of the kidneys, liver, and different reproductive and abdominal organs.

✓ *Yog* therapists also recommend it for the development of concentration, for it helps balance the mind of the practitioners.

✓ Veerasan allows more awareness of the unconscious realms and brings both—physical and mental relaxation—quickly.

✓ This easy pose even benefits those with uncontrolled thoughts because it assists in shaping their thinking process clearly.

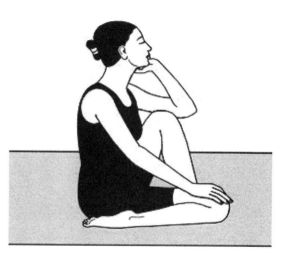

5. Ananda Madirasan (Alcoholic Bliss Pose)

Procedure

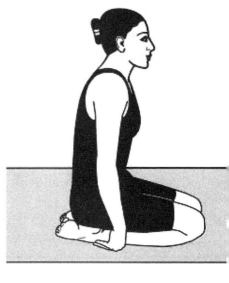

i. Sit down with your legs outstretched and joined together in front; keeping the back erect, place your palms on the floor behind the buttocks, with the fingers pointing backward, i.e. Dandasan (See page 117).

ii. Then, slowly come to Vajrasan (See page 113) by flexing your legs at the knees.

iii. Now, rest your palms on top of the heels.

iv. Make sure your head and spine remain erect.

v. Now, close your eyes and with slow and even breathing, relax the body fully.

vi. Stay in this position for as long as you are comfortable.

Awareness
✧ On the breaths flowing in and out through your nose
✧ On the unbroken recalling of "Radhey Krishna" all the time while breathing

Benefits
✓ Ananda Madirasan, very clear from its name, pacifies the mind—comforting the whole nervous system.
✓ This *asan* relieves one from acidity, gas, constipation, and indigestion.
✓ It also backs in curing chronic maladies like peptic ulcer, piles, menstrual disorder, and hydrocele.

6. Bhadrasan (Gentle Pose)

Procedure

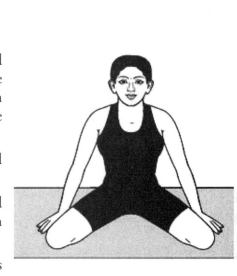

i. Sit down with your legs outstretched and joined together in front; keeping the back erect, place your palms on the floor behind the buttocks, with the fingers pointing backward, i.e. Dandasan (See page 117).

ii. Then, come into Vajrasan (See page 113) and spread your knees as far as you are comfortable.

iii. Make sure your heels are separated a bit and buttocks rest comfortably on the floor in between the feet.

iv. Without any uneasy force, try to separate the knees further and rest the palms on the knees.

v. Gaze at the tip of the nose and maintain the pose for as long as possible with slow and even breathing.

vi. If the eyes get tired, relax them by closing them for a while and again continue the gazing act.

vii. At last, come to Shithil Dandasan (See page 117) and relax.

Awareness

✧ On the breaths flowing in and out
✧ On the tip of your nose
✧ On mentally chanting the Holy Names "Radhey Krishna" with your each breath, and feeling the presence of the sentient Form of "Radhey Krishna" as well

Benefits

✓ Bhadrasan keeps the abdominal muscles and organs in a healthy state.
✓ As the back, arms, and the legs are mainly used, it helps remove stiffness from these parts.

7. Shaithalyasan (Animal Relaxation Pose)

Procedure

i. Sit down with your legs outstretched and joined together in front; keeping the back erect, place your palms on the floor behind the buttocks, with the fingers pointing backward, i.e. Dandasan (See page 117).

ii. Slowly fold your left knee, take your left foot toward the inner part of the right thigh so that the sole of left foot rests against it.

iii. Then, fold your right knee and place the right heel to the outer side of the right buttock, with the inner part of the leg touching the floor.

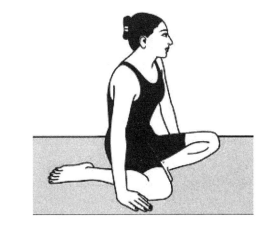

iv. Comfortably, rotate your trunk to the left side and while inhaling (Radhey), gently lift your arms straight over your head.

v. While exhaling (Krishna), bend

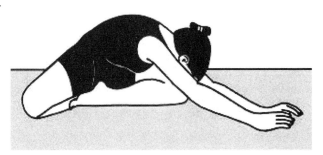

forward over the left knee and touch the forehead to the floor.

vi. Rest in this position for as long as you are comfortable with normal breathing.

vii. Then, come back to the starting position.

viii. Practice on the other side.

ix. Lastly, come into Shithil Dandasan (See page 117) and rest.

Awareness
✧ On the bodily movements and breaths synchronized with them; the stretch of the back
✧ On mentally uttering the Holy Names "Radhey Krishna" in your breath, and feeling Their presence at all times

Benefits
✓ Shaithalyasan exercises the abdominal organs excellently.
✓ It gives a nice stretch to the back, pelvic region, and thighs.
✓ Besides, it also makes the hip joints very flexible.

Contraindications
- Persons suffering from lower back cases should do Shaithalyasan carefully.

8. Namaskarasan (Salutation Pose)

Procedure

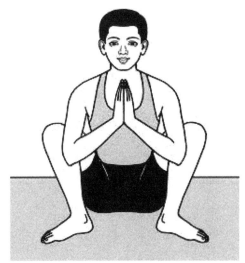

i. Sit down with your legs outstretched and joined together in front; keeping the back erect, place your palms on the floor behind the buttocks, with the fingers pointing backward, i.e. Dandasan (See page 117).

ii. Slowly fold your legs and come to a squatting position with both the feet flat on the floor about 1.5 feet apart.

iii. Make sure your knees remain apart as far as possible, and the elbows rested on the inner sides of the knees.

iv. Join your palms together in front of the chest as though praying and apply force on the inner sides of the knees with the elbows.

v. With an inhalation (Radhey), stretch your head backward, and simultaneously push your knees away as far as possible with the help of biceps.

vi. Now while exhaling (Krishna), straighten your arms in front of the chest, and simultaneously—pushing in with the knees—press the upper arms inside.

vii. In this position, lean the head forward with the chin touching the chest with optimum force.

viii. Ensure there is no tension in the upper back muscles and shoulders.

ix. Stay in this pose for at least five seconds with normal breathing.

x. Now, come back to the squatting position.

xi. This completes one round; repeat for 5-8 rounds likewise.

xii. Finally, come into Shithil Dandasan (See page 117) and relax.

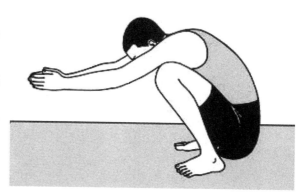

Awareness

✧ On your breaths synchronized with the movements
✧ On the extension of the back of the neck, upper back, chest, and the shoulder muscles
✧ On spontaneously recalling "Radhey Krishna" along with your breaths

Benefits

✓ Namaskarasan mainly increases flexibility in the hips and exercises the nerves.
✓ It also tones up the muscles of the thighs, knees, shoulders, arms, and the neck.

9. Baithak Merudandasan (Sitting Spinal Pose)

Procedure

i. Sit down with your legs outstretched and joined together in front; keeping the back erect, place your palms on the floor behind the buttocks, with the fingers pointing backward, i.e. Dandasan (See page 117).

ii. Keep your back straight and place both arms behind your back.

iii. Bend your left leg, and place the left foot on the kneecap of the right leg.

iv. Inhale (Radhey) in this state.

v. Exhaling (Krishna), gently twist your spine, bringing the left knee toward the ground on the opposite side; and twist your head and neck on the opposite side of your left knee.

vi. Keep your right leg locked on the floor in this state.

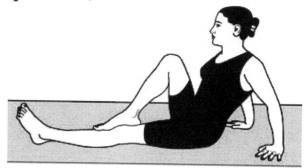

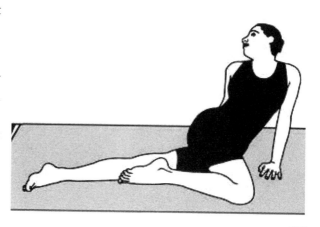

vii. Stay in this pose for 25-30 seconds, breathing normally.

viii. Repeat the pose on the other side.

ix. Finally, get into Shithil Dandasan (See page 117) and relax.

Awareness
- ✧ On the breaths synchronized with the spinal twisting and stretching
- ✧ On mental chanting of the Divine Names "Radhey Krishna" in your breaths, and always feeling Their presence

Benefits
- ✓ Baithak Merudandasan loosens up the spinal column and helps mitigate lower backache.
- ✓ Also, it exercises the internal abdominal organs and helps to increase peristalsis process.

Contraindications
- Those who are suffering from severe back spasms like scoliosis, should not practice this *asan*.

10. Yog Mudrasan (Psychic Union Pose / Yogic Seal Pose)

Procedure
i. Sit in Padmasan (See page 116).

ii. Take both hands behind your back and grasp the wrist of the one hand with the other, and relax the whole body.

iii. Inhale (Radhey) in this position.

iv. Now with an exhalation (Krishna), gently lean forward from your hips.

v. Keeping your trunk erect, move your forehead to the floor.

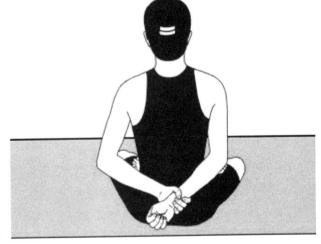

vi. Without any stress, be in this position with normal breathing for as long as possible.

vii. Comfortably, regain the initial position.

viii. Repeat the *asan* with the legs crossed in the alternate way in Padmasan.

Awareness
- ✧ On the breaths and the forward and upward movements synchronized with them

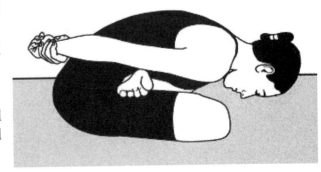

- ✧ On the pressure of the back and abdomen
- ✧ On mentally chanting the Sacred Names "Radhey Krishna" in your breaths

Benefits
- ✓ This relaxing *asan*, Yog Mudrasan, improves elasticity of the spine by exercising the spinal nerves.
- ✓ It also helps root out several diseases associated with the abdominal parts such as constipation and indigestion.

Contraindications
- - Persons with heart maladies, back pain, and poor eye vision should not do it. It would be best if excluded by women in the post-delivery period.

11. Mandukasan (Frog Pose)

Procedure

i. Sit in Vajrasan (See page 113).

ii. Form fists, with the thumbs inside.

iii. Keep your fists together, with the knuckles facing each other.

iv. Place your fists on either side of the navel in such a way that sides of your index fingers touch the navel portion.

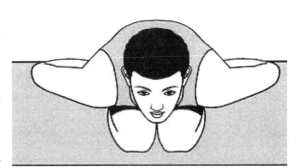

v. Inhale (Radhey) and exhaling (Krishna), lean forward from your waist till your chest touches the thighs.

vi. Next, exert light pressure on the abdomen with your fists and look upward.

vii. Stay in the pose for 15-20 seconds with normal breathing.

viii. Now inhaling (Radhey), gently come back to Vajrasan.

ix. Repeat it twice.

Awareness
- ✧ On your breaths and bodily movements synchronized with them
- ✧ On the pressure around your navel
- ✧ On mentally chanting the Holy Names "Radhey Krishna" in your breaths

Benefits
- ✓ Mandukasan stimulates your pancreas and helps in controlling diabetes.
- ✓ It is effective in curing abdominal ailments.
- ✓ Additionally, it massages the heart properly, and thus helps in curing heart diseases.

12. Singhasan (Lion Pose)

Procedure

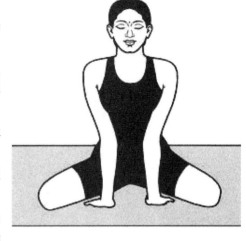

i.   Slowly folding your legs, come to Vajrasan (See page 113) with the knees one foot apart.

ii. Place your hands in the front, on the floor, between the knees, with the fingers spread and pointing toward the body.

iii. Lock your elbows firmly; push the lower back forward and then tighten the neck.

iv. Now, balance your body on the straightened arms, shifting the body-weight on them.

v.   Fixing your eyes on the eyebrow centre, maintain the posture for as long as you are comfortable with normal breathing.

vi. Slowly, return to Vajrasan and then come to Shithil Dandasan (See page 117) and relax.

Awareness

✧ On the stretch of the neck, lower back, and the arms

✧ On realizing the presence of "Radhey Krishna" in front of you while inhaling and exhaling air

Benefits

✓ Singhasan exercises the liver and controls the flow of bile.

✓ The strong pressure on the palms helps remove stress and tension.

✓ In addition, it maintains adequate blood supply and tones up the nerves.

✓ If performed regularly, it helps develop concentration.

13. Singha Garjan Asan (Roaring Lion Pose)

Procedure

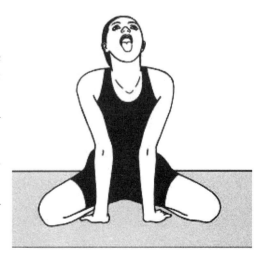

i.   Sit in Vajrasan (See page 113).

ii. Spread your knees about 1-2 feet apart; place the hands on the floor in between the knees with the fingers facing backward.

iii. Keeping your arms locked, lean slightly forward.

iv. Now shifting some of the body-weight onto the hands, raise the head backward.

v.   Arch your back a little bit; gaze at the eyebrow centre and inhale (Radhey) deeply.

vi. While exhaling (Krishna), stick the tongue out as much as possible.

vii. Opening the mouth as wide as possible, produce a roaring sound like that of a lion.

viii. Repeat it 3-5 times in the same manner.

ix. Then, come into Sukhasan (See page 111), and massage the throat with the fingers while swallowing saliva to remove the uneasiness in the throat.

Awareness

✧ On the roaring sound
✧ On the throat
✧ On the gaze
✧ On feeling the omnipresence of "Radhey Krishna" in your breaths

Benefits

✓ Singha Garjan Asan is chiefly recommended for problems related to the ears, nose, and the throat.
✓ It also cures stuttering and stammering problems.
✓ It is useful in tonsils, thyroid, and other throat related cases.
✓ It is also beneficial for those who are neurotic or introverted.

Contraindications

- Persons with heart maladies, back pain, and poor eyesight should not do it. It would be best if excluded by women in the post-delivery period.

14. Udarakarshan Asan (Abdominal Extension Pose)

Procedure

i. Sit down with your legs outstretched and joined together in front; keeping the back erect, place your palms on the floor behind the buttocks with the fingers pointing backward, i.e. Dandasan (See page 117).

ii. Now, come into the squatting position with both the feet about one foot apart.

iii. Then, place your hands on the knees.

iv. Inhale deeply (Radhey); while exhaling (Krishna), place your right knee on the floor, close to the left foot.

v. Try to push your left knee to the right with the help of the left hand, simultaneously turn your head and trunk to the left and gaze over the left shoulder.

vi. Feel the pressure in the abdomen.

vii. Rest the inner side of the right foot on the floor.

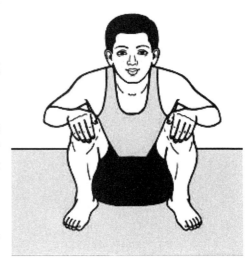

viii. Stay in this position for 15-20 seconds with normal breathing.

ix. Perform with the next leg on the next side to complete one round.

x. Repeat it 3-5 times.

xi. Finally, come into Shithil Dandasan (See page 117) and relax.

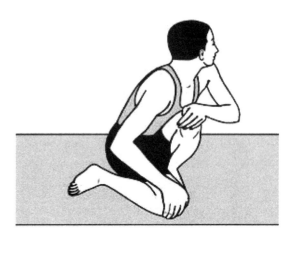

Awareness

✧ On the breaths synchronized with the movements

✧ On the stretch and strain of the abdominal parts

✧ On recalling sentient forms of "Radhey Krishna" along with your breaths

Benefits

✓ Udarakarshan Asan gives relief from abdominal illnesses like constipation, bowel syndromes, etc.

15. Hansasan (Swan Pose)

Procedure

i. Sit in Vajrasan (See page 113).

ii. Slowly kneel on the floor, spreading the knees a bit.

iii. Keep your hands between the knees on the floor, with the fingers pointing backward and both—the elbows and forearms—close to each other.

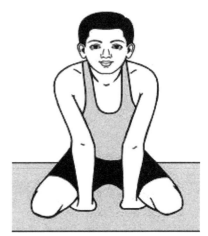

iv. Now, gradually lean forward and rest your abdomen on the elbows—keeping them close to each other on either side of the navel, with the chest resting on the upper arms (triceps portion).

v. Then, lean further down and rest your head on the floor.

vi. Outstretch your legs backward one by one; keep them together and locked, resting the toes on the ground.

vii. As you inhale (Radhey), raise your head and chest upward so that the neck will be

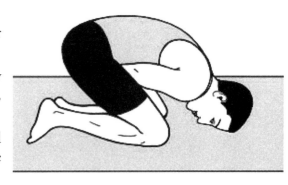

aligned with the trunk.

viii. While exhaling (Krishna), slowly shift the body-weight onto the wrists and hands.

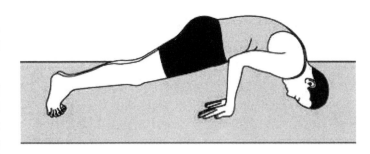

ix. Make sure the feet touching the floor remain at an angle of 30 degrees to the floor when the entire body is balanced on the palms and the toetips.

x. Remain in this position at your ease with normal breathing.

xi. Return to the squatting pose by lowering your legs slowly to the floor and folding them.

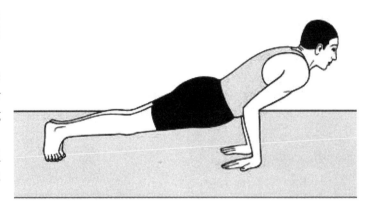

xii. Now come to Vajrasan and finally into Shithil Dandasan (See page 117) and relax.

Awareness

✧ On the breaths flowing in and out
✧ On the abdomen
✧ On spontaneous remembering of "Radhey Krishna" along with your breaths and always feeling Their presence

Benefits

✓ The benefits of Hansasan are more or less similar to Mayurasan (See page 192).
✓ It tones up the abdominal organs by proper massaging.
✓ It increases digestion power and is extremely effectual in the treatment of flatulence, constipation, and malfunction of the kidneys and liver.
✓ It is also helpful in removing worms from the stomach and intestine, and curing dysentery as well.

Contraindications

- Those with high blood pressure, heart ailments, hernia, hyperacidity, and peptic or duodenal ulcer should avoid this *asan*.
- Also, pregnant women, or those who are sick, or physically weak should avoid it.

16. Rajju Karshanasan (Rope Pulling Pose)

Procedure

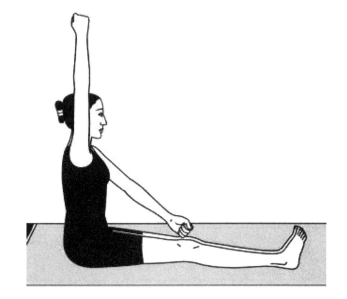

i. Sit down with your legs outstretched and joined together in front; keeping the back erect, place your palms on the floor behind the buttocks, with the fingers pointing backward, i.e. Dandasan (See page 117).

ii. Inhale (Radhey) and raise your right arm vertically, imagining a rope is hanging in front of your body.

iii. Lock your arms at the elbows and look upward.

iv. While exhaling (Krishna), gradually draw your right arm down with force, as if pulling the rope.

v. Make sure that your eyeballs move with the upward and downward movements of the right hand.

vi. Likewise, perform with the other hand, and repeat this *asan* with both the hands (moving up and down) alternatively in a rhythm.

vii. This is one round; perform for 10-15 more rounds.

viii. Eventually, come into Shithil Dandasan (See on page 117) and relax.

Awareness

✧ On the downward movement of the imaginary rope
✧ On the stretch of the upper back and the shoulders
✧ On the Divine Names "Radhey Krishna" along with your breaths

Benefits

✓ Rajju Karshanasan loosens the shoulder joints.
✓ It exercises the upper back muscles.
✓ It tones the breast muscles.

17. Bhu-namanasan (Spinal Twist Prostration Pose)

Procedure

i. Sit down with your legs outstretched and joined together in front; keeping the back erect, place your palms on the floor behind the buttocks, with the fingers pointing backward, i.e. Dandasan (See page 117).

ii. Placing both the hands to the left side of the body, rest them near the left hip and move the left hand a bit away from the buttocks.

iii. Inhale (Radhey) in this state.

iv. While exhaling (Krishna), slowly turn your torso directly to the left; with the support of the hands, gently try to touch the floor (in between the hands near the left hand) with the forehead by leaning the trunk downward.

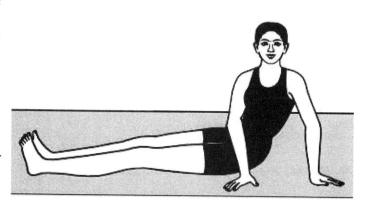

v. Make sure your spine stays straight and both the buttocks act like a base on the floor.

vi. Maintain the position for 15-20 seconds with normal breathing.

vii. Slowly return to the starting position and repeat on the other side.

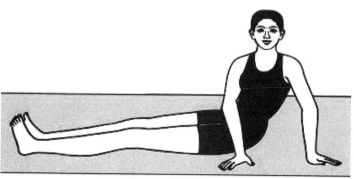

viii. This completes one round; do for two more rounds.

ix. Ultimately, come to Shithil Dandasan (See page 117) and relax.

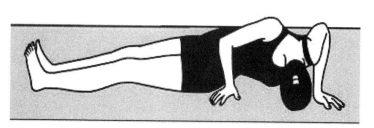

Awareness

✧ On the various bodily movements and the breaths synchronized with them

✧ On the stretching and releasing of the spine, neck, and the shoulders

✧ On spontaneously remembering the Sacred Names "Radhey Krishna" in your breaths and also feeling Their presence at all times

Benefits

✓ A healthy and flexible spine indicates a healthy nervous system. If the nerves are healthy, a man is sound in mind and body.

✓ This *asan* makes the spine and lower back supple and flexible, thus it activates the nerves.

Contraindication

- Women after the second or third month of pregnancy should not practice it.

18. Marjari Asan (Cat Stretch Pose)

Procedure

i. Sit in Vajrasan (See page 113).

ii. Inhale (Radhey); lifting your buttocks off the floor, stand on the knees.

iii. Now with an exhalation (Krishna), slowly lean forward.

iv. Then, place both hands on the floor, in the line of shoulders, with the fingers facing forward.

v. Ensure your arms and thighs remain straight and the hands aligned with the knees.

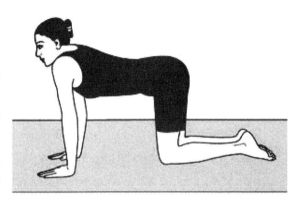

vi. Inhale (Radhey) while depressing (arching) the back and raise the head to look up at the ceiling.

vii. As you exhale (Krishna), raise the spine upward to make it concave; simultaneously pull the stomach muscles in and also bring the chin downward to the chest.

viii. This is one round; try it for up to 5-10 rounds.

ix. Eventually, come to Shithil Dandasan (See page 117) and relax.

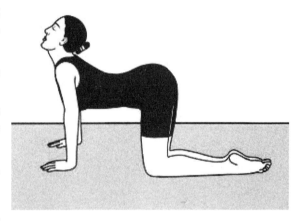

Awareness

◇ On the breaths synchronized with your bodily movements

◇ On spontaneously remembering the sentient forms of "Radhey Krishna" along with your breathing

Benefits

✓ This is a very invigorating *asan* as it makes the spine, neck, and shoulders supple.

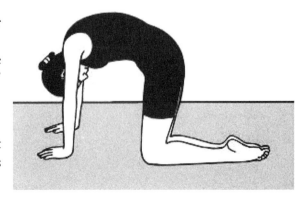

19. Vyaghrasan (Tiger Pose)

Procedure

i. Come into Marjari Asan, iv step, (See page 132) progressively and look ahead.

ii. While inhaling (Radhey), raise your right leg off the floor as high as possible, and then bend your leg at the knee so that the toes will come toward the head.

iii. Simultaneously, bend your head upward and backward, toward the right toes.

iv. In this state, try to touch your head with the right toes without straining.

v. While exhaling (Krishna), straighten your right leg; then bend it at the knee; lowering right knee without touching the floor, bring the right knee toward the chest.

vi. Simultaneously, form a concave shape with the spine; lower your head downward and touch the chin with the right knee.

vii. Repeat the process for upto five times each with both the legs.

viii. Eventually, come to Shithil Dandasan (See page 117) and realx.

Awareness

- ✦ On the breaths synchronized with the various bodily movements
- ✦ On feeling the presence of "Radhey Krishna" in front of you and watching you

Benefits

- ✓ Vyaghrasan keeps the neck, spine, and legs healthy by flexing them nicely.
- ✓ It reduces unnecessary fats from hips and thighs through active movement.
- ✓ It also helps cure sciatica by relaxing the sciatic nerves.
- ✓ Digestion is developed well as due to adequate stretching of the abdominal muscles.
- ✓ In addition, it strengthens the female reproductive system.

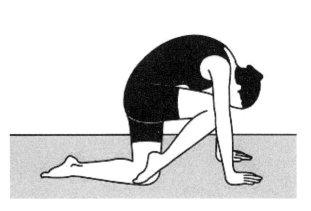
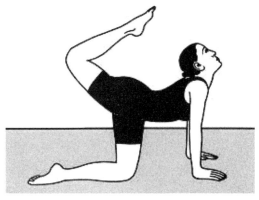

20. Pranamasan (Bowing Pose)

Procedure

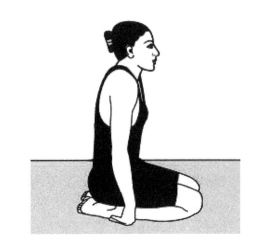

i. Gently come into the final position of Vajrasan (See page 113).

ii. Inhale (Radhey) and grasp your lower calves closer to the ankles.

iii. While exhaling (Krishna), comfortably lean forward and rest the crown on the floor.

iv. Now, raise your buttocks upward until your thighs are perpendicular to the floor.

v. Make sure your hands hold the calves firmly at all times.

vi. Hold this pose for about 15-20 seconds with normal breathing.

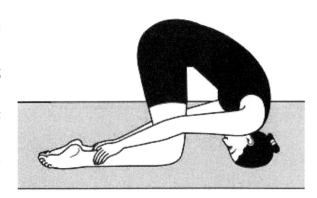

vii. Again return to Vajrasan by lowering the buttocks.

viii. This completes one round; repeat it twice.

ix. Lastly, come into Shithil Dandasan (See page 117) and relax.

Awareness

✧ On the bodily movements and breaths synchronized with them

✧ On mental chanting of "Radhey Krishna" along with your breaths—recalling Them at all times

✧ On the balance in the final step

Benefits

✓ Pranamasan is supportive in asthma as it exercises the lungs and the chest and opens the air passages.

✓ Naturally, it supplies a copious amount of blood to the brain by lowering the head on the floor.

✓ In addition, this pose also decompresses (relaxes) the lower cervical portion, upper and thoracic vertebrae, and the different nerve roots.

Contraindications

- Persons with hypertension (high blood pressure), neck pain, and vertigo (giddiness) should avoid it.

134

21. Kawa Chalasan (Crow Walking)

Procedure

i.   Sit down with your legs outstretched and joined together in front; keeping the back erect, place your palms on the floor behind the buttocks, with the fingers pointing backward, i.e. Dandasan (See page 117).

ii. Comfortably fold your legs and come into the squatting pose with both feet slightly apart and the buttocks on the heels.

iii. Now rest your palms on each knee and take small steps in this position, with each knee touching the floor in turn.

iv. Attempt to keep your legs bent, the buttocks on the heels; then walk either on the toes or the soles.

v.   Try to move at least 50-60 steps with normal breathing.

vi. Ultimately, come to Shithil Dandasan (See page 117) and relax.

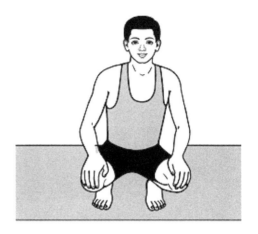

Awareness

✧ On the rhythm of the breaths with the bodily movements

✧ On the effect in the lower back, hips, knees, and the toes or soles

✧ On chanting the Divine Names "Radhey Krishna" and always feeling Their presence

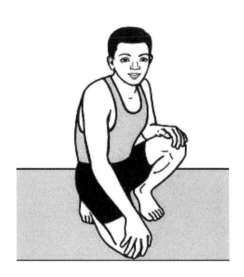

Benefits

✓ Kawa Chalasan is very effectual in constipation problems.

✓ Like Namaskarasan (See page 122) and Vayu Nishkasan (See page 140), it develops suppleness of the legs.

✓ It also rejuvenates the lower portion of the body by enhancing the blood ciuculation in the legs.

Contraindications

-   Those who have the defects in the knees, ankles, and toes should not practice it.

22. Vakrasan (Twist Pose)

Procedure

i. Sit down with your legs outstretched and joined together in front; keeping the back erect, place your palms on the floor behind the buttocks, with the fingers pointing backward, i.e. Dandasan (See page 117).

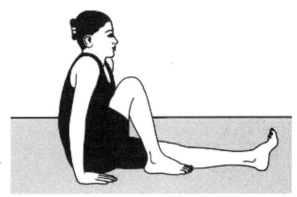

ii. Slowly fold the right leg at the knee and place the foot beside the inner side of the left knee.

iii. Inhale (Radhey); while exhaling (Krishna), try to stretch both—the trunk and head—as much as you can; turn the waist rightward and place your left arm around the right knee and grasp the right big toe.

iv. Slowly move the right arm backward and place the right palm on the ground.

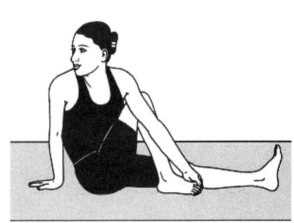

v. Try to keep your trunk erect as much as you can with a proper twist; simultaneously twist your head rightward and look backward.

vi. Hold this position for 15-20 seconds, breathing normally.

vii. Slowly unwind your torso and return to Dandasan.

viii. Repeat similarly on the other side.

ix. Lastly, come into Shithil Dandasan (See page 117) and relax.

Awareness

✧ On the breaths synchronized with the twisting movements of your body parts
✧ On the stretches and strains of the spine, neck, legs, and arms
✧ On feeling relaxation in the spine, neck, legs, and arms, and spontaneously remembering the Names "Radhey Krishna" while breathing

Benefits

✓ Like other body twisting postures, Vakrasan makes the spine flexible as it is twisted laterally.
✓ It massages the lungs and activates the pancreas.

✓ It alleviates constipation, dyspepsia, and diabetes naturally.

23. Gatyatmak Meruvakrasan (Dynamic Spinal Twist Pose)

Procedure

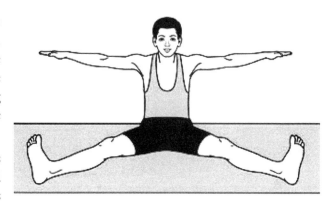

i. Sit down with your legs outstretched and joined together in front; keeping the back erect, place your palms on the floor behind the buttocks, with the fingers pointing backward, i.e. Dandasan (See page 117).

ii. Spread your legs apart as far as possible, and keep your trunk and head perpendicular to the floor, as shown in the figure.

iii. As you inhale (Radhey), slowly extend your hands to the sides at shoulder level.

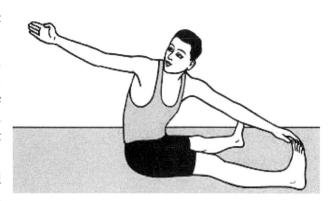

iv. As you exhale (Krishna), comfortably twist (upper body) to the right side and touch the right foot with the left hand, simultaneously moving the right arm behind the back.

v. Also, turn the head rightward and look at the outstretched right hand.

vi. Now, perform the twisting method leftward in the same manner as above.

vii. This finishes one round; repeat this for 10-20 rounds.

viii. Ultimately, come into Shithil Dandasan (See page 117) and relax.

Awareness

✧ On mentally chanting of the Sacred Names "Radhey Krishna" with your each breath
✧ On the spinal twists synchronized with your each breath
✧ On the stretch of the shoulder, upper trunk, neck, and arms

Benefits

✓ Gatyatmak Meruvakrasan loosens the back muscles.
✓ It perfectly tones the nerves of the arms and legs.

Contraindications

- Persons with extreme back problems should not practice this *asan*.

24. Meru Vakrasan (Spinal Twist)

Procedure

i. Sit down with your legs outstretched and joined together in front; keeping the back erect, place your palms on the floor behind the buttocks, with the fingers pointing backward, i.e. Dandasan (See page 117).

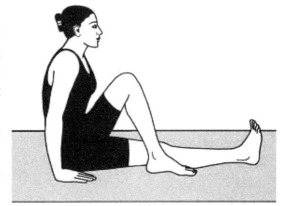

ii. Inhaling (Radhey), slowly place your left foot to the outer side of the right knee.

iii. Exhaling (Krishna), slowly twist your upper body, from the left buttock.

iv. Continuing to exhale (Krishna), slowly place your left hand behind the back—near the right buttock—close to the right hand; make sure legs remain unmoved.

v. Now, try to straighten your spine and twist the head to the right as far as possible.

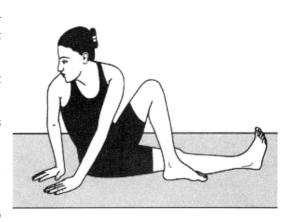

vi. Remain in this position for 15-20 seconds with normal breathing.

vii. Slowly, come back to the starting position.

viii. Repeat similarly on the other side.

ix. This ends one round; perform for two more rounds.

x. Eventually, come into Shithil Dandasan (See page 117) and relax.

Awareness

✧ On the spinal and other movements of your body synchronized with your breaths
✧ On the stretch and strain of the spine, legs, shoulders, and the neck, and always feeling complete relaxation in these parts
✧ On mentally uttering the Divine Names "Radhey Krishna" while breathing

Benefits

✓ This Spinal Twisting Pose exercises the spine by loosening the vertebrae and firming the nerves.
✓ It also helps remove backache, neck pain, lumbago, and sciatica.

Contraindications

- People suffering from excess back problems, hernias, ulcers, or other similar complaints should exclude it from their *Yog* package.

25. Nauka Sanchalanasan (Rowing Boat Pose)

Procedure

i. Sit down with your legs outstretched and joined together in front; keeping the back erect, place your palms on the floor behind the buttocks, with the fingers pointing backward, i.e. Dandasan (See page 117).

ii. Clench both hands (as if holding the oars) to form fists, with both palms facing downward and fists by the chest.

iii. Now inhale (Radhey); exhaling (Krishna), lean forward from your waist, simultaneously moving both hands straight forward and downward the sides of the legs.

iv. Now again inhaling (Radhey), lean backward as far as possible; simultaneously, bring your hands gently to the sides of the chest.

v. Make sure while bending back and forth, your hands form a complete vertical circle (as if you are rowing a boat with imaginary oars).

vi. Also, be sure that your legs remain locked throughout the whole process.

vii. This is one round, do it for up to 5-10 times.

viii. Finally, come to Shithil Dandasan (See page 117) and relax.

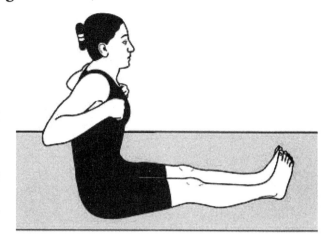
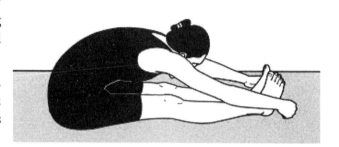
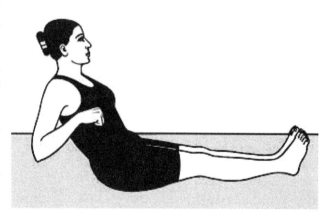

Variation - 1

Nauka Sanchalanasan can be performed with the legs spread too. If this is done, one should row over the legs one by one.

Awareness

✧ On different bodily movements along with the breaths synchronized with them

◇ On the pressure and effect on the lower back and stomach

◇ On mentally uttering the Sacred Names "Radhey Krishna" in your breaths, and always feeling Their presence around you

Benefits

✓ By regular practice of Nauka Sanchalanasan, there is a balanced regulation of energy flow in the abdominal and the pelvic regions.

✓ It also alleviates constipation as the abdominal organs get a good exercise.

✓ For women, it is especially essential for eradicating defects in the reproductive system and post-natal recovery.

26. Vayu Nishkasan (Air Releasing Pose)

Procedure

i. Sit down with your legs outstretched iand joined together in front; keeping the back erect, place your palms on the floor behind the buttocks, with the fingers pointing backward, i.e. Dandasan (See page 117).

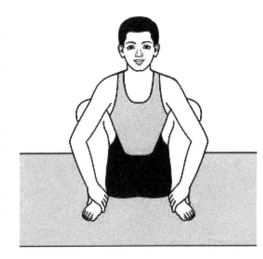

ii. Gently fold your legs and come into squatting pose with both the feet flat on the floor—about two feet apart.

iii. Now, grasp the inner sides of the feet with your fingers below the soles and the thumbs above.

iv. Push the inner knees with your triceps.

v. Keep your elbows slightly bent and make sure your eyes remain open throughout the whole process.

vi. While inhaling (Radhey), move the head slightly back and then look upward.

vii. While exhaling (Krishna), straighten the knees; raising the buttocks, move the head—forward and downward—toward the knees.

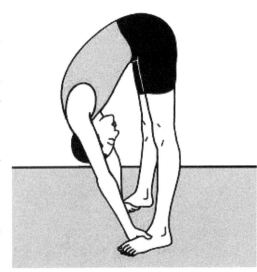

viii. With an inhalation (Radhey), come back to the squatting pose, bringing the head slightly backward.

ix. This is one round; repeat 10-15 times.

x. Finally, come into Shithil Dandasan (See page 117) and relax.

Awareness

⬦ On the breaths synchronized with the forward and upward movements of the body

⬦ On the stretch of the neck

⬦ On bending the spine

⬦ On mentally uttering the Holy Names "Radhey Krishna" while breathing, and also always remembering Them

Benefits

✓ As in Namaskarasan (See page 122), Vayu Nishkasan also increases flexibility in the hips and activizes the nerves.

✓ Similarly, it tones the muscles of the thighs, knees, shoulders, arms, and the neck.

✓ It also massages and stretches the entire spine and the leg muscles perfectly.

✓ As it is very clear from its name, it helps in relieving from flatulence.

27. Dhanurakarshanasan (Archer's Pose)

Procedure

i. Sit down with your legs outstretched and joined together in front; keeping the back erect, place your palms on the floor, behind the buttocks, with the fingers pointing backward, i.e. Dandasan (See page 117).

ii. Now, stretch your arms forward horizontally and keep the right arm on top by crossing the left arm exactly below it.

iii. Leaning a bit forward from the hips, hold your right big toe with left hand and your left big toe with the right hand.

iv. Gently move your right foot up under the right arm; you may rest it on the left thigh.

v. Make sure your right arm remains extended and the spine and head erect.

vi. Inhale (Radhey) in this position.

vii. Exhaling (Krishna), slowly lift the right toe toward the left ear and try to touch the right

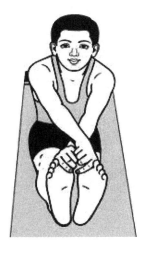

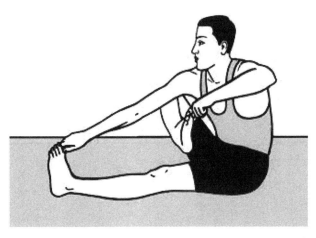

elbow with the right knee.

viii. Try to stay in this posture for 15-20 seconds with normal breathing.

ix. Slowly regain the initial position, and repeat on the other side.

x. This ends one round; repeat the same method for up to three rounds.

xi. Finally, come to Shithil Dandasan (See page 117) and relax.

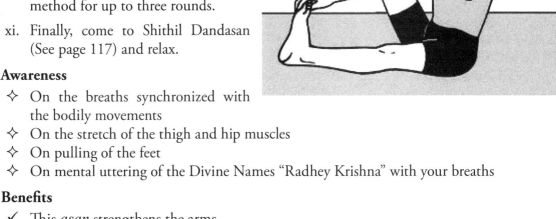

Awareness

✧ On the breaths synchronized with the bodily movements

✧ On the stretch of the thigh and hip muscles

✧ On pulling of the feet

✧ On mental uttering of the Divine Names "Radhey Krishna" with your breaths

Benefits

✓ This *asan* strengthens the arms.

✓ It loosens the hip joints, and thus develops flexibility in the legs.

✓ It not only releases pain in the back and neck, but it also exercises the abdominal parts.

✓ It helps cure hydrocele as well.

Contraindications

- Persons affected with slipped-disc, sciatica, and dislocation of the hip-joints should not include it in their *Yogic* practice.

28. Chakki Chalanasan (Mill Churning Pose)

Procedure

i. Sit down with your legs outstretched and joined together in front; keeping the back erect, place your palms on the floor behind the buttocks, with the fingers pointing backward, i.e. Dandasan (See page 117).

ii. Slowly spread your feet about 3-4 feet sideways.

iii. Raise both arms in front at the shoulder level and interlock the fingers.

iv. Make sure your arms remain stretched

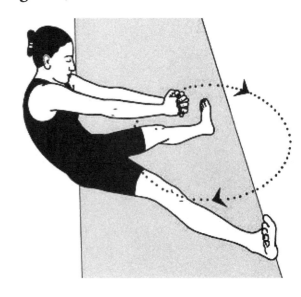

and horizontal throughout the practice.

  v. Shift your interlocked hands above the left leg and inhale (Radhey) in this position.

  vi. Now exhale (Krishna), slowly lean forward from the hips, then swing (rotate) rightward and bring the hands over the right foot.

  vii. Inhaling (Radhey), lean backward swinging from the waist as much as possible.

  viii. Create a circular motion with both—your upper body and arms—as if you are drawing an imaginary circle. Swing to the left and take your interlocked hands over the left toes.

  ix. In this way, repeat in a circular motion, making the buttocks and thighs as the pivotal point while swinging forward, rightward, backward, and leftward.

  x. After practicing for 5-10 times in this direction, perform in the opposite direction.

  xi. At last, come into Shithil Dandasan (See page 117) and relax.

Awareness
✧ On the breaths synchronized with the forward and backward movements of your body
✧ On the churning movement of the stomach
✧ On always recalling the omnipresence of "Radhey Krishna" along with your breathing

Benefits
✓ Chakki Chalanasan tones up the nerves and organs of the abdomen and the pelvis.
✓ This *asan* reduces unnecessary fat from the abdominal area and corrects different menstrual problems.
✓ Women can practice it even during the initial three months of pregnancy.
✓ In addition, it has a good effect on post-natal recovery.

29. Janu Shirasan (Head to Knee Pose)

Procedure
  i. Sit down with your legs outstretched and joined together in front; keeping the back erect, place your palms on the floor behind the buttocks, with the fingers pointing backward, i.e. Dandasan (See page 117).

  ii. Slowly fold your right leg, and place the right sole against the inner left thigh.

  iii. Keep your right knee on the floor; straighten your spine; place your palms on top of the left knee.

  iv. Inhaling (Radhey), raise your arms above the head and turn the palms forward.

  v. Exhaling (Krishna), lean forward from your hips, and attempt to grasp the left toe.

  vi. Continuing to exhale (Krishna), try to touch the left knee with your forehead—stretching the torso; make sure your right leg remains unmoved.

  vii. In the final position, attempt to place the elbows on the floor—on either side of the calf muscles.

viii. Maintain this posture for 15-20 seconds with normal breathing.

ix. As you inhale (Radhey), gently release your hands, and finally come back to the centre.

x. Repeat with the other leg in the same manner.

xi. This is one round; repeat it twice.

xii. Eventually, come to Shithil Dandasan (See page 117) and relax.

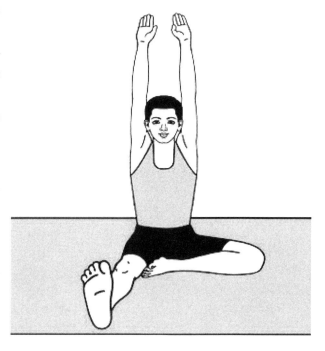

Awareness

✧ On the breaths synchronized with the forward bends and upward movements

✧ On the stretch in the legs, spine, and shoulders

✧ On continuously feeling the presence of "Radhey Krishna" in each breath

Benefits

✓ Janu Shirasan tones and massages the abdominal and pelvic regions including the pancreas, liver, stomach, adrenal glands, and spleen.

✓ It assists in alleviating disorders of the uro-genitals system.

✓ It also controls diabetes, menstrual problems, colitis, kidney troubles, bronchitis, and eosinophilia.

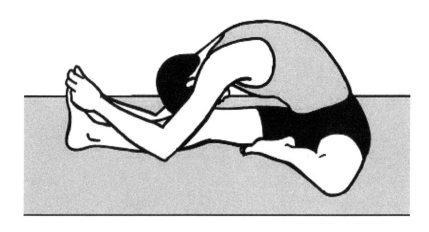

Contraindication

- People with serious back problems should omit it.

30. Gomukhasan (Cow's Head Pose)

Procedure

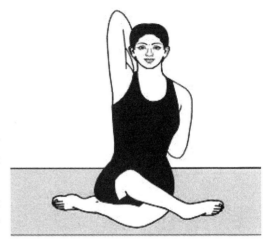

i. Come into Dhyan Veerasan (See page 114) with the right thigh exactly over the left thigh.

ii. Comfortably take your left hand behind the back, from under the left armpit, and place it between the shoulder blades; simultaneously bring the right arm precisely over the right shoulder.

iii. Anchor your fingers of the left and right hands tightly, and place the back of your head against the right elbow.

iv. Make sure your trunk stays erect and the head tilted slightly backward.

v. Hold this position for as long as comfortable with normal breathing.

vi. Slowly, release your hands and come back to Dhyan Veerasan.

vii. Repeat on the other side.

viii. Finally, let go of the legs; come into Shithil Dandasan (See page 117) and relax.

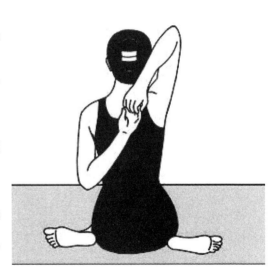

Awareness

✧ On the stretches and strains of the shoulders and arms
✧ On feeling the presence of "Radhey Krishna" both—in your breaths and everywhere

Benefits

✓ Gomukhasan activates the kidneys.
✓ Without any side effect, it alleviates chronic diseases such as diabetes, etc.
✓ Similarly, backache and sciatica are decreased wonderfully with its regular practice.
✓ It relieves one from stiffness of the neck and shoulders as well as provides additional strength to the legs.
✓ If practiced for a longer period, mental benefits like stress, tension, anxiety, and fatigue are naturally rectified.

31. Kashth Takshanasan (Chopping Wood Pose)

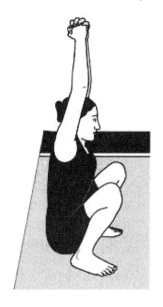
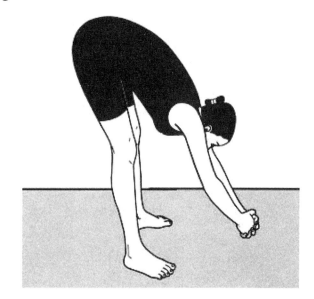

Procedure

i. Sit down with your legs outstretched and joined together in front; keeping the back erect, place your palms on the floor behind the buttocks, with the fingers pointing backward, i.e. Dandasan (See page 117).

ii. Spread your legs about one foot apart, and slowly bending on the knees, come to squatting position.

iii. Drawing the arms forward, interlock your fingers; keep them on the floor in between the feet and make sure that backside of the upper arms (triceps portion) touch the inner knees and that the knees are bent completely.

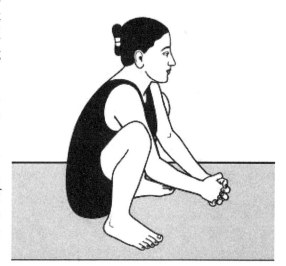

iv. Now, imagine that there is a large and round wooden log in front of you.

v. Slowly, with an inhalation (Radhey), raise your hands as high as possible as if raising an axe above your head.

vi. Now exhale (Krishna) and while making a "Ha" sound, lower the hands down in between your feet—quite rapidly and forcefully, as if chopping the wooden log.

vii. Simultaneously, raise your buttocks backward and upward and also try to lower the head in between the knees.

146

viii. This completes one round; practice 5-10 rounds

ix. Lastly, come to Shithil Dandasan (See page 117) and relax.

Awareness

✧ On your breaths synchronized with the different bodily movements

✧ On the imaginary wooden log

✧ On the stretch of your arms

✧ On mentally chanting the Sacred Names "Radhey Krishna" in your breaths

Benefits

✓ Kashth Takshanasan gives a special effect on the muscles of the back—between the shoulder blades, shoulder joints, and the upper back.

✓ It also flexes the pelvic girdle along with toning the pelvic muscles.

✓ It prepares women for child bearing, so it can be practiced during the first trimester of pregnancy.

32. Santulanasan (Balancing Pose)

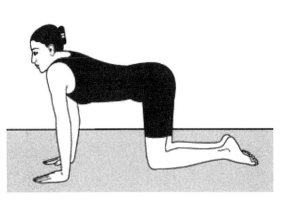
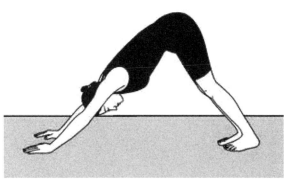

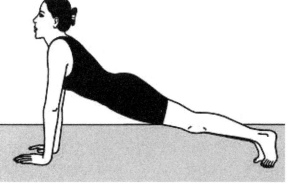

Procedure

i. Slowly come to Marjari Asan, iv step (See page 132), i.e. table pose.

ii. Inhaling (Radhey), raise your buttocks and resting your legs on the toes, stretch out both the legs.

iii. While exhaling (Krishna), gently lean forward and place both palms on the floor (almost like a dog pose).

iv. Continuing to exhale (Krishna), bring your shoulders forward, and let your buttocks go downward until the whole body becomes slanted.

v. Slightly raising the head, comfortably lock your knees and straighten the arms vertically.

vi. Then, concentrate on a fixed point ahead at eye level.

vii. Be in this position at your ease with normal breathing.

viii. Return to the starting pose by following the steps in the reverse order.

ix. Finally, come to Shithil Dandasan (See page 117) and relax.

Variation – 1

i. Come to the final pose of Santulanasan, following the above steps i-v, as mentioned in the main procedure.

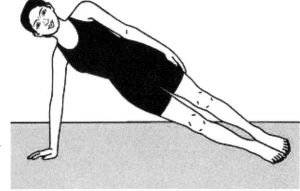

ii. Inhale (Radhey); shift the body-weight on the right arm and balance on it; as you exhale (Krishna), slowly flip your body onto the right side, and simultaneously raise the left arm vertically to place it along the side of the body.

iii. Hold this pose to your capacity with normal breathing.

iv. Return to your initial position, and practice the same method on the other side.

v. Now, return to the starting position by following the steps in the reverse order.

vi. Lastly, come to Shithil Dandasan (See page 117) and relax.

Variation – 2

i. Assume the final pose of Santulanasan, following the above steps i-v, as mentioned in the main procedure.

ii. Concentrate the eyes on a certain point in front of the body.

iii. Comfortably outstretch the right leg and lift it upward as high as possible.

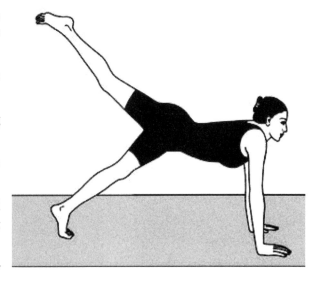

iv. Stay in this pose for a short duration with normal breathing.

v. Now, return to the initial state and perform the same process with the left leg.

vi. Come back to the starting position by following the steps in reverse order.

vii. Finally, come into Shithil Dandasan (See page 117) and relax.

148

Awareness

◇ On the balance

◇ On always feeling the presence of "Radhey Krishna" in front of you

Benefits

✓ This Balancing Pose tones up the muscles of the shoulders, arms, and spine.

✓ By this exercise, one can develop a sense of inner equilibrium and coherence because there is growth in the nervous balance in a natural way.

33. Sasangasan (Rabbit Pose)

Procedure

i. Come into Vajrasan (See page 113).

ii. Slightly raising the buttocks, grip your heels firmly in such a way that the thumbs are on the outer side of the feet.

iii. In this position, inhale (Radhey).

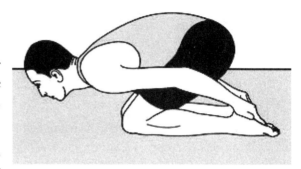

iv. As you lower the chin toward the chest, exhale (Krishna); then slowly curl the trunk until the forehead touches your knees, and the crown touches the floor.

v. Without disjoining your forehead from the knees, raise your spine and buttocks until your thighs become perpendicular to the floor.

vi. Balancing on lower legs, do not shift more weight onto the head.

vii. Hold this position for 15-20 seconds with normal breathing.

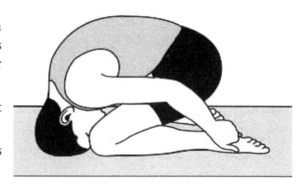

viii. While inhaling (Radhey), come to the Vajrasan and sit on the heels.

ix. This finishes one round; repeat thrice.

x. Lastly, come to Shithil Dandasan (See page 117) and relax.

Awareness

◇ On the various bodily movements and the breaths synchronized with them

◇ On the stretch and strains in the lumbar region, waist, buttocks, and shoulders

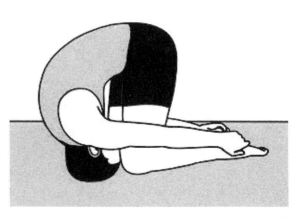

◇ On the Sacred Names "Radhey Krishna" along with breathing, and always feeling Their presence

Benefits
✓ Rabbit Pose brings about manifold advantages like maintaining the mobility and elasticity of the spine and back muscles, increasing digestion power, curing colds, sinus, and chronic tonsillitis.
✓ Its regular practice shows a profound effect on the thyroid and parathyroid glands.
✓ It improves the flexibility of the scapula and trapezius.

Contraindications
- Those with back cases and knee problems should not attempt it.

34. Moolbandhasan (Perineal Contraction Pose)
Procedure
i. Sit in Butterfly Pose (See page 96).

ii. Then, move your heels toward your perineum, keeping the outer sides of the feet completely on the floor.

iii. Now keep the palms on either side of the buttocks on the floor; get support from the palms and lift the buttocks onto the heels in such a way that the heels give pressure to the perineum.

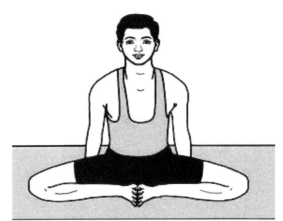

iv. Next, rest both hands on your knees in any *mudra*, with the head and trunk vertical.

v. Make sure your knees touch the floor, there is no strain in the ankles, and also the eyes are concentrated on a fixed point.

vi. Also, keep your spine, neck, and head erect.

vii. Stay in this state for as long as comfortable with normal breathing.

viii. Gently, come into Shithil Dandasan (See page 117) and relax.

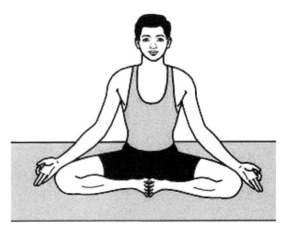

Awareness
◇ On the pressure of the heels at the perineum
◇ On mentally remembering the Divine Names "Radhey Krishna" along with the breathing process

Benefits

- ✓ Moolabandhasan is considered very significant for the preservation of semen.
- ✓ It strengthens the reproductive and excretory organs.
- ✓ It gives good flexibility to the legs and feet.

35. Bhumi Pada Mastakasan (Half-Head Stand)

Procedure

i. Come to Vajrasan (See page 113).

ii. Stand on the knees and inhale (Radhey) in this state.

iii. While exhaling (Krishna), gradually bend forward from the hips and place the palms on the floor, just below each shoulder.

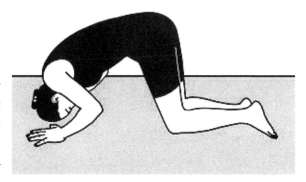

iv. With the support of the hands, gently lower the head and rest it on the floor, in between the hands.

v. Again inhale (Radhey) in this position.

vi. While exhaling (Krishna), slowly outstretch the legs backward, raising the buttocks as high as possible.

vii. Then, raise your heels a bit and lift the arms one by one, and while maintaining balance on the crown and toes, rest your hands on their respective hips.

viii. Ensure your entire body forms a triangle with the floor.

ix. Look at a fixed point and try to maintain balance.

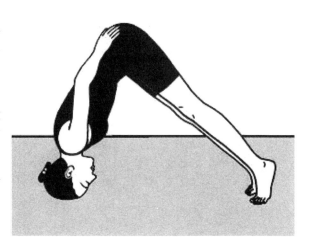

x. Hold the position for 15-20 seconds with normal breathing.

xi. Inhaling (Radhey), gently bring your hands down and use them as a support to lower the buttocks and revert back to the normal position in the reverse order.

xii. This completes one round; repeat twice.

xiii. Finally, come into Shithil Dandasan (See page 117) and relax.

Awareness

- ✧ On the breaths synchronized with the different bodily movements
- ✧ On spontaneously chanting "Radhey Krishna" with your each breath, and always recalling

Their Divine Forms

✧ On the focus of balance in the last state

Benefits

✓ Bhumi Pada Mastakasan is quite beneficial in case of low blood pressure.

✓ In mental regards, it helps increase creativity by balancing the nervous system.

✓ Along with toning the neck and head muscles, it also rejuvenates one's whole body with the supply of adequate amount of blood to the brain.

Contraindications

- Those who are affected with cervical spondylitis, severe asthma, tuberculosis, cold, impure blood, slipped-disc, weak spine, etc. should not perform this *asan*.

- Also, those with high blood pressure, heart ailments, ear problems, poor eyesight, defects of pituitary and thyroid glands, arteriosclerosis, and thrombosis should not perform it.

36. Ardh Navasan (Half-Boat Pose)

Procedure

i. Sit down with your legs outstretched and joined together in front; keeping the back erect, place your palms on the floor behind the buttocks, with the fingers pointing backward, i.e. Dandasan (See page 117).

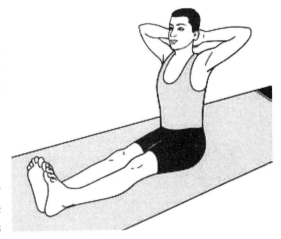

ii. Now, interlock your fingers. Folding your arms, place them on the back of the head, exactly above the neck.

iii. While inhaling (Radhey), recline your trunk backward, and simultaneously raise the legs from the floor with the knees locked and toes pointed upward.

iv. Balance your body on your buttocks, with no other part of the body touching the floor.

v. Keep the legs at an angle of 30-40 degrees with the floor and the head in line with the toes.

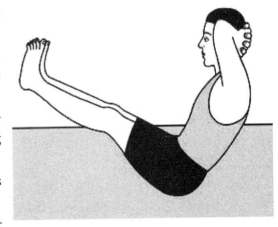

vi. Make sure you don't slouch and your body does not shake or move while maintaining the perfect balance.

vii. Stay in this position for 15-20 seconds with normal breathing.

viii. With an exhalation (Krishna), slowly lower

the legs to the floor and simultaneously bring the trunk back to the centre.

ix. This is one round; do it for up to three rounds.

x. Finally, lower your arms gradually and come into Shithil Dandasan (See page 117) to relax.

Awareness

✧ On the breaths synchronized with the movements
✧ On the stretch and strain of the abdomen and legs
✧ On the balance
✧ On the mentally uttering "Radhey Krishna" in your breaths

Benefits

✓ Ardh Navasan mainly strengthens and provides extra vigor to the back.
✓ It is considered to be very effective on the intestines.
✓ For all child-bearing women, it is a great boon as it tones and massages the womb portion.

37. Dwi Hasta Bhujangasan (Two-Handed Cobra Pose)

Procedure

i. Sit down with your legs outstretched and joined together in front; keeping the back erect, place your palms on the floor behind the buttocks, with the fingers pointing backward, i.e. Dandasan (See page 117).

ii. Bending your legs gently, assume the squatting position on the floor, with the feet about 1.5 feet apart.

iii. Place your palms flat on the floor between the feet, about six inches apart; ensure your fingers remain pointing forward.

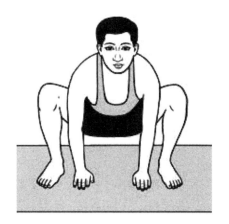

iv. Now, look at a fixed point at eye level; then lift the left foot from the floor, mounting it around the outside of the left arm; next place it on the left upper arm and maintain the balance.

v. Keeping the balance on the arms, shift the body-weight onto them and raise the right leg slowly to place it on the outer side of the right arm, just above the elbow.

vi. Stay in this state for 15-20 seconds with normal breathing.

vii. Comfortably return back to the squatting

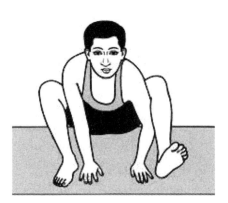

position.

viii. This finishes one round; perform this method for up to three rounds.

ix. At last, come into Shithil Dandasan (See page 117) and relax.

Awareness

◇ On the balance
◇ On pressure on the arms and thighs
◇ On chanting the Holy Names "Radhey Krishna" along with breathing process

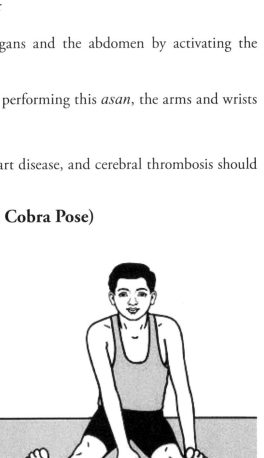

Benefits

✓ Dwi Hasta Bhujangasan helps build the arm muscles and develop suppleness in the shoulder joints and lower back.

✓ It massages and strengthens the visceral organs and the abdomen by activating the pancreas to produce sufficient insulin.

✓ It balances the nervous system.

✓ Due to the dynamic use of both hands while performing this *asan*, the arms and wrists become very strong.

Contraindications

- Those suffering from high blood pressure, heart disease, and cerebral thrombosis should not attempt this *asan*.

38. Ek Hasta Bhujangasan (One-Handed Cobra Pose)

Procedure

i. Sit down with your legs outstretched and joined together in front; keeping the back erect, place your palms on the floor, behind the buttocks, with the fingers pointing backward, i.e. Dandasan (See page 117).

ii. Now, move your feet a bit apart and place the right palm in between the thighs—closer to the right thigh.

iii. Slowly flex your right leg at the knee, and rest it as high as possible on the outer part of the right arm.

iv. Resting both palms flat on the floor, focus on a certain point at eye level.

v. Gently lift your whole body up from the

floor, keeping the left leg parallel to the floor.

vi. Balance on your arms and stay in this position at your ease with normal breathing.

vii. Comfortably, regain the central position.

viii. Perform the same process as above with the other leg.

ix. Eventually, come into Shithil Dandasan (See page 117) and relax.

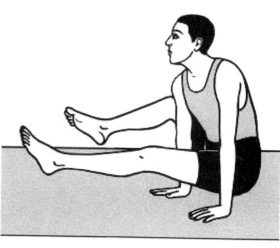

Awareness

✧ On the balance

✧ On the pressure in the arms and the thighs

✧ On always feeling the presence of "Radhey Krishna" with your breaths

Benefits

✓ Ek Hasta Bhujangasan develops the arm muscles; it adds suppleness in the shoulder joints and the lower back.

✓ It massages and strengthens the visceral organs and abdomen, especially by activating the pancreas to produce insulin.

39. Hasta Santulanasan (Balancing on Hands Pose)

Procedure

i. Sit down with your legs outstretched and joined together in front; keeping the back erect, place your palms on the floor—behind the buttocks—with the fingers pointing backward, i.e. Dandasan (See page 117).

ii. Slowly folding your legs at the knees, assume the posture of Padmasan (See page 116).

iii. Rest your palms on the floor—beside the thighs.

iv. Inhale (Radhey).

v. While slowly exhaling (Krishna), raise your body and balance the body on the hands, locking the arms. Make sure your head and spine stay erect.

vi. Maintaining the balance, try to stay in this *asan* for as long as possible with normal breathing.

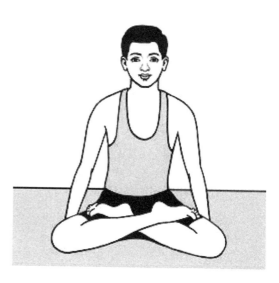

vii. With an inhalation (Radhey), slowly bring your body downward to the floor.

viii. Repeat the pose with the other leg and arm.

ix. Lastly, release your legs; come into Shithil Dandasan (See page 117) and relax.

Variation - 1

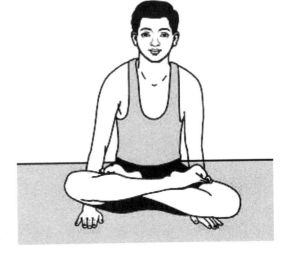

i. Come to the final position of Hasta Santulanasan (steps i-v) progressively.

ii. Now, start swinging your body back and forth between your arms.

iii. Maintaining the balance on your hands, swing as long as possible with normal breathing.

iv. With an inhalation (Radhey), slowly lower your body downward to the floor.

v. Lastly, release your legs; come into Shithil Dandasan (See page 117) and relax.

Awareness

✧ On the breaths synchronized with the different movements
✧ On the balance, and the Holy Names "Radhey Krishna" in your breaths, and simultaneously feeling Their presence all the time

Benefits

✓ Hasta Santulanasan gives good exercise to your arms, wrists, shoulders, and abdominal muscles.
✓ It generates control, dexterity, and concentration.

40. Ardh Ushtrasan (Half Camel Pose)

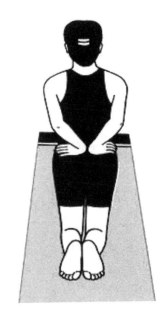

Procedure

i. Come into Vajrasan (See page 113).

ii. Now spread your knees slightly apart.

iii. Comfortably, kneel on the knees and place both hands on your waist, with the fingers pointing forward.

iv. While inhaling (Radhey), straighten the arms to the sides, and raise them upward to bring them at the shoulder level.

v. While exhaling (Krishna), turn your upper body slightly to the right; lean backward gently (slightly arching your spine backward) and try to grip the left ankle with the right hand.

vi. Simultaneously, raise and straighten the left arm in front of the head—almost at the level of the forehead.

vii. Drop the head slightly back and concentrate on the raised hand.

viii. Make sure your abdomen is pushed forward and the thighs remain at the right angle to the floor.

ix. Hold this pose for as long as possible with normal breathing.

x. While inhaling (Radhey), come back to Vajrasan by bringing the buttocks down.

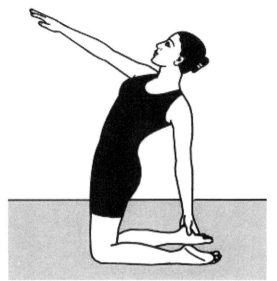

xi. Practice it on the other side.

xii. This ends one round; repeat it for up to three rounds.

xiii. Finally, come into Shithil Dandasan (See page 117) and relax.

Awareness
✧ On the backward and upward movements of the body and breaths synchronized with them
✧ On the stretching and releasing of the back and the neck
✧ On mentally uttering the Holy Names "Radhey Krishna," and spontaneously feeling Their omnipresence

Benefits
✓ One of the main benefits of Ardh Ushthrasan is that it exercise the stomach and intestines that help remove constipation, increase the digestion power, and even tone up different reproductive parts.
✓ It has other versatile functions such as relieving from lumbago, rounded back, and drooping shoulders—particularly by loosening the vertebrae and activating the spinal nerves.

Contraindications
- Persons with cases of backache and enlarged thyroid glands should not do it without the prior consent and counsel of *Yog* experts.

41. Kapotasan (Pigeon Pose)
Procedure
i. Sit in Vajrasan (See page 113) and place your palms on either side of the knees.

ii. Now, inhale (Radhey) and with the support of both arms on the floor, gradually slide your right leg backward until its outer side rests completely on the floor.

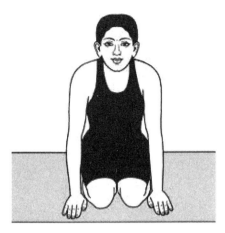
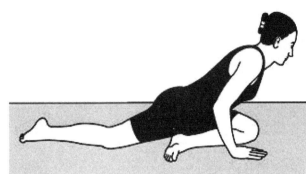

iii. Comfortably tuck your left knee in between the two hands in such a way that the right heel gets aligned with the perineum.

iv. Ensure that the outer sides of the right knee and foot lie along the floor in this state.

v. Now, stretch your spine and neck backward, trying to arch the back as much as possible.

vi. Keep the palms firm on the floor by stretching them as needed.

vii. Remain in this state for as long as possible with normal breathing.

viii. Again, return to the starting position by reversing the process.

ix. Repeat the process with the other leg.

x. Now, return back to Vajrasan.

xi. Finally, come into Shithil Dandasan (See page 117) and relax.

Awareness

✧ On the stretch of the thighs, hips, buttocks, and the lower back
✧ On the unbroken mental chanting of the Divine Names "Radhey Krishna" along with breathing.

Benefits

✓ Kapotasan stretches the hips on either side, and makes the back very supple while creating an arch with it.
✓ As the chest is expanded fully during the *asan*, it refreshes the body and the mind with a plentiful supply of oxygen.
✓ This pose even stretches the thighs and buttocks exceptionally.

Contraindications

- People suffering from peptic ulcer, hernia, or hyperthyroidism should perform this *asan* under the guidance of a *Yog* expert. Similarly, women in second or third month of pregnancy should avoid it.

42. Ardh Matsyendrasan (Half Twist Pose)

Procedure

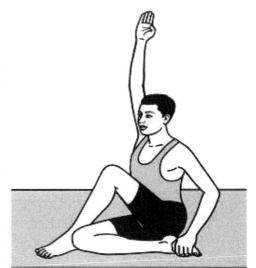

i. Sit down with your legs outstretched and joined together in front; keeping the back erect, place your palms on the floor behind the buttocks with the fingers pointing backward, i.e. Dandasan (See page 117).

ii. Fold the left leg and place the left foot flat on the floor against the outer side of the right thigh (near the right knee).

iii. Fold your right leg and bring your right foot under the left buttock; also make sure the outer side of the lower right leg (especially the outer right foot) touches the floor and also not to sit on the heels.

iv. Inhaling (Radhey), raise your right arm vertically and stretch the shoulders.

v. Exhaling (Krishna), twist the waist to the left and place the right arm on the outer part of the left knee.

vi. Now, catch hold of either the left toes or the left foot with your right hand, resting the right triceps on the outer side of the left knee.

vii. Move your left hand behind the back while twisting the trunk and head leftward, try to

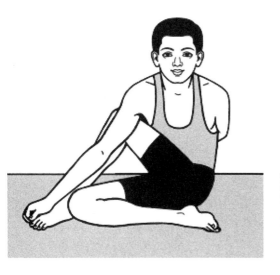
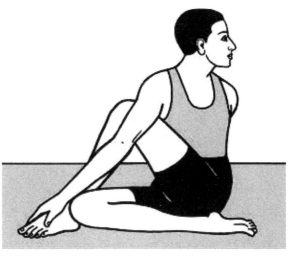

touch the right hip with your left hand.

viii. Maintain the posture for 15-20 seconds with normal breathing.

ix. Slowly letting go of your arms, come back to the starting position.

x. Repeat the method on the other side.

xi. This is one round; do it for three rounds.

xii. Finally, come to Shithil Dandasan (See page 117) and relax.

Awareness
- On the breaths synchronized with your bodily movements
- On the stretches and strains of the spine
- On the movement of the abdomen
- On always feeling the omnipresence of "Radhey Krishna"

Benefits
- Ardh Matsyendrasan tones up the spinal nerves to perfection and makes the back very flexible.
- Basically, it relieves backache and helps prevent the adjoining vertebrae to develop osteophytes.
- It even helps alleviate digestive ailments.
- It is recommended for diabetics as well as it regulates the secretion of adrenaline and bile juice.
- It is also helpful in curing cervical spondylitis, colitis, menstrual disorders, bronchitis, constipation, and sinus related cases, as long as it is done comfortably.
- It is an invaluable aid for rectifying sciatica, peptic ulcer, hernia, hyper thyroid, and slipped-disc condition—if done carefully under the guidance of a *Yog* expert.

Contraindication
- Women who are in the second or third month of their pregnancy should not perform this *asan*.

43. Baddh Konasan (Restrained Angle Pose)

Procedure
i. Come to Titali Asan (See page 96) and grip the toes firmly by interlocking your fingers.

ii. Make sure your outer knees touch the ground completely and that spine remains erect.

iii. Inhale (Radhey) in this position; then while exhaling (Krishna), bend forward from your hips slowly; then rest either the forehead or the chin on the floor.

iv. Hold this pose for 15-20 seconds with normal breathing.

v. Breathing in (Radhey), raise the trunk and regain the sitting pose.

vi. This is one round; repeat twice.

vii. Lastly, release your feet; come into Shithil Dandasan (See page 117) and relax.

Awareness

✧ On the breaths synchronized with various bodily movements

✧ On the stretch and pressure on the lower back, abdomen, and legs

✧ On mentally chanting the Divine Names "Radhey Krishna" in your breaths and always recalling Them

Benefits

✓ Baddh Konasan is helpful in problems related to the pelvis, the abdomen, and the urinary bladder.

✓ A regular practice of this pose supplies sufficient blood to the back and keeps the kidneys and prostrate gland healthy.

✓ It prevents hernia and helps relieve pain and heaviness in the testicles.

✓ It alleviates sciatic pain.

✓ It checks the irregular menstrual periods if coupled with Sarvangasan, and frees pregnant women from delivery pain if done regularly.

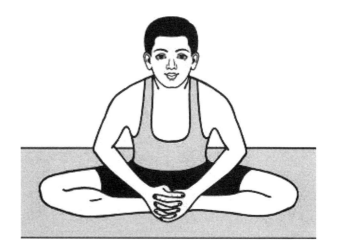

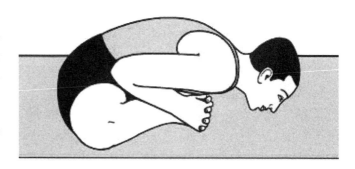

Contraindication

- Those with severe back problems should omit this *asan* from their daily *Yog* package.

44. Meru Dandasan (Spinal Column Pose)

Procedure

i. Sit down with your legs outstretched and joined together in front; keeping the back erect, place your palms on the floor behind the buttocks, with the fingers pointing backward, i.e. Dandasan (See page 117).

ii. Slowly flex your legs at the knees and place your soles flat on the floor in the front.

iii. Now, spread your feet sideways,

about 1.5-2 feet apart.

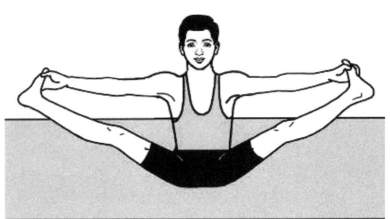

iv. Inhaling (Radhey), catch hold of either of the big toes firmly, and slowly recline backward, and balance your body on the coccyx (the tail bone).

v. As you exhale (Krishna), stretch your legs both ways—sideward and upward.

vi. Steady your body with your spine stretched, and then spread the legs apart—as far as possible.

vii. Maintain the balance in this position, focus on a fixed point at eye level.

viii. Be in this position for 15-20 seconds with normal breathing.

ix. To come back to the central position, first inhale (Radhey); then slowly move the legs together to the centre, bend your legs at the knees and finally lower your feet down to the floor.

x. This is one round; perform two more rounds.

xi. Then, slowly come into Shithil Dandasan (See page 117) and relax.

Awareness

✧ On the breaths synchronized with the bodily movements
✧ On the stretch of the legs and arms
✧ On balancing on the coccyx
✧ On always feeling the presence of "Radhey Krishna" with your breaths

Benefits

✓ Meru Dandasan firms and tones the abdominal organs (particularly the liver) and muscles.
✓ Not only does it assist in eliminating intestinal worms, but it also activates intestinal peristalsis by relieving constipation.
✓ This *asan* strengthens the sympathetic and parasympathetic nervous systems.
✓ It stretches the muscles of the back and helps shape the spine too.

Contraindications

- People with slipped-disc, sciatica, heart illness, and high blood pressure should not include this *asan* in their *Yog* exercise.

45. Mareechyasan (Sage Mareechi's Pose)

Procedure

i. Sit down with your legs outstretched and joined together in front; keeping the back erect, place your palms on the floor behind the buttocks, i.e. Dandasan (See page 117).

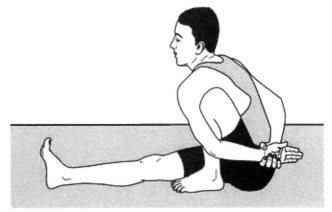

ii. Comfortably fold your left leg at the knee, and place the left sole and the heel flat on the floor.

iii. Make sure your left shin stays vertical and the left heel is placed near the perineum.

iv. Then, place right palm flat on the floor—just beside the right buttock; raise the left arm vertically above your head and shoulder, with the bicep touching the left ear.

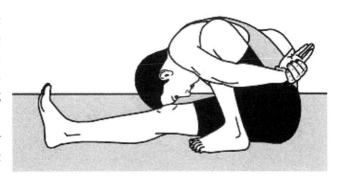

v. Slowly draw your left shoulder forward until the left armpit reaches the upper left shin.

vi. Now, lower the left arm and wrap it around the upper left shin and thigh—flexing it and moving the left forearm behind the back, at the waist.

vii. Also, take your right hand just behind your back, and hold the left hand with it.

viii. Inhale (Radhey) in this position.

ix. Exhaling (Krishna), slowly move your body forward and draw your head closer to the right knee. Make sure your right leg stays unmoved.

x. Maintaining normal breathing, attempt to remain in this position for as long as you are comfortable.

xi. Inhaling (Radhey), slowly let your hands go of freely; then straighten the left leg and ultimately come to Dandasan.

xii. Repeat the above process with the other leg.

xiii. Lastly, come to Shithil Dandasan (See page 117) and relax.

Awareness

✧ On the breaths synchronized with the bodily movements

163

- ✧ On the stretches and strains on the legs, spine, shoulders, and the arms
- ✧ On mentally chanting "Radhey Krishna" with your breaths and always feeling Them standing in front of you and watching you

Benefits

- ✓ Mareechyasan circulates the blood around the abdominal organs, and thus keeps them healthy.
- ✓ The dorsal region of the spine is perfectly exercised.
- ✓ It has other functions like providing extra strength to the fingers and increasing flexibility in the back and legs.

Contraindication

- - People with serious back and knee problems should avoid it.

46. Matsyasan (Fish Pose)

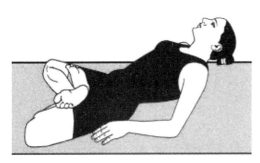
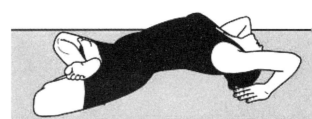

Procedure

i. Come to Padmasan (See page 116) and try to be comfortable for a few seconds.

ii. Inhale (Radhey) and gently recline backward from the hips with the support of your arms and elbows.

iii. Lie on the back in this position.

iv. Place the palms on either side of the head in such a way that all the fingers point toward the shoulders.

v. Exhale (Krishna) in this position.

vi. Then inhale (Radhey) and with the support of the hands, comfortably arch the back.

vii. Then, raise your chest a little; move your head backward and place the crown on the floor.

viii. Now, catch hold of your big toes with the hands.

ix. While resting the elbows on the floor, try to balance on the crown to form shape of an arch with the trunk.

x. Let the whole body remain relaxed with proper balance.

xi. Stay in this position for 15-20 seconds with normal breathing.

xii. This is one round; do it for two more rounds with the legs crossed other way.

xiii. Lastly, come into Shithil Dandasan (See page 117) and relax.

Awareness
✧ On the various physical movements and the breaths synchronized with them
✧ On the stretch and strain of the abdomen and the chest
✧ On recalling the Sacred Names "Radhey Krishna" with your each breath

Benefits
✓ Although Matsyasan seems to be a simple pose, it removes abdominal problems by giving a good exercise to the intestines and abdominal parts.
✓ It helps cure bleeding piles and even benefits those with asthma and bronchitis.
✓ It also invigorates the body with improved blood circulation in the back, and thus helps in solving the cases like backache and cervical spondylitis.
✓ Similarly, it reinforces immune power by activating the thyroid and thymus glands.
✓ It is a great boon for women as it removes defects in the reproductive organs with proper blood circulation.
✓ Besides, it is also considered extremely effectual in sore throat and tonsillitis.

Contraindications
- Persons with heart cases, hernia, peptic ulcers, and back pains should avoid this pose. Also, women at delivery stage should omit it.

47. Parivritti Janu Shirasan (Spiralled Head to Knee Pose)
Procedure

i. Sit down with your legs outstretched and joined together in front; keeping the back erect, place your palms on the floor behind the buttocks, with the fingers pointing backward, i.e. Dandasan (See page 117).

ii. Now, spread your feet about three feet apart, then flex the right leg at the knee and place the right foot against the left thigh with the heel touching the perineum.

iii. Slowly twist your trunk to the right; while inhaling (Radhey), raise the left hand up vertically above the head.

iv. While exhaling (Krishna), comfortably lean

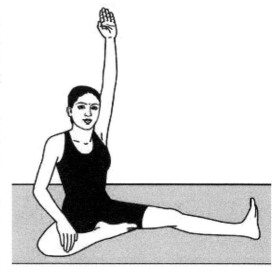

your upper body laterally toward the left leg; grasp the left toes or foot with the left hand, managing to put the left elbow on the floor near inner side of the stretched leg. Place your right hand on the right thigh or hip in this state.

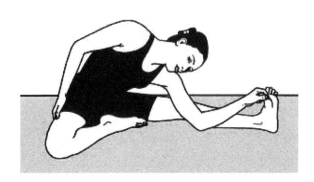

v. Now bring your right arm over the head; catch hold of your left foot or ankle portion and rest the head comfortably under the right arm with the left ear touching the left knee. Also, ensure both of the legs stay unmoved in this position.

vi. Be in this position for as long as comfortable with normal breathing.

vii. Slowly come back to the starting position.

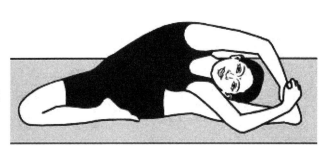

viii. Repeat it on the other side.

ix. Eventually, come to Shithil Dandasan (See page 117) and relax.

Awareness
- ◇ On breathing in and out along with the various movements
- ◇ On the stretch and release of the arms, shoulders, and the knees
- ◇ On recalling the omnipresence of "Radhey Krishna"

Benefits
- ✓ Parivritti Janu Shirasan yields manifold benefits such as toning and massaging the abdominal and pelvic regions—including the pancreas, liver, stomach, adrenal gland, and spleen, which help to eradicate digestive ailments.
- ✓ It assists in alleviating disorders of the uro-genitals system.
- ✓ It controls diabetes, colitis, kidney troubles, bronchitis, and eosinophilia.
- ✓ Parivritti Janu Shirasan makes the mind sound by toning the spinal nerves and making the back extremely flexible.
- ✓ It is also a blessing for relieving backaches and preventing the adjoining vertebrae from developing osteophytes.
- ✓ Many *Yog* practitioners consider it as a useful method to cure cervical spondylitis, menstrual disorders, bronchitis, constipation, and sinus related cases, as long as it is done comfortably.
- ✓ It even heals sciatica, peptic ulcer, hernia, hyperthyroid, and slipped-disc condition when done carefully under the guidance of a *Yog* therapist.

Contraindications

- Women during pregnancy and people with back problems should avoid it.

48. Santulit Marjari Asan (Balancing Cat)

Procedure

i. Sit in Vajrasan (See page 113).

ii. Inhale (Radhey); lifting your buttocks off the floor, stand on the knees.

iii. Now with an exhalation (Krishna), slowly lean forward.

iv. Then, place both hands on the floor, right in the line of shoulders—with the fingers facing forward.

v. Ensure your arms and thighs remain erect and the hands aligned with the knees.

vi. Inhale (Radhey); slowly raise your right arm forward and left foot backward aligned with the trunk, balancing with the left hand and right leg folded at the knee.

vii. Exhale (Krishna) in this state.

viii. Make sure your right arm, left leg, and trunk stay parallel to the floor in this condition.

ix. Stretch both—the right fingers and left toes.

x. Remain in this pose for 15-20 seconds, breathing normally.

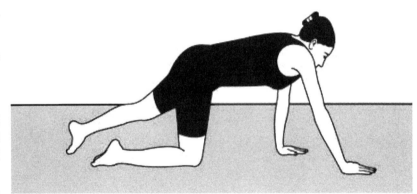

xi. While exhaling (Krishna), come back to the initial state.

xii. Repeat the method other side.

xiii. At last, come into Shithil Dandasan (See page 117) and relax.

Awareness

✧ On the breaths and the various bodily movements synchronized with them

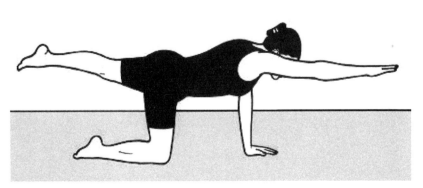

- ✧ On mental chanting of the Sacred Names "Radhey Krishna" in your each breath along with feeling Their presence at all times
- ✧ On the balance in the final position

Benefits

- ✓ Santulit Marjari Asan exceptionally strengthens a range of back muscles by providing a diagonal extension across the back.
- ✓ It develops a wonderful balance between the mind and body.

49. Ushtrasan (Camel Pose)

Procedure

i. Come into Vajrasan (See page 113).

ii. With the support of your hands, stand on the knees with the ankles joined together.

iii. Place your palms on the waist, stretching both, the thighs ribs portion.

iv. As you inhale (Radhey), recline slowly backward and place the right palm over the right heel, and the left palm over the left heel.

v. Make sure your thighs stay vertical and that the upper trunk is pushed toward the thighs and the hips.

vi. With normal breathing, remain in this position for 15-20 seconds.

vii. Exhaling (Krishna), come back to the centre; simultaneously, release your hands one by one and place them on the waist.

viii. This completes one round; repeat it for two rounds.

ix. Finally, come back to Vajrasan and then to Shithil Dandasan (See page 117) and relax.

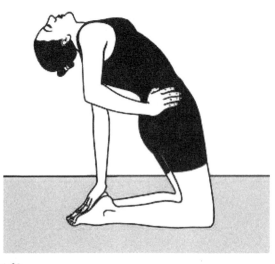
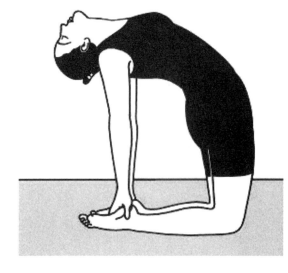

Awareness

⬦ On the physical movements along with breaths synchronized with them

⬦ On the stretch of the arms, shoulders, trunk, buttocks, and the thighs

⬦ On feeling the presence of "Radhey Krishna" with your each breath

Benefits

✓ Ushtrasan is good for those with drooping shoulders and hunched backs.

✓ It also tones up the spine and keeps the brain active by increasing blood circulation to the head.

Contraindications

- People suffering from hernia, acute hypertension, and lower back pain should be careful while doing this *asan*.

50. Pashchimottanasan (Back Stretching Pose)

Procedure

i. Sit down with your legs outstretched and joined together in front; keeping the back erect, place your palms on the floor behind the buttocks, with the fingers pointing backward, i.e. Dandasan (See page 117).

ii. Inhale (Radhey) deeply; slowly raise your arms over the head and turn the palms forward.

iii. Make sure your legs, spine, head, and arms stay fully stretched throughout.

iv. Exhaling (Krishna), slowly bend forward from the hips and grasp the toes.

v. Now, keep your elbows on the floor by the side of the calves, and attempt to touch the knees with the forehead, without giving any strain to the body.

vi. Make sure your feet don't get separated and legs don't get bent.

vii. Maintain this posture for 15-20 seconds, breathing normally.

viii. Inhaling (Radhey), slowly come back to the centre.

ix. This ends one round; practice for two more rounds.

x. Lastly, come into Shithil Dandasan (See page 117) and relax.

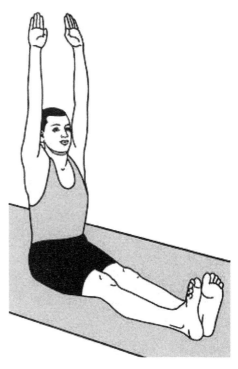

Awareness

⬦ On the breaths flowing in and out and the bodily movements synchronized with them

- ✧ On the stretch of the legs, spine, and shoulders
- ✧ On the spontaneous remembrance of the Holy Names "Radhey Krishna" while breathing

Benefits

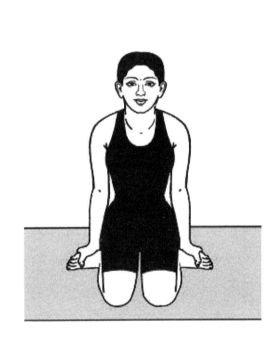

- ✓ Pashchimottanasan helps tone and massage the abdominal and pelvic regions including the pancreas, liver, stomach, adrenal glands, and spleen.
- ✓ It assists in alleviating disorders of the uro-genitals system as well.
- ✓ A regular practice of this *asan* helps control diseases like diabetes, menstrual problems, colitis, kidney troubles, bronchitis, and eosinophilia.

Contraindications

- - People with serious back problems should avoid it.

51. Brahmacharyasan (Celibate's Pose)

Procedure

i. Sit in Vajrasan (See page 113).

ii. Twist both feet to the sides with the support of the hands, and keep the inner side of your heels closer to the buttocks; the left toes point leftward and right—rightward.

iii. Bring your knees as much closer to each other as possible.

iv. Now straighten your trunk and head, making it perpendicular to the floor and place the palms on the knees.

v. make sure both arms remain well extended in this position.

vi. Maintain the position for as long as possible with normal breathing.

vii. Finally, carefully come into Shithil Dandasan (See page 117) and relax.

Awareness

✧ On the stretch of the ankle joints, calves, knees, and thighs

✧ On the breaths flowing in and out and the bodily movements synchronized with them

✧ On always uttering the Divine Names "Radhey Krishna" mentally

Benefits

✓ The chief purpose of Brahmacharyasan is the preservation of sexual energy.

✓ It is extremely advantageous in seminal defects and urinary diseases.

✓ It helps in controlling diabetes.

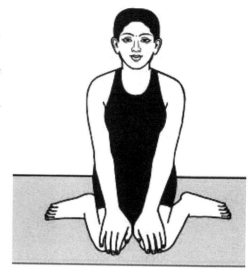

52. Ardh Chandrasan (Half Moon Pose)

Procedure

i. Sit in Vajrasan (See page 113) and stand on your knees.

ii. Now bring both arms to the chest and cross them in such a way that right hand lies under the left armpit and the left hand lies under the right armpit.

iii. While inhaling (Radhey), comfortably recline backward from the waist along with the head and neck until a half moon shape is formed with the body.

iv. Push your hips slightly forward and keep your thighs erect.

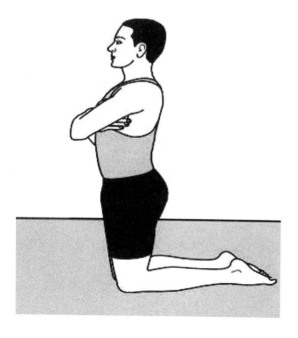
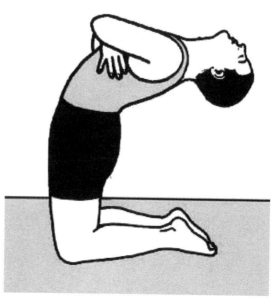

v. Remain in this position for 15-20 seconds with normal breathing.

vi. With an exhalation (Krishna), gently return back to the centre.

vii. This finishes one round; repeat twice.

viii. Lastly, come to Shithil Dandasan (See page117) and relax.

Awareness
✧ On breathing in and out along with the back and forth movements
✧ On the stretch of the lower back and the neck
✧ On realizing the omnipresence of "Radhey Krishna" at all times

Benefits
✓ Ardh Chandrasan makes your spine flexible.
✓ It relieves pain in the lower back.
✓ It helps reduce unnecessary fat from the waist.
✓ It is also beneficial in treating hernia and hypertension, if practiced with a great care.

Contraindications
- People with the history of abdominal or heart operations should be cautious while doing it.

53. Shashank Bhujangasan (Striking Cobra Pose)

Procedure

i. Assume the final position of Shashankasan (See page 117).

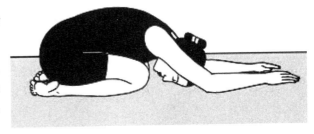

ii. Now, keeping your arms outstretched in front of the shoulders, inhale (Radhey); slowly raise your chest, and move it forward to bring it over the palms.

iii. Lower your pelvis, and try to bring the hips to the floor—as close as possible.

iv. In this position, straighten your arms; arch your back and lift the head without the navel touching the floor.

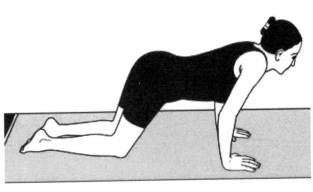

v. Remain in this position for about 15-20 seconds with normal breathing.

vi. While exhaling (Krishna), return to Shashankasan by gently lifting the buttocks, and then coming backward with the arms straight.

vii. Perform two more rounds likewise.

viii. Ultimately, come into Shithil Dandasan (See page 117) and relax.

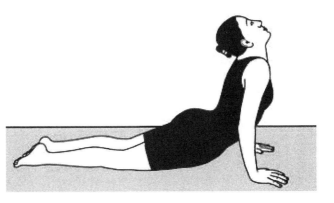

Awareness

✧ On the breaths synchronized with the bodily movements

✧ On always feeling the presence of "Radhey Krishna" in front of you

Benefits

✓ Shashank Bhujangasan naturally firms different reproductive organs, and thus helps in cases of menstrual disorders.

✓ It tightens the abdominal and pelvic parts, activates the functions of the kidney, liver, and different visceral organs.

✓ It releases the practitioners from back pain and spinal stiffness.

✓ As in Shashankasan (See page 117), it is significantly beneficial for the mitigation of constipation, which is a common problem nowadays due to wrong intake of daily foods.

54. Parighasan (Cross Beam Pose)

Procedure

i. Come into Vajrasan (See page 117).

ii. With the support of your hands, stand on your knees with the ankles joined together.

iii. Comfortably extend your right leg to the right, and align it with the trunk and left knee.

iv. Next, turn your right foot to the right (sideways), keeping the right leg locked at the knee.

v. Inhaling (Radhey), raise the arms sideways, making them parallel to the floor.

vi. Exhaling (Krishna), gently bend your trunk and right arm laterally—down to the stretched right leg; place the right hand on the right foot, with the right palm facing downward.

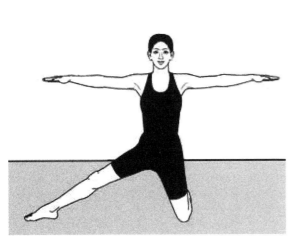

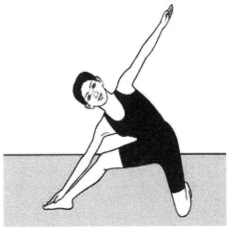

vii. Continuing to exhale (Krishna) as usual, slowly move your left arm over the head—aligning with the right arm; slowly bring the left palm downward and place it just over your right hand.

viii. Ensure your head lies in between your arms in this position.

ix. With normal breathing, stay in this pose for as long as possible.

x. As you inhale (Radhey), bring the trunk and arms back to the centre and bring the right leg to the kneeling position.

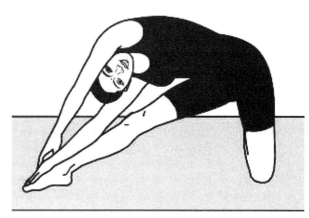

xi. Practice the *asan* with the alternate combination of arms and legs.

xii. Lastly, come into Shithil Dandasan (See page 117) and relax.

Awareness
- ✧ On the breaths synchronized with the movements
- ✧ On the stretch and strain in the sides of the trunk, arms, and legs
- ✧ On mentally chanting Divine Names "Radhey Krishna" along with your breaths
- ✧ On the balance in the final pose

Benefits
- ✓ This sideward bending exercise keeps the abdominal muscles and organs in a healthy condition.
- ✓ Those who desire to have a supple body are largely benefited as it removes stiffness from the back, arms, and legs.

Contraindications
- - Persons suffering from recent or chronic knee, hip, or shoulder injuries or swelling should not attempt this pose.

55. Ardh Baddh Padma Pashchimottanasan (Half-Bound Foot)

Procedure
i. Sit down with your legs outstretched and joined together in front; keeping the back erect, place your palms on the floor behind the buttocks, with the fingers pointing backward, i.e. Dandasan (See page 117).

ii. Slowly come to Half Lotus Pose (See page 111) with the right foot on top of the left thigh and try to touch the floor with the right knee.

iii. Inhale (Radhey); while exhaling (Krishna), gently raise your right arm, move it around the back and grip the right big toe firmly.

iv. Make sure the left leg remains stretched on the floor.

v. Now again inhaling (Radhey), raise the left arm.

vi. With a slow exhalation (Krishna), comfortably lean forward; catch your left big toe with the left hand and then rest the head on the left leg without any stress.

vii. Hold this pose for the duration of 15-20 seconds with normal breathing.

viii. While inhaling (Radhey), come back to the centre raising the left hand upward.

ix. Repeat the same process for twice.

x. Then, release the leg and straighten it.

xi. Perform the method thrice with the other leg.

xii. Finally, come to Shithil Dandasan (See page 117) and relax.

Awareness

✧ On the breaths synchronized with the bodily movements
✧ On always recalling the sentient forms of "Radhey Krishna"
✧ On the stretch of the legs and pressure on the shoulders and the upper torso
✧ On feeling relaxation in the stretched and contracted parts

Benefits

✓ Ardh Baddh Padma Pashchimottasan—one of the difficult *asans*—develops flexibility in the spine.
✓ It stretches the hamstrings.

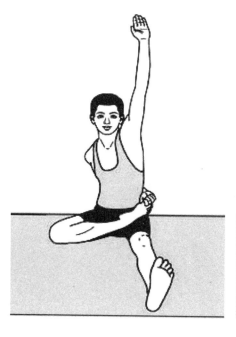
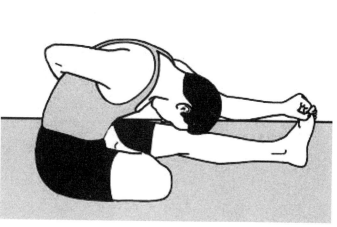

- ✓ Alleviates the enlargement of the liver and spleen, and even cures abdominal distention (swelling because of intense pressure), which is caused by wrong diet and activities.
- ✓ It nourishes the damaged tissues.
- ✓ It roots out constipation by improving the function of the bowels.

Contraindications

- Those who have not perfected Pashchimottanasan and Padmasan should omit this *asan* from their *Yog* package.

56. Ardh Padma Pashchimottanasan (Half Lotus Back Stretching Pose)

Procedure

i. Sit down with your legs outstretched and joined together in front; keeping the back erect, place your palms on the floor behind the buttocks, with the fingers pointing backward, i.e. Dandasan (See page 117).

ii. Fold your right leg at the knee; rest your right foot on top of the left thigh; while stretching the left leg, try to move the right foot as far back as possible.

iii. While inhaling (Radhey), raise the arms up above the head.

iv. While exhaling (Krishna), bend your upper body forward and hold the left big toe with both hands.

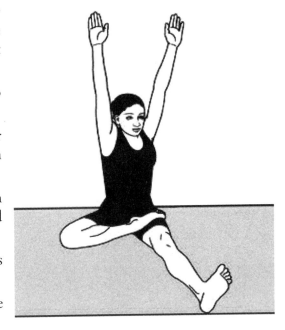

v. Comfortably, try to place the elbows on either side of left leg; stretch the trunk and attempt to touch the forehead to the knee.

vi. Maintain this position for 15-20 seconds with normal breathing.

vii. Make sure your left leg stays locked on the floor.

viii. Also, relax your back muscles.

ix. Gradually, release your left big toe, and raising the upper body, return back to the starting position.

x. Perform the above process with the other leg.

xi. This completes a single round; repeat twice.

xii. Finally, come to Shithil Dandasan

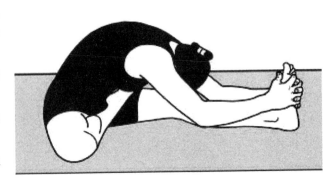

(See page 117) and relax.

Awareness

◇ On the breaths and the bodily movements synchronized with them

◇ On the stretch and strain of the legs, arms, and the upper back

◇ On always remembering the Divine forms of "Radhey Krishna" in your mind

Benefits

✓ The effects of Ardh Padma Pashchimottanasan are same as that of Pashchimottanasan (See page 169).

Contraindication

- People with serious back problems should avoid this *asan*.

57. Pada Prasar Pashchimottanasan (Legs Spread Back Stretched Pose)

Procedure

i. Sit down with your legs outstretched and joined together in front; keeping the back erect, place your palms on the floor behind the buttocks, with the fingers pointing backward, i.e. Dandasan (See page 117).

ii. Spread your feet apart as wide as possible; then move your arms backward, placing them at the centre of the buttocks, and interlock the fingers.

iii. Slowly twist your trunk to the right.

iv. While inhaling (Radhey), raise your arms behind the back, with your palms facing forward.

v. While exhaling (Krishna), bend forward to touch forehead with the right knee.

vi. Ensure the legs and arms remain locked well.

vii. Remain in this position for 15-20 seconds, breathing normally.

viii. Slowly lower the arms; return to the centre.

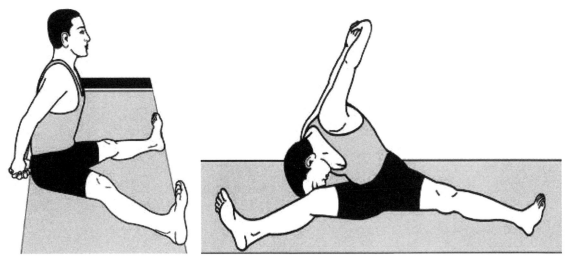

ix. Practice the same process on the other side.

x. This completes one round; practice for two more rounds.

xi. Lastly, come into Shithil Dandasan (See page 117) and relax.

Awareness

✧ On the breaths synchronized with the bodily movements

✧ On the stretch of the shoulder blades and the legs

✧ On the mental chanting of the Divine Names "Radhey Krishna" along with your breaths, and remembering Their Divine forms

Benefits

✓ This *asan* tones and massages the abdominal and pelvic regions that include the pancreas, liver, stomach, adrenal gland, and the spleen.

✓ It assists in alleviating disorders of the uro-genital system.

✓ It benefits the practitioners by helping to control diabetes, menstrual problems, colitis, kidney troubles, bronchitis, and eosinophilia.

Contraindication

- People with serious back ailments should avoid this *asan*.

58. Supt Vajrasan (Sleeping Thunderbolt Pose)

Procedure

i. Sit in Vajrasan (See page 113) and place your hands on the thighs.

ii. While inhaling (Radhey), gently recline backward, taking support of the right elbow first and then the left elbow.

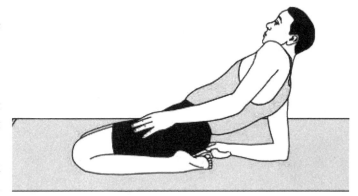

iii. Slowly, lie flat on your back by keeping the arms crossed above the head; make sure the knees remain joined or closed together, touching the ground.

iv. Be in this position for 15-20 seconds with normal breathing.

v. Exhaling (Krishna), slowly come up to the sitting position with the support of the elbows and arms.

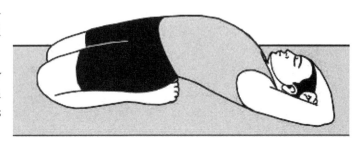

vi. This completes one round; practice for two more rounds.

Awareness
- ✧ On the bodily movements and breaths synchronized with them
- ✧ On the stretch and pressure on the lower back
- ✧ On the abdomen
- ✧ On the unbroken rememberance of "Radhey Krishna" with each breath

Benefits
- ✓ Supt Vajrasan tones up the spinal nerves and gives extra suppleness to the back.
- ✓ It massages the abdominal organs, eliminates different digestive ailments, and constipation.
- ✓ It is extremely advantageous in reducing asthma, bronchial, and other pulmonary problems.
- ✓ It helps redirect sexual energy upward to the brain.

Contraindications
- - Persons with knee complaints, sciatica, sacral infection, and slipped-disc should not do it.

59. Kukkutasan (Cockerel Pose)

Procedure

i. Come into Padmasan (See page 116) and gently insert your hands in between the calves and thighs.

ii. Raising the folded legs slightly, move your forearms downward through the legs—up to the elbows.

iii. Now rest your hands on the floor in such a way that the fingers point forward.

iv. Concentrate the eyes on a fixed point; lock the arms firm on the floor; while inhaling (Radhey), balance on either of the arms, and gently raise your rest of the body up to the level of the elbow.

v. Make sure your head and back remain erect.

vi. Stay in this posture for as long as possible with normal breathing.

vii. Slowly regain the starting position, by lowering your body to the floor

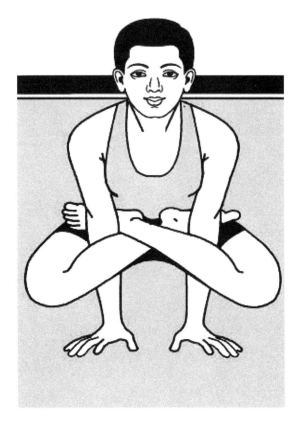

and moving the arms to the sides.

viii. Repeat the procedure with the alternate leg-position in Padmasan.

ix. Finally, come into Shithil Dandasan (See page 117) and relax.

Awareness

✧ On the balance

✧ On spontaneously remembering the sentient forms of "Radhey Krishna"

Benefits

✓ Kukkutasan gives extra strength to the arms, shoulder muscles, and chest.

✓ Legs get flexibility and suppleness.

✓ It helps develop balancing-power and concentration ability.

60. Kashyapasan (Sage Kashyap's Pose)

Procedure

i. Come to the final pose of Santulanasan (See page 147).

ii. Now raise the left arm upward, balancing on the right arm and legs, and slowly flip the whole body onto the right side.

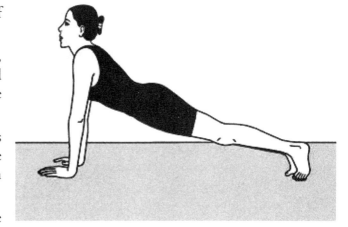

iii. Make sure your left arm is placed along the left side of the body and the left leg lying on the right leg.

iv. Gradually flex your left knee and then rest the left foot on top of the right thigh as in the Half Lotus Pose (See page 111).

v. Carefully, move the left arm behind the back and grasp the left toes.

vi. Hold the position for as long as comfortable with normal breathing.

vii. Now release the left foot, then slowly flip the body back to the centre so that the chest faces downwards and the left hand rests on the floor.

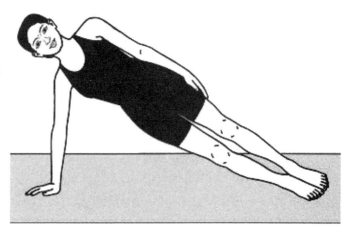

viii. Repeat this process on the other side.

ix. Ultimately, come to Shithil Dandasan (See page 117) and relax.

Awareness

✧ On the balance

✧ On the spontaneous remembrance of the Divine Names of "Radhey Krishna"

Benefits

✔ This *asan* exercises the abdominal muscles, which helps in toning various digestive organs, and also eradicating problems in the large intestine.

✔ It tremendously increases the capacity of both—physical and mental balance, and thus brings good concentration ability.

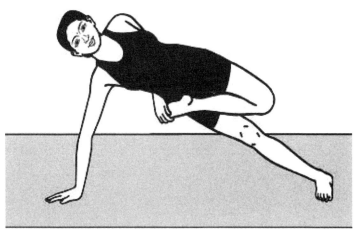

61. Ek Pada Padmottanasan (One Leg Raised To Head Pose)

Procedure

i. Sit down with your legs outstretched and joined together in front; keeping the back erect, place your palms on the floor behind the buttocks, with the fingers pointing backward, i.e. Dandasan (See page 117).

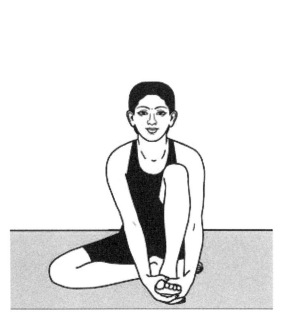

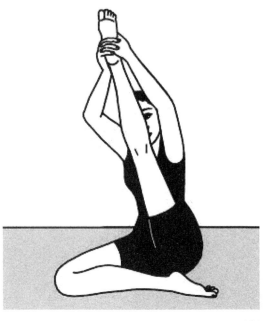

ii. Gently flex your left leg at the knee, bringing it toward the chest; rest the left foot flat on the floor—aligning with the left buttock.

iii. Now while bending your right leg at the knee, touch the left perineum with right heel with the right knee touching the floor.

iv. Bring your hands under the left foot and interlock them around the left sole.

v. Inhale (Radhey) in this position.

vi. Then while exhaling (Krishna), raise the left leg and slowly lock it at the knee.

vii. Keeping the spine erect, try to touch the nose with the left knee.

viii. Stay in the position for 15-20 seconds with normal breathing.

ix. Gradually, come back to the initial position and repeat the same process with the other leg.

x. Practice it up to three times.

xi. At last, come into Shithil Dandasan (See page 117) and relax.

Awareness
- ✧ On the breaths, flowing in and out, along with the physical movements synchronized with them
- ✧ On the stretch of the hamstrings and the upper back
- ✧ On mentally uttering the Holy Names "Radhey Krishna" in your each breath and feeling Their presence at all times

Benefits
- ✓ It flexes your hip joints and hamstring muscles.
- ✓ It tones up the adrenals, which helps cure inflammatory and allergic diseases.
- ✓ If done sincerely, it helps cure disorders of the reproductive system.

Contraindications
- - People with back problems and any defects in the coccyx should omit this *asan*.

62. Baka Dhyanasan (Crane's Meditative Pose)

Procedure

i. Sit down with your legs outstretched and joined together in front; keeping the back erect, place your palms on the floor behind the buttocks, with the fingers pointing backward, i.e. Dandasan (See page 117).

ii. Gently, squat on the floor with both feet slightly apart.

iii. Now balancing on the toes, rest your hands flat on the floor in front of the feet; also keep the fingers pointed forward.

iv. Keep your arms slightly bent, and bend forward so that the inner sides of both knees touch the outer sides of the upper arms (triceps portion).

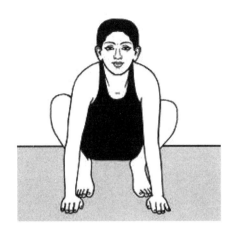
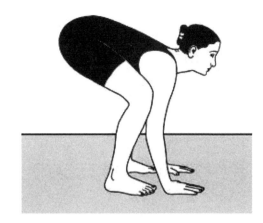

v. Bending further forward; stand up slightly on your legs, then gradually raise your feet off the floor.

vi. Try to balance the body on both—the arms and hands by resting the knees on the upper arms (triceps portion).

vii. Slowly, join the feet together and look at the nose tip to maintain balance.

viii. Stay in this pose for 15-20 seconds, breathing normally.

ix. Gradually, lower your feet to the floor and come back to the squatting position.

x. This is a single round; try up to three rounds.

xi. Finally, come to Shithil Dandasan (See page 117) and relax.

Awareness
✧ On the unbroken remembrance of "Radhey Krishna" flowing through the breaths
✧ On the pressure in the arms
✧ On the balance in the final position

Benefits
✓ Baka Dhyanasan strengthens the arms and wrists.
✓ It develops balance in the nervous system, and thus improves the sense of physical balance.

Contraindications
- Persons suffering from the heart ailments, cerebral thrombosis, and high blood pressure should avoid this *asan*.

63. Ek Pada Baka Dhyanasan (One-Legged Crane Pose)

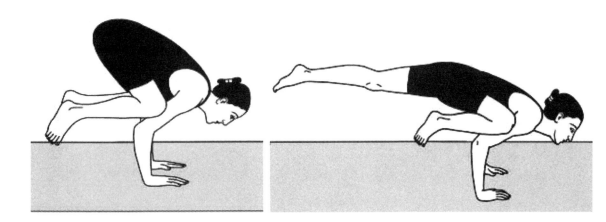

Procedure

i. Assume the final pose of Baka Dhyanasan, steps i-vi (See pages 182 and 183) progressively.

ii. Maintaining the balance with the gaze at the nose tip, gradually outstretch the right leg back until it is almost parallel to the floor.

iii. Make sure your head, neck, and trunk remain aligned and straight—horizontally.

iv. Remain in this position for as long as possible with normal breathing.

v. Slowly bring your right knee back on the upper right arm and lower both the feet to the floor.

vi. Again repeat the process, stretching the other leg.

vii. Finally, come to Shithil Dandasan (See page 117) and relax.

Awareness

✧ On mental chanting of the Divine Names "Radhey Krishna"
✧ On the balance

Benefits

✓ Although Ek Pada Baka Dhyanasan is relatively more challenging than Baka Dhyanasan, its effects of are similar to Baka Dhyanasan (See page 182)

Contraindications

- Persons suffering from the heart ailments, cerebral thrombosis, and high blood pressure should not include this *asan* in their *Yog* package.

64. Gupt Padmasan (Hidden Lotus Pose)

Procedure

i. Sit in Padmasan (See page 116).

184

ii. Leaning slightly forward, place both hands on the floor—on the outer sides of the knees.

iii. With an inhalation (Radhey), first take support of the arms and lean further forward, ensuring your hands stay static.

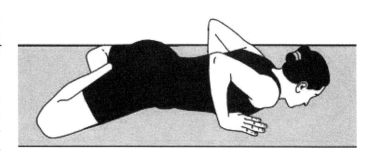

iv. Now raising the buttocks, lean your upper body forward; shift your arms quickly under the shoulders so that you can kneel on the knees.

v. Now with an exhalation (Krishna), take 2-3 more forward steps with your hands and comfortably lower the trunk downward

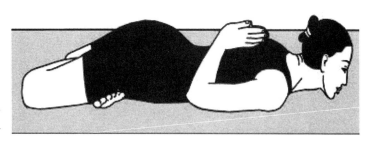

until the front part lies completely on the floor, with the chin or forehead resting on the floor.

vi. Then inhaling (Radhey), simultaneously move both hands behind the back.

vii. Also, try to form Namaste Mudra at the back of your body by joining all the fingers of your hands.

viii. Stay relaxed and stay in this position with normal breathing.

ix. Practice the *asan* once more by altering the leg position in Padmasan.

x. At last, come to Shithil Dandasan (See page 117) and relax.

Awareness

✧ On the various physical movements and the breaths synchronized with them
✧ On the unbroken recalling of "Radhey Krishna" with your each breath
✧ On relaxing the whole body in the last state

Benefits

✓ Gupt Padmasan is very supportive in postural defects of the spine.
✓ It is also effectual in releasing the mind from tension and anxiety.

Contraindications

- Persons with fractured legs and fractured arms should not attempt it without the counsel of a *Yog* therapist.

65. Ardh Padma Padmottanasan (Half-Lotus Leg Stretched Pose)

Procedure

i. Sit down with your legs outstretched and joined together in front; keeping the back erect, place your palms on the floor behind the buttocks, with the fingers pointing backward, i.e. Dandasan (See page 117).

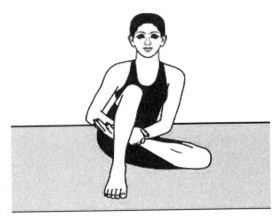

ii. Flex your left knee and place the left foot on top of the right thigh, just as in the half-lotus position (See page 111).

iii. Gently, flex the right knee, drawing it closer to the chest; rest the right foot flat on the floor with the toes pointing forward.

iv. Now, place your arms under the right thigh, from either side, and hold it firmly.

v. Inhale (Radhey) and fix your eyes on any point ahead; move slightly backward onto the coccyx (tail bone); while exhaling (Krishna), comfortably lift the right leg up—in front of the chest—by stretching it upward.

vi. Maintain the balance on the back portion of the buttocks and simultaneously move the stretched leg closer to the head; try to keep the back and head erect.

vii. Remain in this position for 15-20 seconds with normal breathing.

viii. While inhaling (Radhey), carefully return to the centre by lowering the right foot to the floor and come into Dandasan again.

ix. Repeat with the other leg.

x. This ends one round; attempt for two more rounds.

xi. Finally, come into Shithil Dandasan (See page 117) and relax.

Awareness

✧ On the bodily movements and your breaths synchronized with them

✧ On mentally uttering the Divine Names "Radhey Krishna" in your breaths, and feeling Their presence as well

✧ On the balance on the buttocks in the final state

Benefits

✓ Ardh Padma Padmottanasan gives sterling elasticity to the legs; so it is really a beneficial

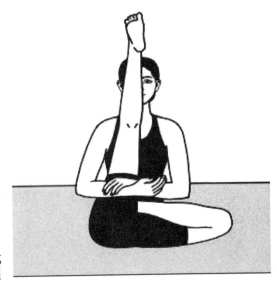

pose for those who desire to sit in Lotus Pose.

- ✓ It also plays an immense role in the stimulation of intestinal peristalsis as it considerably helps remove constipation.
- ✓ Performing this *asan* daily, greatly helps balance the nervous system.

Contraindications

- - Persons suffering from the heart ailments, cerebral thrombosis, and high blood pressure should not attempt it without the counsel of *Yog* experts.

66. Kurmasan (Tortoise Pose)

Procedure

i. Sit down with your legs outstretched and joined together in front; keeping the back erect, place your palms on the floor behind the buttocks, with the fingers pointing backward, i.e. Dandasan (See page 117).

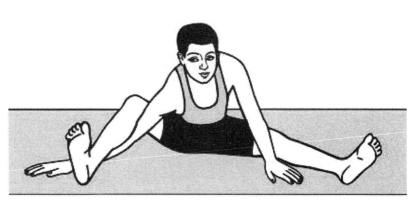

ii. Now, spread your feet about three feet apart and lift your knees slightly upward by folding them a bit.

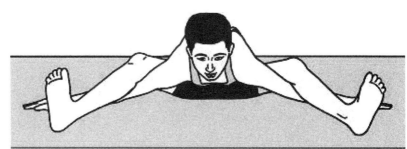

iii. Inhale (Radhey) in this position; while exhaling (Krishna), slightly bend the trunk forward, and extend your arms apart one by one through under the knees.

iv. Stretching your arms completely, rest the shoulders

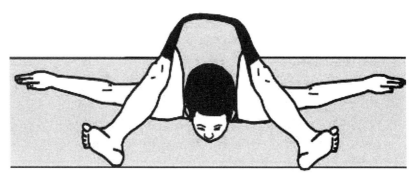

on the floor with the palms facing downward.

v. Now, extend your trunk further and stretch the neck; place your forehead or chin and finally the chest down to the floor.

vi. Make sure your knees settle around the armpits and the back of the knees on the upper arms.

vii. Increasing the extension gradually, stretch the legs fully and push the heels downward.

viii. Hold the position about 15-20 seconds with normal breathing.

ix. Comfortably, return to the central position.

x. This is one round; repeat twice.

xi. Eventually, come into Shithil Dandasan (See page117) and relax.

Awareness
- ✧ On the breaths synchronized with the bodily movements
- ✧ On the stretch and strain of the legs, spine, arms, and neck
- ✧ On mental utterance of the Divine Names "Radhey Krishna" along with your breaths

Benefits
- ✓ Kurmasan tones up the spine and stimulates the abdominal organs extremely.
- ✓ Those who feel inactiveness and tiredness due to either bodily weakness, or other reasons can get sufficient energy as its practice frees their minds from the emotions of passion, fear, anger, and pains.

Contraindications
- Only those people with normal health and outstanding flexibility should try this.

67. Niralamb Pashchimottanasan (Unsupported Back Stretching Pose)

Procedure

i. Sit down with your legs outstretched and joined together in front; keeping the back erect, place your palms on the floor behind the buttocks, with the fingers pointing backward, i.e. Dandasan (See page 117).

ii. Fold your knees gradually by bringing them toward the chest, and keeping the feet flat on the floor.

iii. Then, gently move your arms from outside of the legs, and catch hold of the soles firmly.

iv. Gazing at a fixed point in front at the eye level, inhale (Radhey) and recline a little bit backward—onto the coccyx.

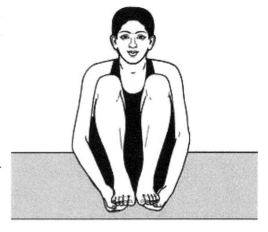

v. Exhale (Krishna); balancing on the buttocks, slowly raise your legs and then straighten them.

vi. Now, draw the knees toward the head and then without force, pull the arms back.

vii. Attempt to remain in this pose for 15-20 seconds with normal breathing.

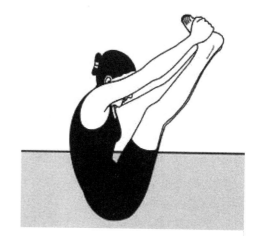

viii. While inhaling (Radhey), flex the knees gently and lower the feet to the floor and let go of the soles.

ix. While exhaling (Krishna), bring your trunk to the centre.

x. This finishes one round; do it for two more rounds.

xi. Finaly, come to Shithil Dandasan (See page 117) slowly and relax.

Awareness

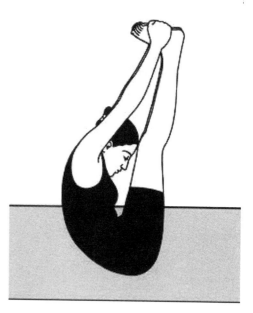

✧ On the different bodily movements and the breaths synchronized with them

✧ On the balance

✧ On mental chanting of the Divine Names "Radhey Krishna" with your breaths and spontaneously remembering Them

Benefits

✓ Niralamb Pashchimottanasan tones and massages the abdominal and pelvic regions including pancreas, liver, stomach, adrenal gland, and spleen.

✓ It effectively assists in allaying disorders of the uro-genitals system.

✓ Niralamb Pashchimottanasan can even control diabetes, menstrual problems, colitis, kidney troubles, bronchitis, and eosinophilia.

✓ From a mental perspective, it has a great impact on balancing the whole nervous system.

Contraindications

- People with heart ailments, high blood pressure, slipped-disc, sciatica, and sacral infections should avoid this *asan*.

68. Purvottanasan / Setu Asan (Front Intense Stretch Pose)

Procedure

i. Sit down with your legs outstretched and joined together in front; keeping the back erect, place your palms on the floor behind the buttocks, with the fingers pointing backward, i.e. Dandasan (See page 117).

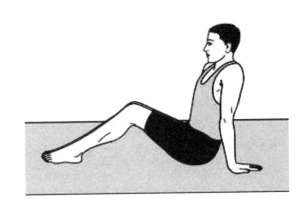

ii. Gently flex your knees; keep both soles and heels on the ground as shown in the figure.

iii. Now shift the body-weight onto the arms and feet.

iv. With a continuous inhalation (Radhey), raise your body slowly upward.

v. Keep both the arms and the legs straight with the knees and elbows firm in this state.

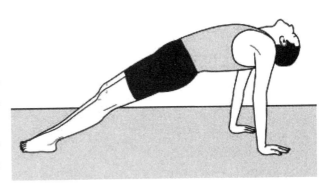

vi. Try to make the arms perpendicular to the ground and trunk parallel to the ground.

vii. Without any strain, stretch your neck and drop your head—as much as possible.

viii. Be in this state for as long as possible with normal breathing.

ix. Eventually, while exhaling (Krishna), come back to Shithil Dandasan (See page 117) and relax.

Awareness
✧ On the bodily movements and the breaths synchronized with them
✧ On the stretch in the arms, legs, neck, shoulders, stomach, and back
✧ On mentally uttering the Divine Names "Radhey Krishna" along with your breaths, and realizing Them standing in front of you and watching you

Benefits
✓ Setu Asan makes the wrists and ankles very powerful.
✓ It exercises the shoulder joints.
✓ It widens the chest.
✓ It strengthens the heart, anus, spinal column, and waist—slowly and effectively.
✓ It relieves fatigue caused by various forward bending poses.

Contraindications
- Those with high blood pressure, heart disease, stomach ulcers, or weak wrists should not practice this *asan*.

69. Baddh Padmasan (Locked-Lotus Pose)

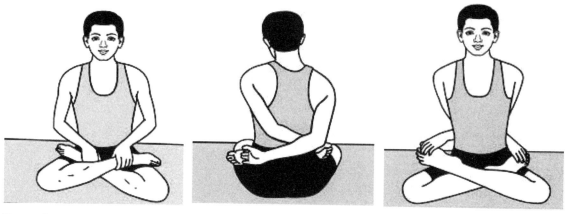

Procedure

i. Come to Padmasan (See page 116).

ii. Stretch your folded legs, bringing the feet as far back as possible so as to almost touch the waistline.

iii. Slowly take your arms behind the back and cross them.

iv. Now lean slightly forward, grasp your right big toe with the right hand first, and then the left big toe with the left hand.

v. Make sure your spine, neck, and the head remain erect and perpendicular to the floor.

vi. Be in this position for as long as comfortable, with slow and deep breathing.

vii. Gently, release the hands and come back to Padmasan.

viii. Repeat the *asan* with the alternate leg-position in Padmasan.

ix. Finally, return to Shithil Dandasan (See page 117) and relax.

Variation – 1

i. Come to the final position of Baddh Padmasan (steps i-iv).

ii. Inhale (Radhey) deeply.

iii. With an exhalation (Krishna), lean forward into Yog Mudrasan (See page 124).

Note: Do not attempt this variation before perfecting Baddh Padmasan.

Awareness

✧ On the breaths flowing in and out

✧ On mentally chanting the Holy Names "Radhey Krishna" with your each breath and always recalling the presence of Them

Benefits

✓ Baddh Padmasan helps eliminate aches in the shoulders, hands, and spine.

✓ With its diligent practice, the chest becomes widened.

✓ The internal organs are massaged well if practiced with Yog Mudrasan (See page 124).

70. Mayurasan (Peacock Pose)

Procedure

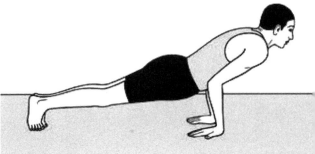

i. Slowly come to the final position of Hansasan (See page 128).

ii. Inhale (Radhey) in this position.

iii. As you exhale (Krishna), move forward on the toetips to lift the legs off the ground; slowly shift the body-weight onto the wrists and upper arms, and simultaneously stretch your trunk and head upward.

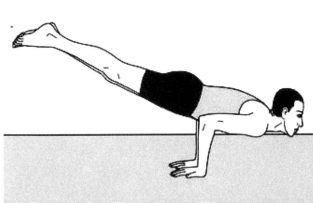

iv. You may lift the legs either one by one, or both at the same time, but make sure the feet remain together in the final position.

v. Also ensure the head, trunk, and legs stay parallel to the floor when the whole body is lifted on the palms of the hands.

vi. Stay in this position for as long as possible with normal breathing.

vii. Come back to the initial position by lowering the legs and trunk gradually to the floor.

viii. Finally, come into Shithil Dandasan (See page 117) and relax.

Awareness

✧ On the balance

✧ On recalling the sentient forms of "Radhey Krishna" with your each breath

Benefits

✓ Mayurasan tones up the abdominal organs and helps circulate blood well through the whole body as the elbows exert pressure against the abdominal aorta.

✓ It especially increases appetite by growing digestive power, cures ailments of the stomach and spleen, and even prevents the accumulation of toxins as they are burnt inside the body.

✓ It is very beneficial in the treatment of flatulence, constipation, diabetes, and malfunctions of the liver and kidneys.

✓ It develops both—mental and physical balance—thus bringing harmony among the glands of the endocrine system.

Contraindications

- Those with high blood pressure, heart problems, hernia, hyperacidity, and peptic or duodenal ulcer should best avoid this *asan*. Also, pregnant women, or those who are sick, or physically weak should not try it.

71. Padma Mayurasan (Lotus Peacock Pose)

Procedure

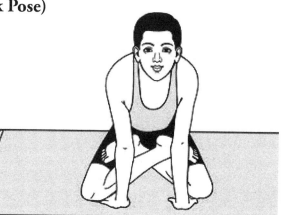

i. Sit in Padmasan (See page 116) progressively.

ii. Leaning forward, take support of the two arms, lift the body off the floor and balance the body-weight on the knees.

iii. Now, slightly lean forward and rest the two palms on the floor in front of the body, keeping the fingers pointing backward.

iv. Gently fold your arms, keep them close to each other; then slowly lean the upper body further forward and rest the elbows on the sides of the abdomen.

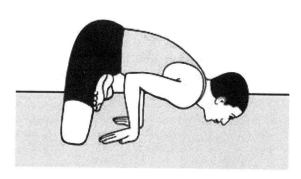

v. Leaning still further downward, rest the chest on the backside of the upper arms (deltoids and triceps) and find an approximate balance point of the body.

vi. Now, leaning even further downward, carefully try to raise your legs in Padmasan from the ground legs in Padmasan—without any strain.

vii. In the final step, make sure the trunk, head, and legs stay in a single line.

viii. Stay in this position for as long as possible with normal breathing.

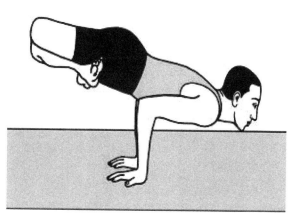

ix. Then, come back to the initial position by gently bringing the knees down to the floor and releasing the legs from Padmasan.

x. Perform one more round by changing leg-position in Lotus Pose.

xi. Finally, come to Shithil Dandasan (See

page 117) and relax.

Awareness
- ✧ On the balance
- ✧ On unbroken mental chanting of "Radhey Krishna"

Benefits
- ✓ The effects of this pose are exactly the same as that of Mayurasan (See page 192); the difference here is only of the cross legged position.

Contraindications
- - Same as that of Mayurasan (See page 192).

72. Garbhapindasan (Embryo in the Womb Pose)

Procedure

i. Sit in Padmasan (See page 116).

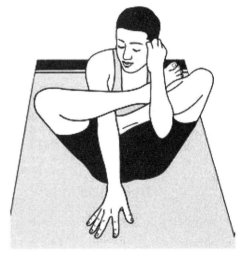

ii. Now, insert both arms in between the thighs and the calves, each on its own side.

iii. Inhale (Radhey); then exhaling (Krishna), bend your arms through the inner thighs and calves.

iv. Now balancing your body with the support of the right arm and buttocks, gradually raise your left arm along with the knee and catch hold of the left ear.

v. Now shifting the balance on the coccyx (tail bone), slowly lift your right arm along with your right knee and catch hold of your right ear.

vi. Remain in this position for as long as possible with normal breathing.

vii. Make sure your back and neck remain as erect as possible.

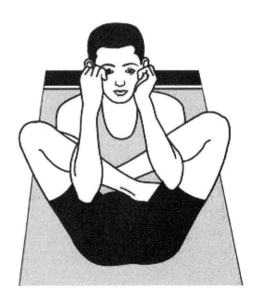

viii. With an inhalation (Radhey), release the ears; gradually lower your legs and then release your arms from the legs one by one.

ix. Repeat the process with the alternate leg-position in Padmasan.

x. Finally, unfolding the legs, come to Shithil Dandasan (See page 117) and relax.

Awareness

✧ On the breaths synchronized with the different movements
✧ On the balance
✧ On the stretch and effort in the arms, neck, and the legs
✧ On mentally chanting the Divine Names "Radhey Krishna" with your each breath and always feeling Their presence

Benefits

✓ This *asan* removes nervous disorders.
✓ It exercises and tones the abdominal parts, and increases digestive fire, thus resulting in the increase of appetite.
✓ It not only soothes an excited mind, but also enhances concentrating capacity.

Contraindication

- Prior to gaining good flexibility of the body, one should not attempt this *asan*.

73. Hanumanasan (Hanuman's Pose)

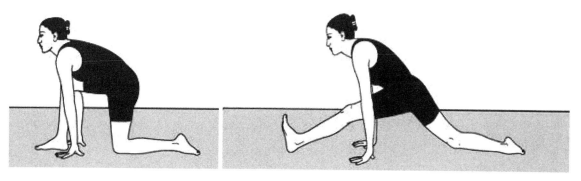

Procedure

i. Sit in Vajrasan (See page 113).

ii. Then, stand on the left knee, folding your right leg at the knee, ground it in front with the thigh parallel and shin perpendicular to the floor.

iii. Rest your palms on the floor on either side of the right foot.

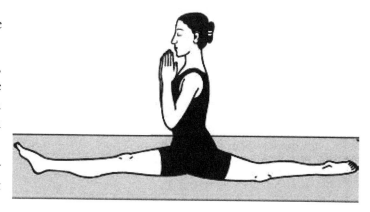

iv. Simultaneously balance the body-weight on the hands.

v. Now, stretch both the legs by sliding the right foot forward and the left foot backward as far as possible without any strain.

vi.   Next, lower your buttocks to the floor so that both the legs will be totally on the floor.

vii. Ensure your trunk and head remain erect.

viii. Then stretch the body, join the palms to make Namaste Mudra and look ahead.

ix.   Stay in this position to your comfort with normal breathing.

x.   Gradually, come back into Vajrasan and try the pose on the other side.

xi.   Ultimately, come to Shithil Dandasan (See page 117) and relax.

Awareness
- ✧ On the stretch of the leg muscles
- ✧ On mentally remembering the Names "Radhey Krishna" and always realizing Their presence

Benefits
- ✓ Hanumanasan tones up the leg muscles.
- ✓ It relaxes the thigh muscles.
- ✓ It massages the abdominal organs.
- ✓ It helps alleviates sciatica and other leg related problems.
- ✓ It exercises the female reproductive organs, and thus aids in preparing pregnant women for childbirth.
- ✓ It gives elasticity to the legs.

Contraindications
-   Persons who suffer from the cases like slipped-disc, sciatica, hernia, and the dislocation of the hip joints should avoid this pose.

74. Gorakshasan (Yogi Gorakhnath's Pose)

Procedure

i.   Come to Butterfly Pose (See page 96).

ii.   Now, slide your heels toward the perineum.

iii. Twisting your lower leg, turn your heels up; the toes will be on the floor.

iv.   Make sure your hands lie behind the buttocks in such a way that the fingers point downward.

v.   Push your body forward till your feet become completely vertical.

vi.   Ensure your knees touch the floor, and you do not use any uneasy force on any part of the body.

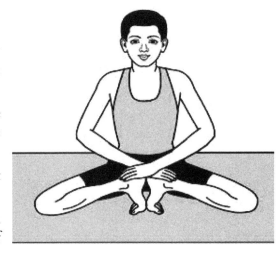

vii. Now bring your arms in front of the navel, and cross the wrists to hold the left heel with the right hand and right heel with the left hand as shown in the figure.

viii. Make sure your spine remains erect and face frontward; try to fix your eyes on a certain point.

ix. Maintain this position with ease and normal breathing.

x. Finally, come into Shithil Dandasan (See page 117) and relax.

Awareness

✦ On maintaining your balance
✦ On the pressure in your feet and knees
✦ On remembering the Divine Names "Radhey Krishna"

Benefits

✓ Like Moolabandhasan (See page 150), Gorakshasan also tones up the legs and feet, giving exceptional suppleness.
✓ The reproductive glands are exercised well and the retention of semen is made possible.
✓ It even benefits in the disease of wet-dreams and cases related to bladder and menstruation.
✓ It soothes the waist pains.

Contraindications

- Obese people and those with heart ailments should omit this exercise from their daily *Yog* package.

75. Padma Parvatasan (Lotus Mountain Pose)

Procedure

i. Sit in Padmasan (See page 116).

ii. Leaning your upper body slighty forward, gradually extend your arms on either side of the knees and rest the palms on the floor, fingers facing forward.

iii. Inhaling (Radhey), gently raise your hips with the support of the arms; move the hips slightly forward.

iv. Stretch your trunk and head vertically and raise your thighs to stand on the knees.

v. While balancing the body, slowly raise the hands up to the chest level and join the palms together in front of the chest to form Namaste Mudra; ensure the the head and neck stay erect.

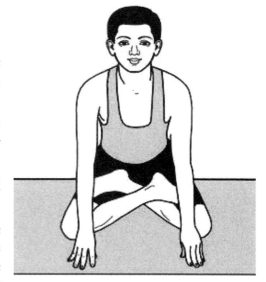

vi. Maintain the posture as long as possible with normal breathing.

vii. Exhaling (Krishna), gently lower the hands to the floor and also lower the hips downward, taking the support of the hands.

viii. Repeat the *asan* by the alternate combination of the legs in Padmasan.

ix. Finally, unfold the legs and come to Shithil Dandasan (See page 117) and relax.

Awareness

✧ On the breaths synchronized with the bodily movements

✧ On chanting the Holy Names "Radhey Krishna" in your breaths and always realizing Their presence in front of you—watching you

✧ On the balance in the final position

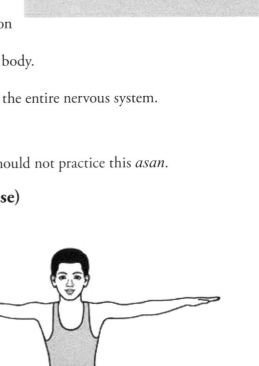

Benefits

✓ Padma Parvatasan develops concentration power.

✓ It brings coordination between the mind and body.

✓ It makes the knees extremely strong.

✓ It stimulates respiratory function and soothes the entire nervous system.

✓ It strengthens the buttocks and back.

Contraindications

- People with the problems in the knee joints should not practice this *asan*.

76. Upavishth Konasan (Seated Angle Pose)

Procedure

i. Sit down with your legs outstretched and joined together in front; keeping the back erect, place your palms on the floor behind the buttocks, with the fingers pointing backward, i.e. Dandasan (See page 117).

ii. Slowly spread your feet apart as far as possible in this position.

iii. Keep your hands on top of the knees, or slightly below the knees, with the head and torso well erect and chest outstretched.

iv. Inhaling (Radhey) deeply, raise your both arms at the shoulder level.

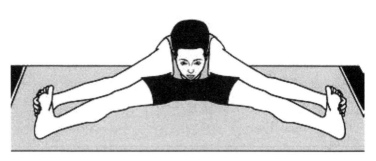

v. Exhaling (Krishna) slowly, lean forward and grasp the outer sides of your feet with your hands.

vi. Continuing to exhale (Krishna), slowly lean further forward from the hips and place the head/chin on the floor.

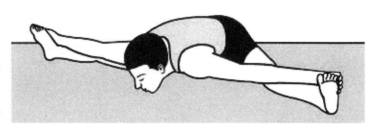

vii. Ensure your legs remain locked at the knees while catching hold of your feet properly.

viii. Try to remain in this pose as long as possible with normal breathing.

ix. Inhaling (Radhey), release the feet from the hands and lift your trunk back to the centre.

x. Finally, come to Shithil Dandasan (See page 117) and relax.

Awareness

✧ On the forward and upward movements and the breaths synchronized with them
✧ On the extension of the arms, spine, and the legs
✧ On mentally uttering the Sacred Names "Radhey Krishna" along with your breaths

Benefits

✓ Upavishth Konasan stretches the hamstrings and the pelvic joints and also prevents hernia.
✓ It eliminates sciatic pains, and helps control and regularize menstrual flow.
✓ It is also helpful in developing the elasticity of the body.

Contraindications

- People with serious back cases, sciatica, and knee problems should avoid it.

77. Vasishthasan (Sage Vasistha's Pose / Side Plank Pose)

Procedure

i. Come to the final pose of Santulanasan, following the steps i-iii (See page 147).

ii. Inhale (Radhey); shift the body-weight onto the right arm and balance on it; as you

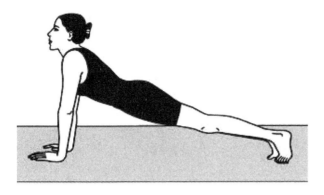

exhale (Krishna), gently flip your body onto the right side, and simultaneously raise the left arm vertically to place it along the side of the body.

iii. Fold your left leg at the knee and catch hold of the left big toe with the left hand.

iv. Now stretch your left leg; raise your leg upward vertically and while turning the head slowly, attempt to concentrate on the raised left big toe.

v. Maintain balance with the legs and arms extended completely.

vi. Maintain this pose as long as possible with normal breathing.

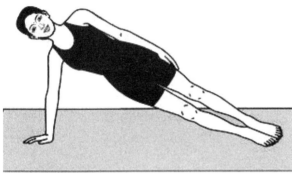

vii. Return to the initial position and repeat on the other side.

viii. Finally, come into Shithil Dandasan (See page 117) and relax.

Awareness

✧ On the balance
✧ On the stretch of the legs and the arms
✧ On remembering the Divine Names "Radhey Krishna" with the breaths

Benefits

✓ Vasishthasan, one of the balance poses, tones the arms the lower back, and abdomen by maintaining elasticity in the leg muscles.
✓ Besides this, it develops the balance in the nervous system and thus, improves the sense of physical balance.
✓ It can develop your sense of equanimity, trust, and open-mindedness.

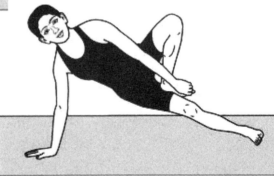

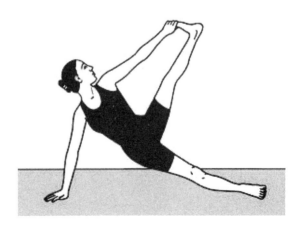

Contraindications

- People with fractured arms or legs should not attempt this pose.

78. Ek Pada Shirasan (One Foot to Head Pose)

Procedure

i. Sit down with your legs outstretched and joined together in front; keeping the back erect, place your palms on the floor behind the buttocks, with the fingers pointing backward, i.e. Dandasan (See page 117).

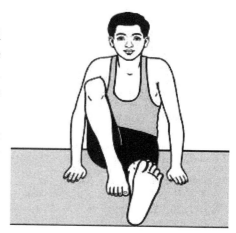

ii. Gradually fold your right leg; keep your right foot on the floor, near the left knee, and slant your right leg slightly rightward.

iii. Now, intertwine the right arm around the right leg—through the inner side—to grasp the outer side of the right ankle.

iv. Also, with your left hand, catch your right foot from the outside.

v. Now slowly lift your right leg, using your arms and hands. Lean your trunk forward, twisting it a bit to the left.

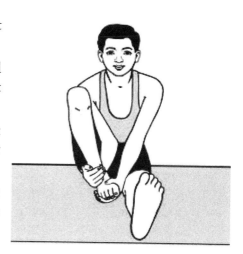

vi. Rest the right leg comfortably on the right shoulder—without any strain; then release either of the arms.

vii. Try to move your right leg higher with your left hand by pushing the thigh backward with the right upper arm.

viii. Now, rest the right foot exactly behind the head—at the nape of the neck.

ix. Also, attempt to make the spine and head erect.

x. Then, bring your hands down in front of the chest in Namaste Mudra.

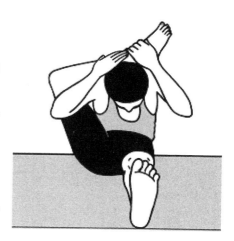

xi. Make sure your head remains in the centre and erect, as much as possible.

xii. Maintain this position as long as you can with normal breathing.

xiii. Then, come back to the initial position by lowering the right leg from the shoulder with the help of your arms and hands.

xiv. Perform the same method above on the other side.

xv. Finally, come into Shithil Dandasan (See page 117) and relax.

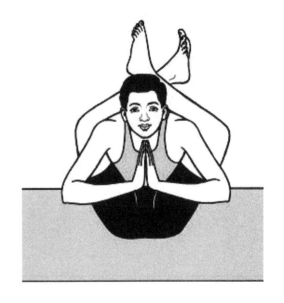

Awareness

- ✧ On the balance
- ✧ On remembering the sentient forms of "Radhey Krishna" with the breaths

Benefits

- ✓ Ek Pada Shirasan has multiple functions like exercising the abdominal organs, and activating peristalsis, thus helping in the elimination of constipation.
- ✓ It is a blessing pose for ladies as it strengthens the reproductive organs.
- ✓ It also supplies copious blood to the legs and spine and increases blood hemoglobin levels, which assists in energizing both—the body and the mind.

Contraindications

- Those who suffer from slipped-disc, sciatica, and hernia should omit it from their *Yogic* exercise.

79. Dwi Pada Shirasan (Two Feet To Head Pose)

Procedure

i. First come into the final position of Ek Pada Shirasan, steps viii and ix (See page 201), progressively.

ii. Take a few breaths in this position; then slowly lift the left leg over the left shoulder by intertwining the left arm around the left leg—through the inner side, and grasp the outer side of the left ankle; then repeat rest of the same process for the right leg too.

iii. Without any strain, lock the feet exactly behind the neck by crossing them.

iv. Now, keep the hands on floor by the

sides of the thighs and try to balance on the coccyx (tail bone).

v. Also move your hands one by one to the chest, and join both of your palms together to form Namaste Mudra.

vi. Make sure your head remains in the centre and erect.

vii. Maintain the pose as long as comfortable with normal breathing.

viii. As you come back to the central position, carefully come to Shithil Dandasan (See page 117) by reversing the process above and relax.

Awareness

✧ On the breaths flowing in and out along with the spontaneous chanting of "Radhey Krishna" in your mind

✧ On the balance in the final position

Benefits

✓ This advanced *asan* massages the adrenal glands and solar plexus.

✓ It firms the abdominal and pelvic organs, which contribute for the development of the efficiency of the digestive, reproductive, and excretory systems.

✓ It provides superb control of the nervous system.

Contraindications

- Persons with back-pain and without extra elasticity should omit this *asan*.

80. Utthan Ek Pada Shirasan (Standing Foot to Head Pose)

Procedure

i. First come into the final position of Ek Pada Shirasan, steps viii and ix (See page 201), progressively.

ii. Then, place both the palms on the floor to form a support with the hands and arms.

iii. Lean little bit backward, come into a squatting pose with the left leg; inhale (Radhey) and balancing on the left leg, gently raise your body and stand up unhurriedly.

iv. Place both the palms together in front of the chest in Namaste Mudra.

v. Without any stress, maintain balance in the standing pose as long as you are comfortable.

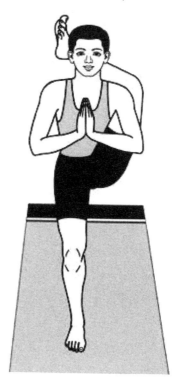

vi. Slowly and with care, sit down so that you can come back to the initial position by lowering the right leg from the shoulder.

vii. Repeat the above process with the other leg.

viii. Finally, return to the central position, go into Shithil Dandasan (See page 117) and relax.

Awareness
✧ On feeling the spontaneous omnipresence of "Radhey Krishna" throughout while breathing in and out
✧ On the balance in the final position

Benefits
✓ Utthan Ek Pada Shirasan exercises the internal organs excellently due to the pressure on both sides of the abdomen, thus helps in eradicating constipation and activizing the peristalsis process.
✓ It firms the reproductive organs and maintains plentiful blood circulation in the legs and spine.
✓ It increases the amount of hemoglobin in the blood, which equally energizes both—the body and the mind.

Contraindications
- Persons with slipped-disc, sciatica, or hernia should omit this *asan*.

81. Purna Matsyendrasan (The Full Twist Pose)

Procedure
i. Come to Ardh Padmasan (See page 111) with the right knee touching the floor.

ii. Now, fold your left leg at the knee and bring your left foot on the outer side of the right thigh near the right knee.

iii. Inhaling (Radhey), raise your right arm vertically and stretch the shoulder.

iv. Exhaling (Krishna), twist the waist to the left and place the right arm over to the outer part of the left knee.

v. Now, firmly catch hold of the left toes with the right hand, resting the right triceps on the outer side of the left knee.

vi. Take your left hand behind the back, and twisting the trunk and head to the left, try to touch the right thigh.

vii. Maintain this posture for 15-20 seconds with normal breathing.

viii. Slowly, come back to the starting position.

ix. Repeat the same process on the other side.

x. This is one round; repeat it for up to two more rounds.

xi. Finally, come into Shithil Dandasan (See page 117) and relax.

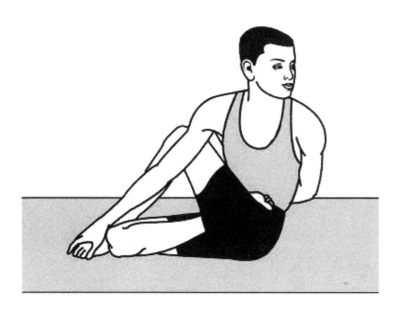

Awareness

- ✧ On the breaths synchronized with the bodily movements
- ✧ On the stretch and strain of the legs, spine, and arms
- ✧ On realizing sentient forms of "Radhey Krishna" in your breaths and always feeling Their presence around you

Benefits

- ✓ This arduous pose, Purna Matsyendrasan, supplies the spinal nerves with adequate supply of blood, increases gastric activity, and thereby helps to digest food, and remove toxins from the body as well.
- ✓ Like Ardh Matsyendrasan, it increases muscle flexibility, stretches the spine and disc, and frees the nerves from anxiety and tension, thus curing neck pain or headaches.
- ✓ It massages the internal parts, and thus is helps cure abdominal ailments like constipation, dyspepsia, and diabetes.
- ✓ And besides, it balances the secretion of adrenaline, which aids in increasing vitality and calmness.

Contraindication

- - Women who are in second or third month of their pregnancy should not do this *asan*.

E. Prone Poses

1. Simple Prone Pose
Procedure

i. Lie down on your abdomen; keep your legs together so that the toes point outward and the soles of the feet face upward.

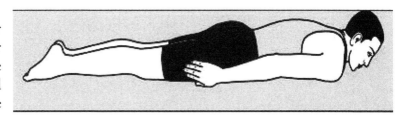

ii. Make sure your chin touches the floor.

iii. Now, stretch your arms and place them on either side of the body in such a way that the palms touch the thighs.

iv. As you stretch the whole body, maintain the position, for a while with normal breathing.

Note: This is the initial position for all the prone postures.

2. Balasan (Child's Pose)
Procedure

i. Lie flat on your stomach, legs together and palms touching the outer sides of your thighs with your chin on the floor, i.e. Simple Prone Posture.

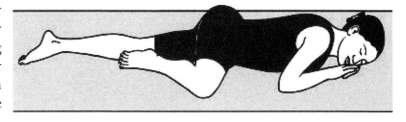

ii. Now, fold your left arm and place the head over your left elbow.

iii. Next, place your right palm above your left hand, fold your right leg at the knee and then bring it closer to the chest, keeping the knee on the ground.

iv. Move your right elbow slightly to the right side.

v. Adjust the position of your head according to your comfort.

vi. Take a few slow and deep breaths, and relax the whole body.

vii. Mentally chant "Radhey" while inhaling, and "Krishna" while exhaling.

viii. Be in this state for a minute with somewhat slow and deep breathing.

ix. In the same way, repeat on the other side.

Awareness
✧ On feeling relaxation of the whole body

✧ On the breaths synchronized with the mental chanting of the Holy Names "Radhey Krishna"

Benefits

✓ Balasan activates the digestive peristalsis by exercising the intestines.
✓ It also alleviates constipation.
✓ It soothes sciatic pain by relaxing the nerves of the legs.
✓ It is a perfect relaxing pose for pregnant women of the later period as they can either sleep, rest, or practice Subtle Body Relaxation (See page 347) in this pose.

3. Advasan (Reversed Corpse Pose)

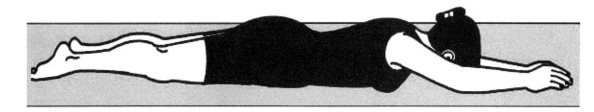

Procedure

i. Lie flat on your stomach, legs together and palms touching outer sides of your thighs with your chin on the floor, i.e. Simple Prone Posture (See page 207).

ii. Extend your arms over the head, keeping your palms flat on the floor.

iii. Make sure your forehead lies on the floor.

iv. Close your eyes so that you can relax both—the entire body and the mind.

v. Remain in this state for 30-60 seconds with slow and consistent breathing.

Awareness

✧ On the relaxation of the whole body
✧ On always feeling the presence of "Radhey Krishna" along with your breathing

Benefits

✓ This relaxing pose, Advasan, acts as an all-curing medicine for those who have slipped-disc, stiff neck, and stooping or hunched body.

4. Shithil Makarasan (Relaxing Crocodile Pose)

Procedure

i. Lie flat on your stomach, legs together and palms touching the sides of your thighs with your chin on the floor, i.e. Simple Prone Posture (See page 207).

ii. Now, spread your feet apart, as wide as possible, with the inner parts of the legs resting on the floor and also the heels facing each other.

iii. Gradually, fold your arms at the elbows, and then place both palms on the opposite biceps.

iv. Rest the chin on the crossed forearms and gently close your eyes.

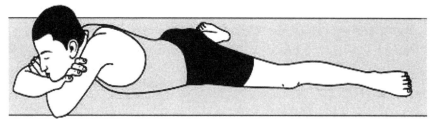

v. Taking some slow and deep breaths, relax the whole body.

vi. Mentally chanting "Radhey" while inhaling and "Krishna" while exhaling, stay in this pose for at least 2-3 minutes.

Awareness

✧ On feeling relaxation of the whole body
✧ On the breaths synchronized with mental uttering of the Divine Names "Radhey Krishna"

Benefits

✓ As it relaxes the entire body, Shithil Makarasan removes fatigue.
✓ It is considerably supportive for those who are affected with slipped-disc, sciatica, lower back pain, and other spinal defects.

5. Matsya Kreedasan (Swimming Fish Pose)

Procedure

i. Lie flat on your stomach, legs together and palms touching the sides of your thighs with your chin on the floor, i.e. Simple Prone Posture (See page 207).

ii. Now interlocking your fingers of the hands, place them precisely under the head.

iii. Slowly flex your left leg, drawing the left knee closer to the chest.

iv. Shifting the face and arms to the left, touch the left knee with the left elbow without any strain.

v. Now, place the right side of the head on the right lower arm.

vi. In the final position, take slow and deep breaths, and then completely relax the whole body.

vii. Mentally chanting (Radhey) while inhaling and (Krishna) while exhaling, attempt to be in this position for a minute.

viii. Lastly, come back to the starting position; repeat the *asan* on the other side.

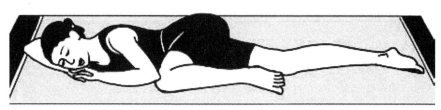

Awareness

✧ On feeling relaxation of the whole body
✧ On the natural breathing along with mental chanting of "Radhey Krishna" with every breath

Benefits

✓ The bebefits of Matsya Kreedasan are the same as that of Balasan (See page 207).
✓ It relaxes both—the body and the mind.
✓ People with backache may practice this pose as a counter pose after doing backward bending poses.
✓ Also, in the later stage of pregnancy, lying on the back may burden different veins and disturb the blood circulation. In such cases, this pose is perfect for relaxing, sleeping, or practising Subtle Body Relaxation.

6. Jyeshthikasan (Superior Pose)

Procedure

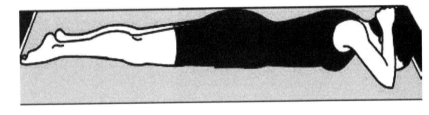

i. Lie flat on your stomach, legs together and palms touching the sides of your thighs with your chin on the floor, i.e. Simple Prone Posture (See page 207).

ii. Stretch your legs and then place the forehead on the floor.

iii. Interlock the fingers of both hands and rest the palms on the back side of the head.

iv. Make sure your elbows lie on the floor.

v. Close the eyes in this position.

vi. Breathe slowly and evenly and relax the whole body, with the focus on the natural and rhythmic breathing process.

vii. Be in this *asan* for one to two minutes.

Awareness

✧ On the breathing process
✧ On the relaxation of the whole body
✧ On always reminding the Sacred Names "Radhey Krishna," flowing with your breaths

Benefits

✓ Jyeshthikasan mainly helps alleviate various spinal complaints such as cervical spondylitis, stiff neck, and the upper back.
✓ It offers relief from herniated discs.

7. Makarasan (Crocodile Pose)

Procedure

i. Lie flat on your stomach, legs together and palms touching the sides of your thighs with your chin on the floor, i.e. Simple Prone Posture (See page 207).

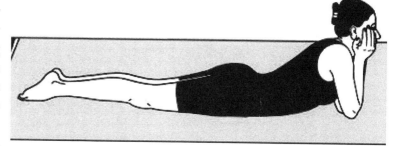

ii. Gradually, raise your head and shoulders, fold your arms and place your elbows in front of the chest; keep them together; rest the chin on the palms.

iii. Keep your elbows close to each other and in line with the neck to form an arch-like shape with the spine.

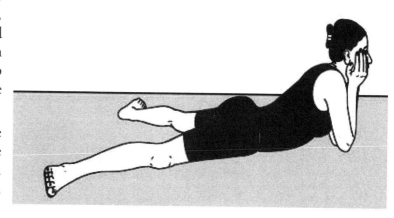

iv. Now, separate your feet as far as possible, with the toes pointing sideward, and the inner part of the legs touching the floor.

v. In the final posture, feel a relaxing effect on the back.

vi. Stay in this position, with deep breathing, for up to five minutes.

vii. Finally, return to the central position by lowering your upper body and bringing your arms by the sides of your thighs.

Variation - 1

i. Follow steps i to iii, as mentioned in the main procedure, progressively.

ii. Now, join your legs, keeping them straight.

iii. Then inhale (Radhey); bend the left leg and try to touch the left buttock with the left heel.

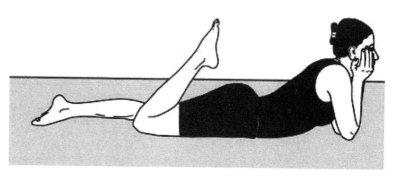

iv. While exhaling (Krishna), straighten the left leg and simultaneously bend the right leg at the knee.

v. Try to touch the right buttock with your right heel in this state.

vi. Maintain a perfect rhythm while raising and/or lowering the legs; to the degree one leg is raised, the other will be lowerd.

vii. Practice this *asan* for about five minutes in the same way.

viii. Finally, return to the central position by lowering your upper body and bringing your arms by the sides of your thighs.

Variation - 2

i. Follow steps i to iii, as mentioned in the main procedure, progressively.

ii. Now, join the legs together, keeping them locked at the knees.

iii. While inhaling (Radhey), bend both the legs simultaneously and try to touch your buttocks with the heels.

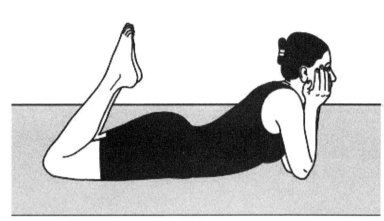

iv. While exhaling (Krishna), lower your legs to the floor.

v. Continue this *asan* for about five minutes.

vi. Finally, return to the central position by lowering your upper body and bringing your arms by the sides of your thighs.

Note: Noramally, the elbows is palced below the neck. Moving the elbows forward increases pressure on the upper back along with the neck and the shoulders; and bringing them back to the chest gives more pressure to the lower back.

When the elbows are joined, further pressure develops on the respective parts. It is necessary to understand that the pressure heals that particular part.

Awareness
  ✧ On the relaxation of the backbone
  ✧ On the movement of your legs in the variations and the breaths synchronized with them
  ✧ On always mentally remembering "Radhey Krishna" flowing with your breaths

Benefits
  ✓ Makarasan is a great medicine for those who are suffering from slipped-disc, sciatica, lower back pain, and other spinal defects.

- ✓ A long stay in this *asan* even helps the vertebral column to regain its normal shape and release compression of the spinal nerves.
- ✓ Additionally, it is quite helpful in curing asthma if performed regularly for 15 minutes before sleeping.

8. Sphinx Asan

Procedure

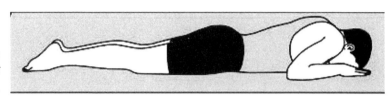

i. Lie flat on your stomach, legs together and palms touching the sides of your thighs with your chin on the floor, i.e. Simple Prone Posture (See page 207).

ii. Straighten your whole body; place the forehead on the floor, with the feet joined together and the toes pointing backward.

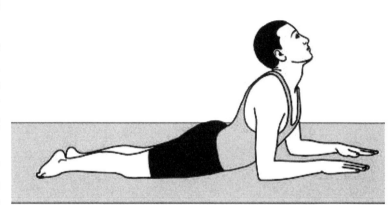

iii. Gently folding your arms at the elbows, keep your forearms on the floor in such a way that they touch either side of the chest.

iv. Make sure your palms rest on the floor—on either side of the head.

v. With an inhalation (Radhey), comfortably raise your head, shoulders, and chest with the support of the forearms and the palms.

vi. Now make the upper arms perpendicular to the floor, try to raise the trunk as high as possible and also stretch the neck backward.

vii. Maintain this state for about 15-20 seconds with normal breathing.

viii. Now while exhaling (Krishna), gently lower the trunk and the head back to the floor.

ix. This completes one round; do it for two more rounds.

x. Lastly, come into Balasan (See page 207) or Matsya Kreedasan (See page 209) and relax.

Awareness

- ✧ On feeling relaxation in the whole body
- ✧ On natural breathing along with mental chanting of "Radhey Krishna" with every breath

Benefits

- ✓ Sphinx Asan is quite beneficial for the recovery of slipped-disc, rejuvenating the spine, and removal of stiffness from the back.
- ✓ It is equally good for persons with lumbago and sciatica.
- ✓ It benefits women by toning up their ovaries and uterus, and also by alleviating various menstrual and gynecological disorders.
- ✓ It helps activate the appetite, eliminates constipation, and tones up the abdominal organs such as the liver and kidneys.

9. Bhujangasan (Cobra Pose)

Procedure

i. Lie flat on your stomach, legs together and palms touching the sides of your thighs with your chin on the floor, i.e. Simple Prone Posture (See page 207).

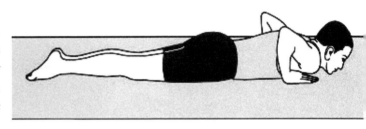

ii. Now, stretch your legs with both feet together; also stretch the toes, keeping them pointed backward.

iii. Place your palms beside the lower chest—just below the shoulders—so that the fingers lie under them.

iv. With an inhalation (Radhey), raise your head, shoulders, and the chest until your navel is nearly 3 cms above the ground.

v. Ensure the pelvic area rests on the floor.

vi. Simultaneously, attempt to arch your dorsal spine and neck backward, as far as possible.

vii. Comfortably, bear the whole weight on the lower part of the body with just nominal support from the hands.

viii. Hold the pose for about 15-20 seconds with normal breathing.

ix. With an exhalation (Krishna), gradually return to the initial pose by bending the arms and then resting the trunk on the floor.

x. Repeat the process twice.

xi. Lastly, come to Balasan (See page 207) or Matsya Kreedasan (See page 209) and relax completely.

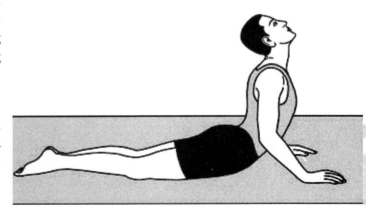

Awareness

✧ On the breaths synchronized with the physical movements
✧ On the stretches and strains of the back
✧ On the Sacred Names "Radhey Krishna" flowing with each breath

Benefits

✓ Bhujangasan has versatile effects like, recovery from slipped-disc, rejuvenation of the spine, alleviation of stiff back problems, and giving natural relief in lumbago and sciatica.
✓ It also provides elasticity to the lungs by expanding the chest, which mainly results in proper blood circulation in the pelvic region.
✓ Bhujangasan is a blessing pose for women as it tones up the ovaries and uterus, and helps alleviate menstrual and various gynecological disorders.
✓ Additionally, it activates the appetite, eliminates constipation, and is tremendously useful for the abdominal organs such as liver and kidneys too.

Contraindications

- Persons with peptic ulcer, hernia, intestinal tuberculosis, or hyperthyroidism should not practice this *asan*.
- Those who have undergone abdominal surgery should avoid this *asan* for at least two months post-surgery.

10. Tiryak Bhujangasan (Twisting Cobra Pose)

Procedure

i. Lie flat on your stomach, legs together and palms touching the sides of your thighs with your chin on the floor, i.e. Simple Prone Posture (See page 207).

ii. Now, spread your feet about 1.5-2 feet.

iii. Next, stretch your legs and rest the feet on the toes.

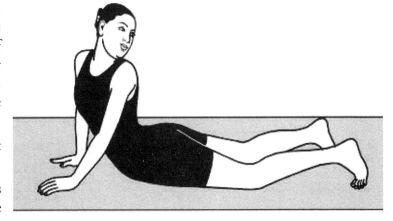

iv. Place your palms next to the lower chest—below the shoulders—so that your fingers come under the shoulders.

v. With an inhalation (Radhey), raise the head, shoulders, and the chest until the navel is approximately 3 cms above the ground.

vi. Make sure the pelvic area rests on the floor and the weight of the lower part of the body is borne with minimal support from the hands.

vii. Look ahead, unlike arching backward as in Bhujangasan.

viii. While exhaling (Krishna), gently twist both—the head and the upper trunk—rightward in order to bring the chin over the left shoulder.

ix. Also, try to fix your eyes on top of the right heel in this position.

x. Keep your arms locked or bent a bit when the body and shoulders are twisted in the final position.

xi. Make sure your navel stays as much closer to the floor as possible.

xii. Remain in the final position for 15-20 seconds with normal breathing.

xiii. Inhaling (Radhey) continuously, gradually return to the centre and twist to the other side in the same manner.

xiv. As you exhale (Krishna), slowly return to the initial pose by bending the arms at elbows and then resting the trunk on the floor.

xv. This finishes one round; perform two more rounds.

xvi. Eventually, return to Balasan (See page 207) or Matsya Kreedasan (See page 209) and relax.

Awareness

◇ On twisting upper trunk, shoulders, and head and on breaths synchronized with them

◇ On the extension of the muscles of the back and the intestines

◇ On mental remembrance of the Holy Names "Radhey Krishna" with every breath

Benefits

✓ Twisting Bhujangasan provides wonderful elasticity to the lungs with the expansion of the chest, which mainly helps in the proper blood circulation in the pelvic region.

✓ As Sphinx Pose (See page 213), it helps one recover from slipped-disc; it rejuvenates the spine, removes the stiffness from the back, and heals lumbago and sciatica as well.

✓ It tones up the ovaries and uterus and helps alleviate all menstrual and gynecological disorders.

✓ Chiefly, it is found to increase appetite, eliminate constipation, and invigorate the abdominal organs such as the liver and kidneys.

Contraindication

- Persons with peptic ulcer, hernia, intestinal tuberculosis, or hyperthyroidism should not practice this *āsan* without the counsel of *Yog* instructors.

11. Sarpasan (Snake Pose)

Procedure

i. Lie flat on your stomach, legs together and palms touching the sides of your thighs with your chin on the floor, i.e. Simple Prone Posture (See page 207).

ii. Gently, place your hands on the buttocks and interlock the fingers.

iii. In this position, make sure your chin rests on the floor.

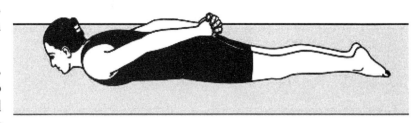

iv. Inhale (Radhey), and taking the help of the abdominal muscles, raise your chest from the floor.

v. Make sure your legs remain joined together throughout.

vi. Push your shoulders backward and raise your interlocked hands away from the buttocks, as high as possible;

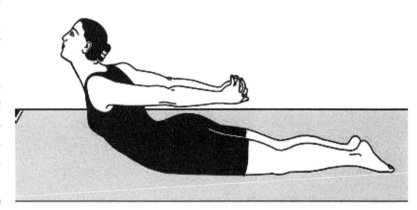

vii. Wait for 15-20 seconds in this position, breathing normally.

viii. Now while exhaling (Krishna), lower your upper body and arms comfortably, and gradually come down to the floor.

ix. This is one round, do it for two more rounds.

x. Finally, come into either Balasan (See page 207) or Matsya Kreedasan (See page 209) and relax.

Awareness
- ✧ On breathing in and out along with the physical movements
- ✧ On the stretch of the shoulders and arms
- ✧ On spontaneously feeling the omnipresence of "Radhey Krishna" with your breaths

Benefits
- ✓ Sarpasan not only strengthens the muscles of the spine, but it also makes the spine very flexible, helps cure slipped-disk, and cervical and back pain.
- ✓ As it massages the heart, the amount of oxygen in the blood streams gets increased by opening out the inactive alveoli.
- ✓ It also wonderfully massages the abdominal organs.
- ✓ It helps in asthmatic cases too.
- ✓ It strengthens the chest and shoulders.

Contraindications

- Those who have been suffering from heart ailments and high blood pressure should perform it only under the supervision of *Yog* therapists.

12. Saral Dhanurasan (Simple Bow Pose)

Procedure

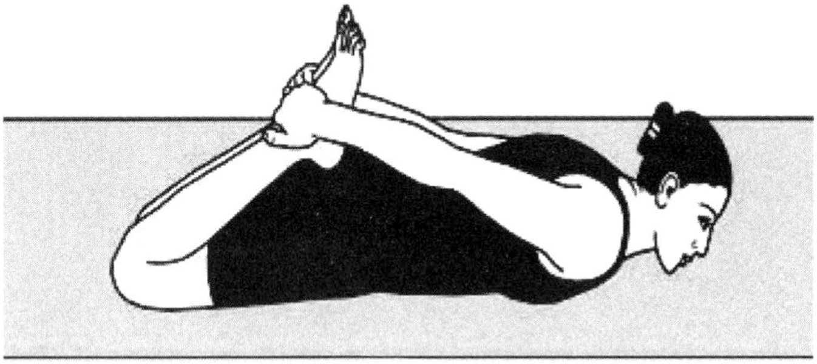

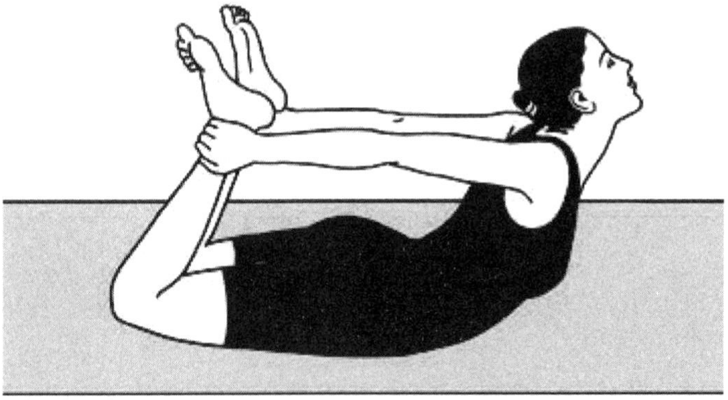

i. Lie flat on your stomach, legs together and palms touching the sides of your thighs with your chin on the floor, i.e. Simple Prone Posture (See page 207).

ii. Now flex your legs, move the heels near the buttocks and hold the ankles with the hands firmly.

iii. Make sure your knees and thighs remain flat on the ground and the arms locked at the elbows throughout the *asan*.

iv. With an inhalation (Radhey), raise your head, shoulders, and chest upward—to your capacity; stretch the neck backward—as far as possible.

v. Stretch your legs sideward and backward and let the knees be separated to raise the trunk as high as possible.

vi. Try to stay in the final position for 15-20 seconds with normal breathing.

vii. With an exhalation (Krishna), return to the initial pose by gradually lowering your chest and head.

viii. This is one round; practice the *asan* for two more rounds.

ix. Finally, come into either Balasan (See page 207), or Matsya Kreedasan (See page 209) and relax.

Awareness

✧ On the bodily movements and the breaths synchronized with them
✧ On the stretch of the abdominal region and the back
✧ On always realizing the presence of "Radhey Krishna" along with your each breath

Benefits

✓ The benefits of this exercise are similar to those of the Dhanurasan (See page 221).

13. Utthan Prishthasan (Lizard Pose)

Procedure

i. Lie flat on your stomach, legs together and palms touching the sides of your thighs with your chin on the floor, i.e. Simple Prone Posture (See page 207).

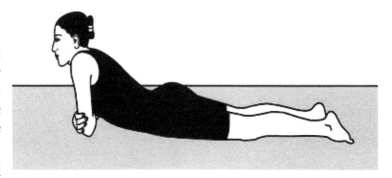

ii. Now, cross your arms and rest them exactly under the chest with the hands holding the upper arms.

iii. Keep a slight distance between your feet, with the sole facing upward and then look frontward.

iv. Ensure you take support of the elbows by keeping them fixed throughout the practice.

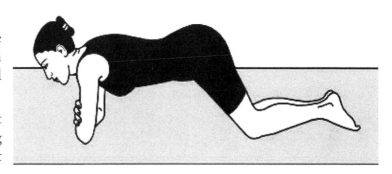

v. Now inhale (Radhey); then slowly raise the trunk and buttocks, taking support of the elbows and knees, and finally stretch the upper body backward.

vi. In this position, keep your chin and chest either on the floor or close to the floor as much as possible.

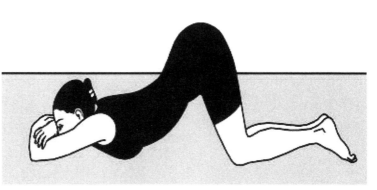

vii. Try to be in this pose for 15-20 seconds with normal breathing.

viii. With an exhalation (Krishna), slowly return to the base position.

ix. This is one round; perform two more rounds.

x. Finally, return to either Balasan (See page 207) or Matsya Kreedasan, (See page 209) or Relaxing Crocodile Pose (See page 208) and relax.

Awareness

- ✧ On the bodily movements and the breaths synchronized with them
- ✧ On the pressure on the back
- ✧ On mentally uttering the Sacred Names "Radhey Krishna" with your each inhalation and exhalation

Benefits

- ✓ Utthan Pristhasan, an easy but effective pose, stretches and firms the diaphragm.
- ✓ It exercises the whole back.
- ✓ It is also incredibly beneficial in removing stiffness between the two shoulder blades.

14. Ardh Shalabhasan (Half Locust Pose)

Procedure

i. Lie flat on your stomach, legs together and palms touching the sides of your thighs with your chin on the floor, i.e. Simple Prone Posture (See page 207).

ii. Place your arms under the body as close to each other as possible, with the palms on the floor, exactly under the thighs.

iii. Stretch the chin a bit forward and keep it held to the floor throughout the *asan*.

iv. Make sure your legs remain locked at the knees at all times.

v. Now while inhaling (Radhey), gradually raise the left leg as high as possible, making sure the right leg remains locked and in contact with the floor.

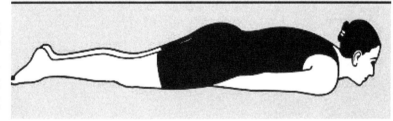

vi. Hold the pose for 15-20 seconds with normal breathing.

vii. With an exhalation (Krishna), unhurriedly lower the left leg to the floor.

viii. Repeat the same process with the other leg.

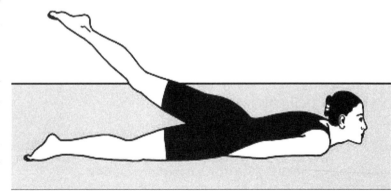

ix. This is one round; try two more rounds.

x. Eventually, come into Balasan (See page 207), or Matsya Kreedasan (See page 209) and relax for a while.

Awareness

✧ On the bodily movements and the breaths synchronized with them

✧ On the pressure on the lower back and the abdomen

✧ On the Holy Names "Radhey Krishna" flowing with your breaths

Benefits

✓ Ardh Shalabhasan is tremendously beneficial in *Yog* therapy for the cure of sciatica and slipped-disc.

✓ It assists in the elimination of constipation.

✓ It helps in improving blood circulation throughout the body.

✓ It tones up the thighs, hips, and buttocks by reducing unwantd fat.

✓ If practiced daily, this pose can even control diabetes.

✓ Women with problems related to ovaries and uterus can benefit from this pose.

Contraindications

- People with hernia and cardiac cases should not practice this pose. Also, pregnant women should not try this pose.

15. Dhanurasan (Bow Pose)

Procedure

i. Lie flat on your stomach, legs together and palms touching the sides of your thighs with your chin on the floor, i.e. Simple Prone Posture (See page 207).

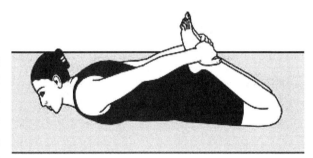

ii. Now bend your legs at knees; catch hold of the left ankle with the left hand and the right ankle with the right hand.

iii. While inhaling (Radhey), gently pull your legs up by lifting the knees above the floor, and simultaneously raise the chest and look ahead.

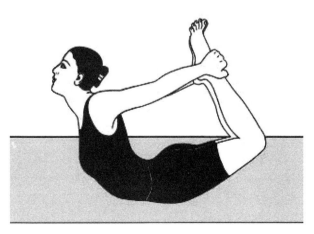

iv. Raise your head and draw it backward—without any strain.

v. Make sure your abdomen bears the body-weight.

vi. Let the knees be separated so that the

body can be raised higher and also try to arch the back as much as possible.

vii. Stay in this pose for 15-20 seconds, with normal breathing.

viii. With an exhalation (Krishna), gradually lower your legs and trunk, and return to the floor.

ix. Repeat the process twice.

x. Finally, come into either Balasan (See page 207), or Matsya Kreedasan (See page 209) and relax.

Awareness

✧ On your bodily movements and the breaths synchronized with them

✧ On the stretch of the abdominal region and the back

✧ On unbroken rememberance of "Radhey Krishna" with every breath, and feeling Their presence everywhere

Benefits

✓ Dhanurasan keeps the liver, kidneys, and abdominal organs and muscles healthy by massaging them well.

✓ It tones up the pancreas and adrenal glands to maintain the balance in their secretions.

✓ It improves the functionality of the digestive and reproductive organs.

✓ It even assists in rooting out gastrointestinal disorders, dyspepsia, chronic constipation, and the poor functioning of the liver.

✓ Many *Yog* experts believe it as a very beneficial posture for the treatment of diabetes, incontinence, colitis, menstrual disorders, and even cervical spondylitis.

✓ The spinal column is realigned properly.

✓ Besides, it alleviates urinary disorders, which are a common concern nowadays.

Contraindications

- People with a weak heart, high blood pressure, hernia, colitis, peptic or duodenal ulcers should avoid this *asan*. One should not do it before sleeping as it activates the adrenal glands and the sympathetic nervous system.

16. Shalabhasan (Locust Pose)

Procedure

i. Lie flat on your stomach, legs together and palms touching the side of your thighs with your chin on the floor, i.e. Simple Prone Posture (See page 207).

ii. Place your arms under the body as close to each other as possible, with the palms on the floor just under the thighs.

iii. Stretch the chin a bit forward and keep it held to the floor throughout the *asan*.

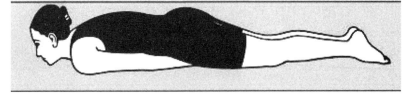

iv. Make sure your legs remain locked at the knees at all times.

v. Now while inhaling (Radhey), gradually raise both the legs together as high as possible, keeping them joined together throughout the *asan*.

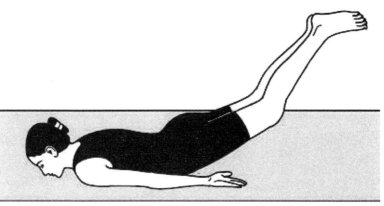

vi. Hold the pose for 15-20 seconds with normal breathing.

vii. With an exhalation (Krishna), unhurriedly lower both the legs to the floor.

viii. This is one round, try two more rounds.

ix. Eventually, come into Balasan (See page 207), or Matsya Kreedasan (See page 209) and relax for a while.

Awareness

✧ On breathing in and out along with the movements
✧ On the pressure on the lower back and abdomen
✧ On mentally chanting "Radhey Krishna" with every breath

Benefits

✓ It is extremely useful in the lessening spinal problems.
✓ It boosts the nervous system.
✓ It stimulates the digestive fire in the stomach.
✓ It helps alleviate abdominal ailments.
✓ It balances the whole digestive system.

Contraindications

- People with high blood pressure, heart maladies, hernia, ulcer, and diabetes should not do this *asan*.

17. Nakrasan (Preying Crocodile Pose)

Procedure

i. Lie flat on your stomach, legs together and palms touching the sides of your thighs with your chin on the floor, i.e. Simple Prone Posture (See page 207).

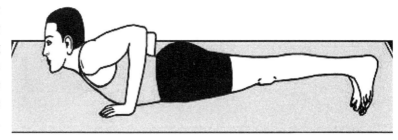

ii. Spread your feet apart with a distance of one foot between them.

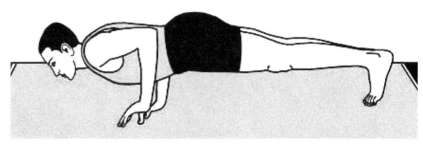

iii. Fold your arms at the elbows and rest the palms flat on the floor by the sides of the waist.

iv. Inhale (Radhey); while exhaling (Krishna), lift the whole body a few inches above the floor with the balance of the palms and the toes.

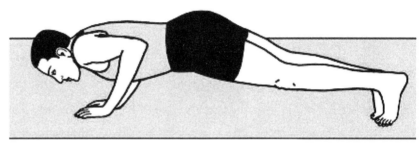

v. Trying to balance on the toes and the palms, straighten the body; lock the knees firmly and keep the body parallel to the floor.

vi. Take a few breaths and while exhaling (Krishna), plunge forward the whole body about one foot forward by quickly lifting both the hands and feet simultaneously off the floor.

vii. Again take a few breaths, and then with an exhalation (Krishna), plunge (jump) forward with force.

viii. Practice this process around 5-6 times.

ix. Reverse the movements, and with exhalations (Krishna), keep plunging (jump) back nearly one foot till you come back to the starting point.

x. Lastly, come into either Balasan (See page 207), or Matsya Kreedasan (See page 209) and rest on the floor.

Awareness

✦ On the back and forth movements and the breaths synchronized with them
✦ On the balance
✦ On the pressure on both—the hands and arms
✦ On spontaneously recalling "Radhey Krishna" along with your breathing

Benefits

✓ Nakrasan makes your wrists extremely powerful.
✓ It removes lethargy from your body and tension from the brain.
✓ It also has wonderful rejuvenating powers over the entire body, and thus makes one feel very energetic and vibrant.

Contraindications

- Persons with either weak arms or defects in the hands should not try this *asan*.

18. Purna Bhujangasan (Full Cobra Pose)

Procedure

  i. Come to the final position of Bhujangasan, steps iv-vii (See page 214).

 ii. Slowly flex your legs and lift the feet toward the head.

iii. Now straightening the hands more, stretch your head, neck, and shoulders backward.

 iv. Then, attempt to touch the crown or back part of the head with the toes or soles.

  v. Be in this position at your ease with normal breathing.

 vi. While exhaling (Krishna), come back to the starting position by gently lowering the legs, the trunk, and the head.

vii. Finally, come into either Balasan (See page 207), or Matsya Kreedasan (See page 209) and relax.

Awareness

 ✧ On the physical movements and the breaths synchronized with them
 ✧ On feeling relaxation in the spine
 ✧ On the stretch around the chest and abdominal areas
 ✧ On the presence of "Radhey Krishna" in your breaths and always recalling Their omnipresence

Benefits

 ✓ The advantages of it are similar to Bhujangasan (See page 214).

Contraindications

- Only those who are either expert in doing different *asans* or children above 12 years with flexible body should attempt it.

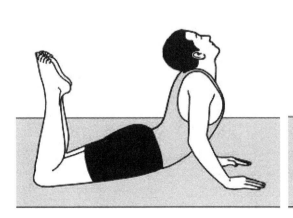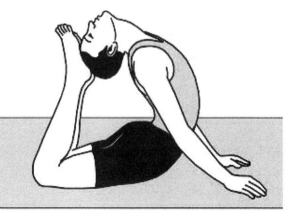

19. Purna Dhanurasan (Full Bow Pose)

Procedure

i.   Lie flat on your stomach, legs together and palms touching the side of your thighs with your chin on the floor, i.e. Simple Prone Posture (See page 207).

ii. Like in Dhanurasan (See page 221), bend your knees; firmly catch hold of the left big toe with the left hand and the right big toe with the right hand.

iii. Now inhaling (Radhey) deeply, pull up the legs by lifting the knees above the floor, and meanwhile raise the chest too.

iv. Gently lift your head, draw it backward and try to bring your legs and head toward each other—as close as possible, till the elbows face upward.

v.   Separate both knees to raise the body higher, and using the abdomen as a pivotal point (as it bears the whole body-weight in the final position), try to catch hold of the right big toe with the right fingers and left big toe with the left fingers.

vi. Remain in this pose for as long as comfortable with normal breathing.

vii. With an exhalation (Krishna), lower the legs, head, and trunk comfortably to the floor.

viii. Finally, let go of your legs, then come into Balasan (See page 207) or Matsya Kreedasan (See page 209) and relax.

For Other Details: See Dhanurasan (See page 221).

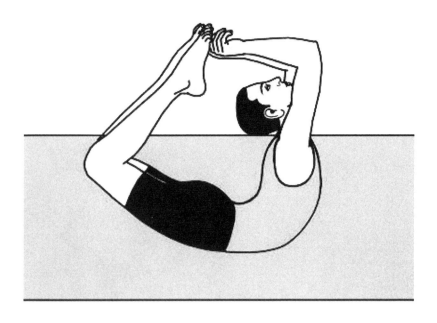

F. Supine Postures

1. Simple Supine Pose

Procedure

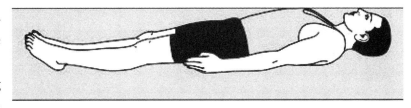

i. Lie down on your back, keeping the legs together.

ii. Now outstretching the whole body, extend your arms along the sides of the body with palms touching the thighs.

iii. Maintain the position with normal breathing.

Note: This is the initial position for all the supine postures.

2. Shavasan (Corpse Pose / Dead Man's Pose)

Procedure

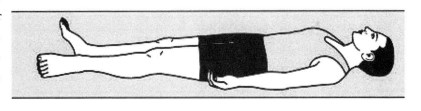

i. Lie flat on your back with both of your legs together and touch the outer sides of the thighs with your palms, i.e. Simple Supine Pose.

ii. You may place a thin pillow underneath your head.

iii. Keep a distance of about one foot between your feet and place both of your hands about six inches away from the body, with both palms facing upward.

iv. Let your fingers curl naturally like that of a corpse.

v. Now, close your eyes and also make sure that your head is not tilted any side.

vi. There should not be any tension in the muscles or feeling of discomfort in any part of your body.

vii. Stop any kind of external movement as it is very important to relax the whole body.

viii. Mentally chant (Radhey) while inhaling, and (Krishna) while exhaling.

ix. Be in this position for a minute with slow and deep breathing.

x. With every breath, be aware of every part of your body and try to relax yourself.

xi. Also, be alert to avoid sleepiness, as you may fall asleep while doing this *asan*.

Awareness

- ◇ On breathing in and out along with the movements
- ◇ On the relaxation of the whole body
- ◇ On feeling the presence of "Radhey Krishna" in your breaths

Benefits

- ✓ Shavasan is a relaxing posture to invigorate the body and mind.
- ✓ It may be practiced either before going to bed, or during, or at the end of the *yogasan* session.
- ✓ If practiced along with Subtle Body Relaxation, it helps mitigate both—physical and mental tension.
- ✓ It develops the awareness of the mind by increasing body awareness.

Note: Get into Shavasan as a final position after each Supine Pose in order to relax your body. You should avoid any external and/or internal movement during the *asan* as a small movement would disturb the whole process.

3. Ananda Balasan (Happy Baby Pose)

Procedure

i. Lie flat on your back with both your legs together and touch the outer side s of the thighs with your palms, i.e. Simple Supine Pose (See page 227).

ii. Gradually, folding your legs at the knee joints, try to touch your chest with the knees and while keeping the whole back flat on the floor, move your knees a bit sideways, to the sides of the torso.

iii. Now, bring your feet directly over the knees so that the soles of the feet face upward and catch hold of the outer sides of the feet tightly with your hands by keeping the elbows near the inside of the knees.

iv. With some adjustments, relax the back comfortably and attempt to rock a few inches from side to side.

v. Maintain this position for 30-40 seconds with normal breathing.

vi. Slowly, return to the initial position in the reverse order.

Awareness

- ◇ On realizing the Divine presence of "Radhey Krishna" around you and everwhere as you breath in and out
- ◇ On the sideward movements of the body in the final condition

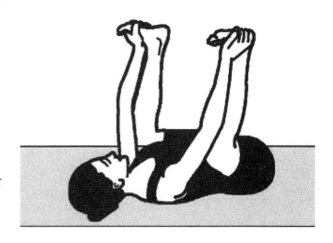

Benefits

- ✓ Ananda Balasan stretches and tones the muscles of the lower back.
- ✓ It helps those who want to sit in a cross legged position.
- ✓ It exercises your hips and gently stretches both—the groins and lower back.
- ✓ It also helps in relieving fatigue and stress from both—the body and the mind.

4. Supt Pada Utthanasan (Sleeping Legs Raised Pose)

Procedure

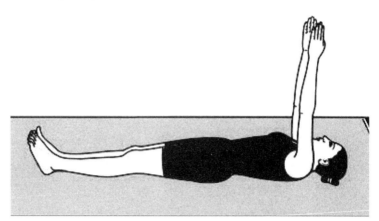

i. Lie flat on your back with both your legs together and touch the outer side s of the thighs with your palms, i.e. Simple Supine Pose (See page 227).

ii. Slowly, move your feet closer to the buttocks and keep the arms on either side of them.

iii. Comfortably, raise both of your knees closer to the chest.

iv. Keep the sacrum and lower back flat on the floor in this position.

v. Now, stretch your neck forward and tuck the chin a bit to stretch the back of the neck.

vi. Inhaling (Radhey), raise the legs and arms until they are perpendicular to the floor.

vii. Hold the posture for 15-20 seconds with normal breathing.

viii. Exhaling (Krishna), lower your knees closer to the chest, then straighten the legs on the floor, and simultaneously drop the arms on either side of the body.

ix. This ends one round; attempt up to three rounds.

x. Finally, extend your legs into Shavasan (See page 227) and relax.

Awareness

- ✧ On the breaths synchronized with different movements of your body

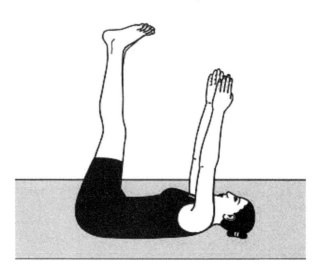

- ✧ On realizing the Divine presence of "Radhey Krishna" around you and everwhere as you breath in and out
- ✧ On the balance in the final position

Benefits

- ✓ This is immensely beneficial for the stimulation of the whole body for it helps in linking gravity and blood flow.
- ✓ As the hips are not raised above the rest of the torso, it can also be practiced by women even during menstruation.

5. Urdhwa Prasarit Padasan (Upright Extended Foot Pose)

Procedure

  i. Lie flat on your back with both your legs together and touch the outer sides of the thighs with your palms, i.e. Simple Supine Pose (See page 227).

 ii. Gently, bring your arms over the head and extend them straight.

iii. Now, with a continuous and slow inhalation (Radhey), lift the legs upward gently till they are perpendicular to the floor.

 iv. Fixing the buttocks on the floor, hold the position for 20-30 seconds with normal breathing.

  v. Again exhaling (Krishna), slowly return to the initial position by lowering the legs to the floor.

 vi. This ends one round; perform up to three rounds.

vii. Ultimately, come to Shavasan (See page 227) and relax.

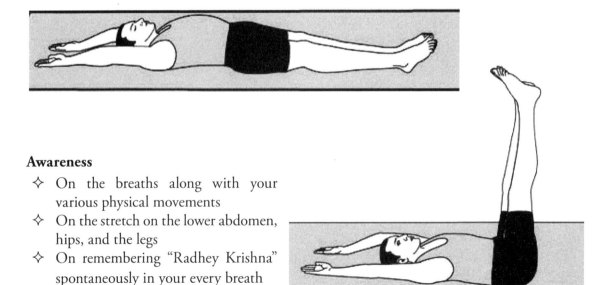

Awareness

- ✧ On the breaths along with your various physical movements
- ✧ On the stretch on the lower abdomen, hips, and the legs
- ✧ On remembering "Radhey Krishna" spontaneously in your every breath

Benefits

✓ Urdhwa Prasarit Padasan provides an excellent exercise for reducing fat around the abdomen.

✓ It firms the lumbar region of the back.

✓ As it exercises the abdominal organs, it relieves one from flatulence and gastric troubles.

6. Padangushth Nasasparshasan (Touching the Nose with the Big Toes)

Procedure

i. Lie flat on your back with both legs together and touch the outer sides of the thighs with your palms, i.e. Simple Supine Pose (See page 227).

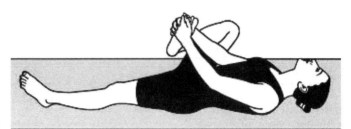

ii. Inhaling (Radhey), gently fold your right leg and hold your right foot by interlocking the fingers of your both hands together.

iii. Now exhaling (Krishna), lift your head slightly upward and pull your right foot toward your head.

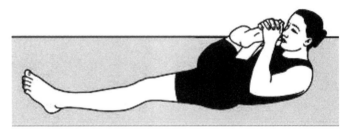

iv. Attempt to touch your nose tip with the right big toe.

v. Make sure that your left leg remains well stretched in this state.

vi. Be in the final position for 15-20 seconds with normal breathing.

vii. In the same manner, repeat the *asan* with the other leg.

Variation – 1

i. Lie flat on your back with both legs together and touch the outer sides of the thighs with your palms, i.e. Simple Supine Pose (See page 227).

ii. Gradually fold your knees, and bring your heels close to your buttocks.

iii. Inhaling (Radhey), gently lift your knees and draw them closer to your chest.

iv. Try to form Namaste Mudra with your legs, by joining the soles against each other.

v. Now slowly bend your arms and adjusting the elbows in the space created between either of the inner-thighs and calves, grasp your soles firmly.

vi. Make sure that both the elbows stay rooted in the corresponding inner-thighs.

vii. Exhaling (Krishna), gradually lift your head a bit and attempt to touch your big toes with

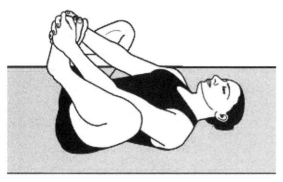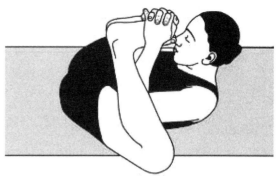

your nose tip.

viii. Be in the final position for 15-20 seconds with normal breathing.

ix. Continuing to exhale (Krishna), release your both feet from the hands by reversing the procedure unhurriedly.

x. Repeat the *asan*, once more, in the similar manner.

Awareness

✧ On the movements synchronized with your breaths

✧ On the compression around abdominal area

✧ On the pressure in the thighs and the arms

✧ On always chanting the Sacred Names "Radhey Krishna" with your each breath, and recalling Them all the time

Benefits

✓ Padangushth Nasasparshasan is very effectual for correcting the problems related with navel.

✓ As it massages the abdominal organs, it is very effectual in the alleviation of flatulence, stomach pain, constipation, weakness, and lethargy.

✓ It also increases digestive fire as it exercises the abdominal portion superbly.

Contraindications

- Those who have undergone a recent abdominal operation should not practice this *asan*.

7. Supt Pawan Muktasan (Leg Locked Air Releasing Pose)

Procedure

i. Lie flat on your back with both your legs together and touch the outer sides of the thighs with your palms, i.e. Simple Supine Pose (See page 227).

ii. Gently bend your right leg and bring the right knee over your abdomen.

iii. Interlock the fingers and place them around the right shin, closer to the knee.

iv. Inhale (Radhey); while exhaling (Krishna), pull the knee to the chest; raise your head and shoulders and try to touch the right knee with your nose.

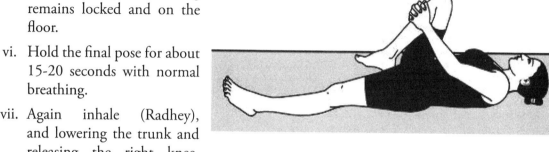

v. Make sure your left leg remains locked and on the floor.

vi. Hold the final pose for about 15-20 seconds with normal breathing.

vii. Again inhale (Radhey), and lowering the trunk and releasing the right knee, return back to the starting position.

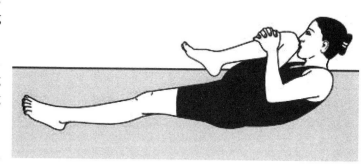

viii. Practice it up to three times, and then come to the starting position again by releasing the right leg.

ix. Repeat the same process up to three times with the other leg.

x. Finally, come to Shavasan (See page 227) and relax.

Variation - 1

i. Lie flat on your back with both your legs together and touch the outer sides of the thighs with your palms, i.e. Simple Supine Pose (See page 227).

ii. Comfortably bend both knees and bring them over the abdomen.

iii. Interlock your fingers and keep them around both the shins, just below the knees.

iv. First inhale (Radhey) deeply, and with a slow exhalation (Krishna), slowly pull both the knees toward the chest.

v. Simultaneously, lift the head and shoulders upward, and attempt to keep the nose between the two knees.

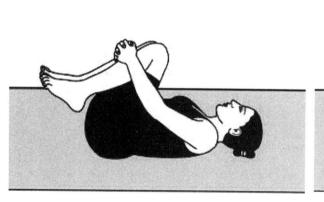 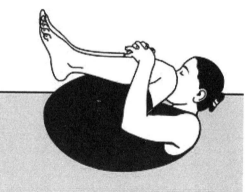

233

vi. Remain in this pose for about 15-20 seconds with normal breathing.

vii. As you return to the centre, inhale (Radhey) and lowering the trunk and head gradually to the floor, release the knees.

viii. Do this process for three times.

ix. Lastly, come to Shavasan (See page 227) and relax.

Awareness
- ✧ On your bodily movements along with the breaths synchronized with them
- ✧ On the pressure on your abdomen
- ✧ On the Holy Names "Radhey Krishna" flowing with your breaths

Benefits
- ✓ Supt Pawan Muktasan is a very invigorating pose as it strengthens your lower back muscles and makes the spinal vertebrae flexible.
- ✓ The main purpose of this pose is to remove gas and constipation, by massaging the abdomen and digestive organs.
- ✓ It is very effectual in rooting out impotence, sterility, and menstrual problems for it also massages the pelvic muscles and reproductive organs.

Contraindications
- - Persons with high blood pressure and acute back cases like sciatica and slipped-disc should avoid it.

8. Supt Udarakarshanasan (Sleeping Abdominal Stretch Pose)

Procedure

i. Lie flat on your back with both your legs together and touch the outer sides of the thighs with your palms, i.e. Simple Supine Pose (See page 227).

ii. Spread your arms sidways at shoulder level, with the palms facing downward.

iii. Flex your legs at the knees and move the feet toward the buttocks, with both the soles on the floor and the heels nearly touching the buttocks.

iv. Make sure your knees and feet stay together throughout.

v. Now inhale (Radhey); exhaling (Krishna), twist rest of the body rightward, keeping the chest still, ensuring the right side of the leg touches the floor.

vi. Ensure your legs stay together and the arms stretched out throughout.

vii. Also, turn the head in the direction opposite (left side) to the legs'

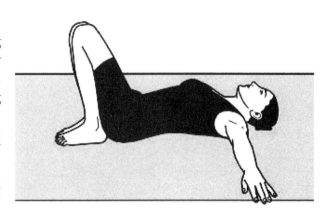

direction and look at the left hand.

viii. Remain in this state for 15-20 seconds with normal breathing.

ix. Now, inhale (Radhey) and return back to the centre.

x. Likewise, perform the pose on the other side.

xi. Practice three times in either direction.

xii. Finally, come into Shavasan (See page 227) and relax.

Awareness

◇ On the breaths synchronized with the movements
◇ On the stretch of both—para-spinal and abdominal muscles
◇ On feeling relaxation in both—para-spinal and abdominal muscles
◇ On the Divine Names "Radhey Krishna" flowing with each inhalation and exhalation

Benefits

✓ By Supt Udarakarshanasan, the abdominal muscles and organs are perfectly stretched, which results in the improvement of digestion and the removal of constipation.
✓ Also, it is an all-curing therapy for those suffering from strain and stiffness of the back as it stretches the spinal muscles and gently twists the vertebral joints.
✓ It tones up the legs.
✓ It assists in slimming the waist and hip portion, which also results in weight loss.

9. Shav Udarkarshanasan (Universal Spinal Twist)

Procedure

i. Lie flat on your back with both your legs together and touch the outer sides of the thighs with your palms, i.e. Simple Supine Pose (See page 227).

ii. Spread your arms sideways, keeping them at the shoulder level with the palms facing downward.

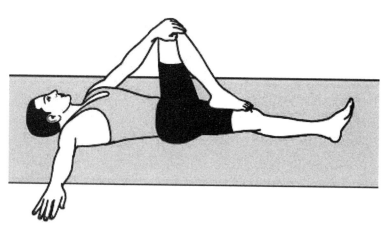

iii. Fold your right leg at the knee; gently place the right sole on top of the left thigh and catch hold of the right knee with the left hand.

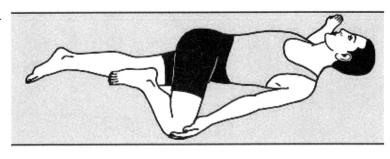

iv. Now inhale (Radhey); while exhaling (Krishna), slowly pull your right knee to the left side and try to touch the floor on the left side with the right knee.

v. Now turn your head to the right and look at the right hand.

vi. In this pose, the arms should remain locked and straight, and the left leg should not be bent at the knee.

vii. Hold this pose for 15-20 seconds with normal breathing.

viii. Again, inhale (Radhey) and returnal back to the central position.

ix. Do it thrice in the same way and then straighten the right leg.

x. Likewise, practice on the other side.

xi. Ultimately, come to Shavasan (See page 227) and relax.

Awareness
✧ On breathing in and out along with the movements
✧ On the stretch of the back
✧ On mentally chanting the Sacred Names "Radhey Krishna" with your every breath and trying to realize the omnipresence of Them all the time

Benefits
✓ Shav Udarkarshanasan relieves body ache.
✓ It strengthens the digestion system and also releases *prāṇic* energy.

Contraindications
- Persons with any disorders of the hip joints and sciatica are advised to avoid this pose.

10. Spinal Rocking

Procedure
i. Lie flat on your back with both of your legs together and touch the outer sides of the thighs with your palms, i.e. Simple Supine Pose (See page 227).

ii. Gradually, draw both feet toward the buttocks, folding both of your legs at the knees.

iii. Now lifting the feet slightly, insert your arms between the legs so that you can grasp both the feet around the ankle portion.

iv. Also, raise your head upward and the upper back a bit forward to maintain the position of a rocking chair.

v. First inhale (Radhey); while exhaling (Krishna), slowly rock forward, shifting the weight from the mid-back to the lower back.

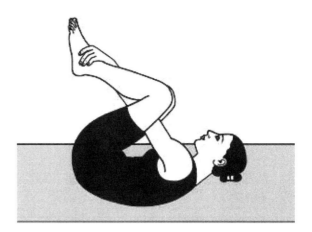

vi. While inhaling (Radhey), rock backward shifting the weight from lower back to mid-back in the reverse order, like the to and fro motion of a rocking chair or a pendulum clock.

vii. Some of the portions of the spine will act like the curved base of a rocking chair as they are in constant contact with the floor.

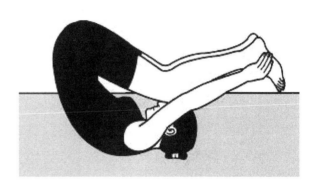

viii. With smooth and gentle motion, repeat the pose for 10-20 times.

ix. Lastly, come into Shavasan (See page 227) and relax.

Awareness

✧ On your breaths synchronized with different physical movements
✧ On the rocking movements in the final position
✧ On the mental chanting of the Revered Names "Radhey Krishna" in your breaths and always trying to realize Them everywhere

Benefits

✓ This swinging exercise stretches and strengthens the muscles of the lower back by giving an excellent massage to them.
✓ It facilitates sitting in the cross-legged pose.
✓ It massages all the vertebrae around the neck and spinal area.
✓ It aids in overcoming lethargy, drowsiness, and stiffness that people often feel on waking up in the morning time.
✓ It also relaxes the entire nervous system, thus helps in establishing a wonderful link between the central nervous system and the rest of the body.

11. Jhulan Lurhakan Asan (Rocking and Rolling)

Procedure

i. Lie flat on your back with both your legs together and touch the outer sides of the thighs with your palms, i.e. Simple Supine Pose (See page 227).

ii. Gently fold both the legs at the knees and bring them over your abdomen.

iii. Now, interlock your fingers and place them around both the shins, exactly below the knees.

iv. Also bring your chin closer to the knees and start rocking forward and backward as long as possible.

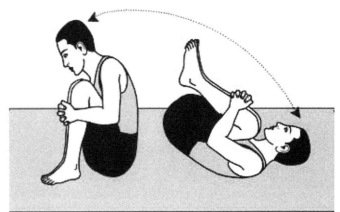

v. While rocking forward, come up to squat (keeping legs joined) on your feet, and then rock backward so that each part of the spine touches the floor.

vi. Repeat this process for 5-10 rounds and return to the central position.

vii. Now, start rolling sideways, taking the support of your elbows.

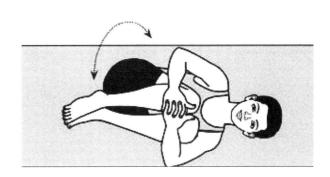

viii. Try to maintain the position of your chin, touching the knees at all times.

ix. Roll for 5-10 rounds actively.

x. Finally, come into Shavasan (See page 227) so that you can relax.

Awareness

✧ On co-ordinating the rocking and rolling movements
✧ On the effect on the back and the buttocks
✧ On the mental chanting of the Revered Names "Radhey Krishna" along with breathing and always trying to realize Them everywhere

Benefits

✓ Due to the movements in the back portion of the body, there is adequate massage on your back, hips, and buttocks.
✓ It removes unnecessary fat from the waist area.
✓ It produces invigorating feeling in the morning after a brisk walk.

Contraindications

- Persons who have severe back problems and/or have undergone abdominal surgery should avoid it. Also, women at second or third trimester of pregnancy best omit it from their *Yogic* exercise.

12. Uttan Padasan (Stretching Out the Legs with the Face Upward)

Procedure

i. Lie flat on your back with both your legs together and touch the outer sides of the thighs with your palms, i.e. Simple Supine Pose (See page 227).

ii. Now bending your arms at the elbows, place your palms on either side of the ears in such a way that your fingers point toward the shoulders and elbows point upward.

iii. As you inhale (Radhey), lift the back off the floor with the support of the arms; also try to form an arch by stretching the neck and dropping the head backward till the crown rests on the floor.

iv. Then, stretch the neck and draw the head backward by raising the chest.

v. Exhale (Krishna); while stretching the back; again inhale (Radhey).

vi. Now, raise both the legs to form a 45-50 degrees angle with the floor.

vii. Lift the arms, making them parallel to the raised legs; make Namaste Mudra by joining the palms.

viii. Ensure your legs and arms remain outstretched and joined together in the final state.

ix. Balancing on the buttocks and the crown, hold the position for as long as you are comfortable with normal breathing.

x. Following the steps in the reverse order, come back to the centre.

xi. This finishes one round; repeat twice in the same way.

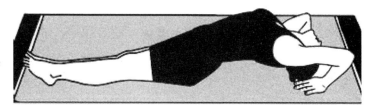

xii. Finally, come into Shavasan (See page 227) and relax.

Awareness

✧ On the breaths flowing in and out synchronized with the different physical movements

✧ On the stretch of the chest and lumbar region

✧ On the tension on the neck

✧ On the balance

✧ On always feeling the presence of "Radhey Krishna" in your breaths

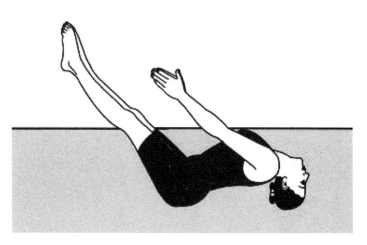

Benefits

✓ The main purpose of this pose is to expand the chest fully and give adequate elasticity to the dorsal portion of the spine.

✓ The abdominal muscles are well exercised by stretching and activizing them; hence it is very beneficial in improving digestion, alleviating constipation, and controlling diabetes.

✓ Particularly it tones up the neck and back, and thus helps regulate the activity of the thyroids with copious supply of oxygenated blood.

✓ Not only wonderful for belly reduction, but it also assists in the working of the inner organs like the intestines, pancreas, and liver.

Contraindications

- Persons suffering from a spinal injury should best omit this pose. Also those with high blood pressure should perform it only under the supervision and counsel of a *Yog* expert.

13. Jathara Parivartanasan (Belly Turning Round Pose)

Procedure

i. Lie flat on your back with both your legs together and touch the outer sides of the thighs with your palms, i.e. Simple Supine Pose (See page 227).

ii. Extend your arms sideways in a single line with the shoulders as if your body is like a cross. Also make sure they remain locked throughout.

iii. While inhaling (Radhey), raise the legs together till they are perpendicular to the floor.

iv. Ensure your legs remain locked and joined toghether.

v. While exhaling (Krishna), move your legs leftward and down to the floor till the left toes rest on the extended left hand.

vi. Try to keep the lumbar region of the back comfortably on the floor, trying to turn the legs only from the hips.

vii. Now staying in this position, slightly twist the abdomen to the right, to increase the pressure.

viii. Stay in this posture for 15-20 seconds with normal breathing.

ix. While inhaling (Radhey), bring the legs to the centre.

x. Repeat the procedure on the right side.

xi. This ends one round; repeat it twice.

xii. Lastly, lower your legs down to the floor and relax fully in Shavasan (See page 227).

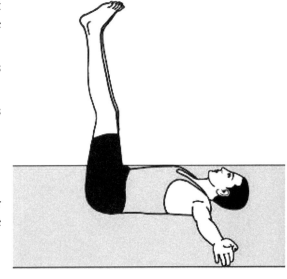

Awareness

✧ On different bodily movements synchronized with your breaths
✧ On the pressure around the abdominal area
✧ On the stretch in the legs
✧ On always recalling "Radhey Krishna" with each inhalation and exhalation

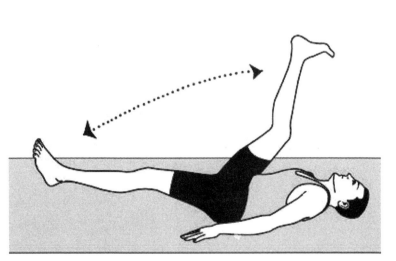

Benefits

✓ This Pose is extremely beneficial for decreasing unnecessary fat.
✓ It aids in firming and rooting out poor functioning of the liver, spleen, and pancreas.
✓ It is helpful in the treatment of gastritis and exercising the intestines.
✓ It relieves sprains and catches in the lower back and the hip regions, and also realigns and stretches the spine.
✓ It brings flexibility and elasticity to the spine.
✓ It improves digestion.

Contraindications

- Those with high blood pressure, suffering from the heart ailments, and recent or chronic injury to the knees, hips, or back should not do this *asan*.

14. Pada Kainchi (Legs' Scissoring)

Procedure

i. Lie flat on your back with both your legs together and touch the outer sides of the thighs with your palms, i.e. Simple Supine Pose (See page 227).

ii. Straighten your arms and place the hands by the side of the thighs, with the palms flat on the floor.

iii. Keep a slight distance between the two feet to facilitate their smooth raising.

iv. Make sure your head, trunk, and hands lie flat on the floor throughout the practice.

v. Now inhale (Radhey); while exhaling (Krishna), lift your left leg upward—as high as possible, keeping it either straight, or slightly bent in case of difficulty.

vi. With a quick inhalation (Radhey), lower it down to the floor, and simultaneously with an exhalation (Krishna), raise the right leg upward—as high as possible.

vii. Ensure both the feet are lowered and/or raised in a perfect rhythm, i.e. to the degree one leg is raised, the other is lowered.

viii. Repeat the process for around 20-30 times.

ix. Finally, get into Shavasan (See page 227) and relax.

Awareness
- ✧ On your each breath synchronized with the movements of the legs
- ✧ On the pressure in the abdomen, hips, thighs, and lower back
- ✧ On the breaths flowing in and out and mental chanting of "Radhey Krishna" along with each breath

Benefits
- ✓ Pada Sanchalanasan strengthens the abdominal and back muscles.
- ✓ It also helps reduce obesity.
- ✓ It helps remove constipation and acidity—thus stimulates the digestive fire in the stomach.

Contraindications
- - Those with a recent history of an abdominal operation, or back problems should not do this with both legs together.
- - As it creates tremendous pressure in the stomach, it should not be practiced by the patients with the heart ailments and blood pressure.
- - Also, women at second or third trimester of pregnancy should not attempt this pose.

15. Utthan Padasan (Lifted Legs Pose)

Procedure

i. Lie flat on your back with both your legs together and touch the outer sides of the thighs with your palms, i.e. Simple Supine Pose (See page 227).

ii. Place your hands by the sides of the body on the floor.

iii. Now inhale (Radhey) and slowly raise both legs to 30 degrees, keeping the knees locked.

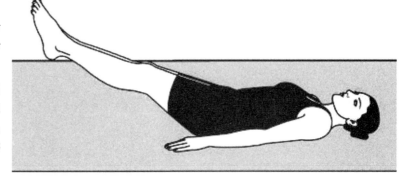

iv. Remain in this position for 10-15 seconds, with normal breathing.

v. With a slow exhalation (Krishna), return back to the base position by lowering the legs gently.

vi. This is one round; repeat the *asan* for up to three times.

vii. Ultimately, come into Shavasan (See page 227) and relax.

Awareness

✧ On the breaths along with the movement of your legs
✧ On the stretch of the legs
✧ On pressurizing the abdomen
✧ On mentally uttering "Radhey Krishna" while breathing

Benefits

✓ As in Naukasan, Utthan Padasan strengthens the abdominal muscles and the back.
✓ It stimulates digestive fire in the stomach, which is necessary for a sound health.

Contraindications

- People with high blood pressure, heart problems, hernia, and peptic ulcer should not attempt this pose.
- Also, women at the stage of pregnancy (second or third trimester) and menstrual period best omit this pose.

16. Naukasan (Boat Pose)

Procedure

i. Lie flat on your back with both your legs together and touch the outer sides of the thighs with your palms, i.e. Simple Supine Pose (See page 227).

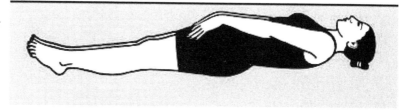

ii. Keep your toes together and place the palms lightly on the thighs.

iii. While inhaling (Radhey), slowly raise your legs, arms, trunk, and head off the floor.

iv. Without any strain, balance your body on

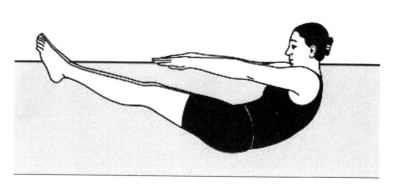

the buttocks and fix the eyes on the toes.

v. In the final position, ensure that your head, hands, and toes stay at the same level, with both the legs and arms locked.

vi. Remain in this pose for 15-20 seconds with normal breathing.

vii. While exhaling (Krishna), slowly return to the base position by lowering the head, body, and legs to the floor and the hands on the thighs.

viii. Repeat this *asan* twice.

ix. Lastly, come to Shavasan (See page 227) and relax.

Awareness

✧ On the breaths synchronized with the movements
✧ On the stretch and pressure around the abdomen
✧ On realizing the presence of "Radhey Krishna" everywhere and always watching you

Benefits

✓ Naukasan is very useful for women for it helps correct various menstrual problems.
✓ As it helps reduce unwanted fat from the abdominal area, it keeps one slim and healthy.
✓ Mainly, it massages and tones up the internal organs like the intestines, pancreas, stomach, etc.
✓ It supplies extra oxygen to the lungs and heart—thus plays a vital role in making one healthier.

17. Pada Sanchalanasan (Cycling)

Procedure

i. Lie flat on your back with both your legs together and touch the outer sides of the thighs with your palms, i.e. Simple Supine Pose (See page 227).

ii. Straighten your arms and place them by the sides of the body, with the palms flat on the floor.

iii. Slowly fold the legs and raising the them into the air, begin cycling, making perfect vertical circles with both the feet—one by one.

iv. Inhale (Radhey) when you straighten the leg; exhale (Krishna) when you flex the knee and bring your thigh closer to the chest.

v. Repeat 20 times clockwise and counterclockwise.

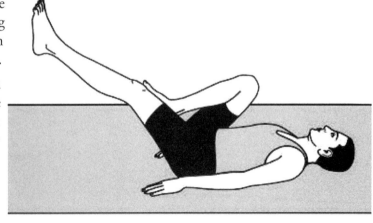

vi. Finally, come to Shavasan (See page 227) and relax.

Variation - 1

i. Lie flat on your back with both your legs together and touch the outer sides of the thighs with your palms, i.e. Simple Supine Pose (See page 227).

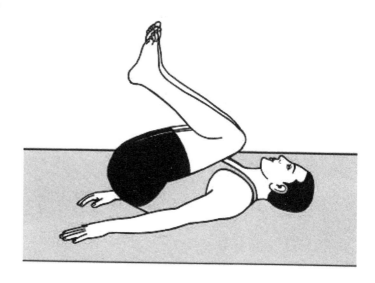

ii. Straighten your arms and place them by the sides of the body and the palms flat on the floor.

iii. Make sure that the legs remain joined together and the head on the floor throughout.

iv. Raising both the legs in the air, slowly bend them; now begin cycling, making perfect vertical circles.

v. Inhale (Radhey) when the legs are straight; exhale (Krishna) when the legs are bent toward the chest.

vi. Repeat 10 times clockwise and counterclockwise.

vii. Finally, come to Shavasan (See page 227) and relax.

For Other Details: See Pada Kainchi (See page 241).

18. Pada Vrittasan (Leg Rotation)

Procedure

i. Lie flat on your back with both your legs together and touch the outer sides of the thighs with your palms, i.e. Simple Supine Pose (See page 227).

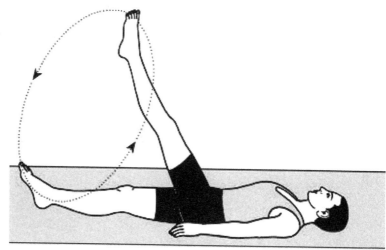

ii. Keep your palms flat on the floor on either side of the body.

iii. Gently, raise the right

245

leg and rotate it sideways as if you are creating several vertica circles in the air.

iv. Make sure the other leg remains straight throughout the *asan*.

v. Inhale (Radhey) during the lower half circle and exhale (Krishna) during the upper half circle.

vi. Repeat 10 times in either direction—clockwise and counterclockwise.

vii. Then comfortably, lower the leg down to the floor.

viii. Now, repeat the same method with the left leg and rotate 10 times in either direction.

ix. Lastly, come into Shavasan (See page 227) and relax.

Variation - 1

i. Lie flat on your back with both your legs together and touch the outer side of the thighs with your palms, i.e. Simple Supine Pose (See page 227).

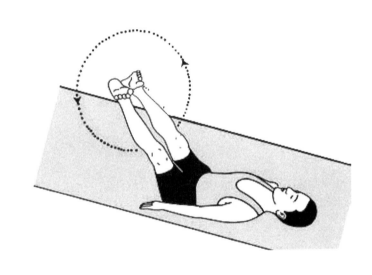

ii. Keep your palms flat on the floor on either side of the body.

iii. Gradually, raise both the legs and rotate them sideways as if you are creating several vertical circles in the air.

iv. Inhale (Radhey) during the lower half circle; exhale (Krishna) during the upper half circle.

v. While bringing the legs upward, do not raise the back.

vi. Make sure the legs remain locked at the knees throughout the practice.

vii. Repeat 10 times in either direction—clockwise and counterclockwise.

Awareness

✧ On the rotation of the legs synchronized with breathing in and out
✧ On the effects on the hips and abdomen
✧ On chanting the Sacred Names "Radhey Krishna" with your each breath

Benefits

✓ Pada Vrittasan is quite useful for developing flexibility of the hip joints.
✓ It makes the body slim by reducing fat.
✓ It also gives exercise to the abdominal, spinal, and thigh muscles.
✓ It is highly effectual for sciatic patients.

Contraindications

- Patients with high blood pressure, heart ailments, peptic ulcer, and abdominal surgery should not try it.
- Also, females at second and third trimesters of pregnancy, and those passing through a menstrual period should also avoid this pose.

19. Poorva Halasan (Preliminary Plough Pose)

Procedure

i. Lie flat on your back with both your legs together and touch the outer sides of the thighs with your palms, i.e. Simple Supine Pose (See page 227).

ii. Now, bring your arms close to the body with the palms facing downward; keep them just under the buttocks.

iii. With a continuous inhalation (Radhey), slowly raise the legs upward until they become perpendicular to the floor.

iv. Make sure your buttocks lie on the floor in this state.

v. Now with a slow exhalation (Krishna), lower your legs toward the head till they make an angle of 45 degrees with the upper body.

vi. Make sure your legs remain locked and stable in this state.

vii. Attempt to maintain a proper balance with the support of the back on the floor.

viii. Stay in this position at your ease with normal breathing.

ix. Come into the supine position by reversing the process.

x. Finally, come into Shavasan (See page 227) and relax.

Awareness

✧ On the breaths synchronized with the various physical movements
✧ On the stretch of your back
✧ On always realizing the sentient forms of "Radhey Krishna" everywhere

Benefits

✓ Poorva Halasan, an invigorating posture, exercises the pelvis by stretching it properly.
✓ It regulates the function of the kidneys superbly.
✓ It stimulates both the intestines.
✓ It even helps slimming down the body by reducing the unnecessary weight.

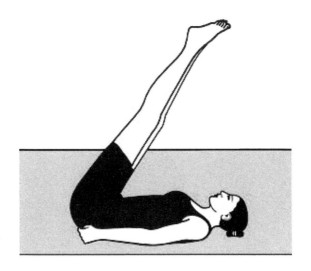

Contraindications

- Those who are either old, or suffering from sciatica and slipped-disc should avoid this *asan.*

20. Anantasan (Lord Vishnu's Pose / Vishnu's Serpent Pose)

Procedure

i. Lie flat on your back with both your legs together and touch the outer sides of the thighs with your palms, i.e. Simple Supine Pose (See page 227).

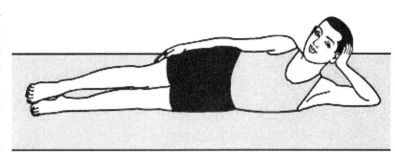

ii. Now flip onto the left in such a way that your left side of the body rests completely on the floor and the right leg rests precisely over the inner left leg.

iii. Then fold your left arm, with the left elbow as a support on the floor, and comfortably raise the upper torso and head.

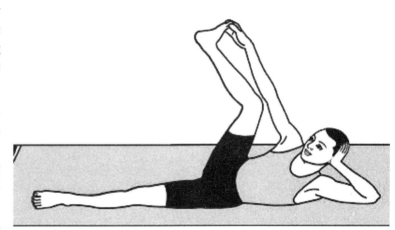

iv. Now rest your head—just above the ear—on the left palm.

v. Make sure your right arm stays along the outer side of the right thigh in this state.

vi. Then, flex the right leg at the knee and catch hold of the right big toe with your right hand.

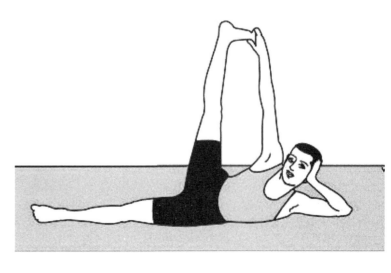

vii. Inhale (Radhey); with an exhalation (Krishna), outstretch both—the

248

right arm and right leg—vertically.

viii. Ensure both—the right arm and right leg—remain locked in the final position.

ix. Be in this pose for as long as you are comfortable, with normal breathing.

x. While coming back to the centre, gently bend your right knee, and lower it by letting it go of from the right hand.

xi. Perform the *asan* on the other side with the alternate combination of the legs and arms.

xii. Ultimately, come into Shavasan (See page 227) and relax for some time.

Awareness

✧ On breathing along with various physical movements
✧ On the stretch in the hips and the lifted leg
✧ On the bodily balance
✧ On always realizing the omnipresence of "Radhey Krishna"

Benefits

✓ Anantasan tones up the pelvic region and tones the hamstring, inner thighs, and abdominal muscles.
✓ Those who are suffering from backaches are given natural relief.
✓ It also decreases weight from the hips and thighs.
✓ It improves balancing capability.
✓ It excercises the hamstrings and calves by stretching, thus helps in blood circulation.
✓ It even heals any sort of muscle pull.
✓ It prevents the growth of hernia.

Contraindications

- Those who have slipped-disc, sciatica, and cervical spondylitis should not perform this *asan*.

21. Halasan (Plough Pose)

Procedure

i. Lie flat on your back with both your legs together and touch the outer sides of the thighs with your palms, i.e. Simple Supine Pose (See page 227).

ii. Place both arms by the sides of the thighs with the palms flat on the floor.

iii. While inhaling (Radhey), raise your legs till they come into a vertical position.

iv. While exhaling (Krishna), slowly raise the buttocks, letting the legs go over the head, and then lower the toes to the

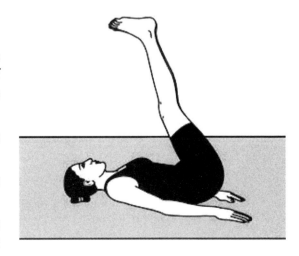

floor—a bit away from your head.

v. Either interlock the fingers or keep the palms on the floor, behind your shoulders and facing downward.

vi. Straighten your arms firmly for support; straighten the legs and try to push the buttocks as much forward as possible.

vii. Remain in this posture for as long as you are comfortable with normal breathing.

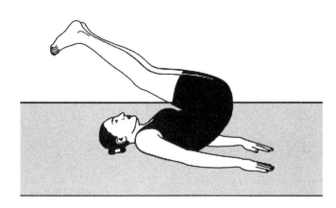

viii. While returning to the central position, again inhale (Radhey); then slowly lower the buttocks to the floor, bringing the legs to vertical position; while exhaling (Krishna), lower the legs down to the floor.

ix. This finishes one round; do two more rounds.

x. Finally, come into Shavasan (See page 227) and relax.

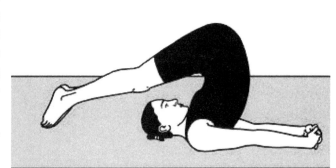

Awareness

✧ On breathing in and out along with the different movements
✧ On the pressure in your abdomen
✧ On relaxing the muscles
✧ On mentally chanting the Holy Names "Radhey Krishna" with your each breath

Benefits

✓ The movement of the diaphragm in Halasan massages all the abdominal and chest organs, activates digestion, increases insulin production in the pancreas, and also improves the function of both—the liver and kidneys.

✓ A healthy and flexible spine indicates a healthy nervous system. If the nerves are healthy, a person is comfortable both—physically and mentally. Therefore, along with strengthening the abdominal muscles, it tones the spinal nerves.

✓ It is found to regulate the activities of the thyroid gland, which balances the body's metabolic rate and stimulates the thymus gland—thus helping to increase immunity in the body.

✓ It also helps increase height.

Contraindications

- Persons with high blood pressure, hernia, arthritis of the neck, spinal problems like cervical spondylitis, and slipped-disc should not do this *asan*.

22. Karnapidasan (Ear Pressure Pose)

Procedure

i.   Follow the steps i-v progressively as mentioned in Halasan.

ii. Then, inhale (Radhey) slowly; exhaling (Krishna), comfortably fold your legs and rest the knees by the sides of the ears.

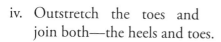
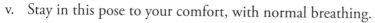

iii. Ensure both the knees rest on the floor.

iv. Outstretch the toes and join both—the heels and toes.

v.   Stay in this pose to your comfort, with normal breathing.

vi. Come back to Halasan, and then to the starting position by reversing the order.

vii. This ends one round; try this for two more rounds.

viii. Ultimately, come to Shavasan (See page 227) and relax.

Awareness

✧ On inhalations and exhalations along with the different movements of your body
✧ On the pressure on your abdomen
✧ On relaxing the muscles
✧ On the mental chanting of the Divine Names "Radhey Krishna" with your each breath and feeling the Their omnipresence

Benefits

✓ It has the same benefits as those of Halasan.
✓ Besides, it helps in curing ear problems like pain in the ear, tinnitus (ringing in the ear), transient deafness, etc.
✓ It assists in curbing obesity and increasing height of the growing ones, as in Halasan (See page 249).

Contraindications

- Persons with high blood pressure, hernia, arthritis of the neck, spinal problems like cervical spondylitis, and slipped-disc should not do this *asan*.

23. Gatishil Pashchimottanasan (Dynamic Back Stretch Pose)

Procedure

i. Lie flat on your back with both your legs together and touch the outer sides of the thighs with your palms, i.e. Simple Supine Pose (See page 227).

ii. Slowly raise your arms just over the head and keep them on the floor with the palms facing upward.

iii. Relax the whole body in this position and inhale (Radhey).

iv. Now exhaling (Krishna), lift your trunk to the sitting pose, straightening both—the hands above your head and the spine.

v. Continuing to exhale (Krishna), bend forward into Pashchimottanasan (See page 169) without a pause; do not make any hasty movements.

vi. Stay in this posture for a few seconds with normal breathing.

vii. As you inhale (Radhey), again return to the sitting position without folding the arms and slowly recline backward until returning to the initial state.

viii. This completes one round; try 5-10 rounds following the same process.

ix. Finally, come into Shavasan (See page 227) and relax.

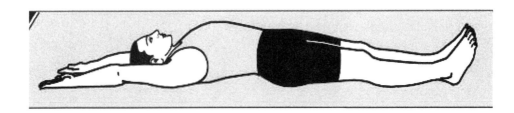

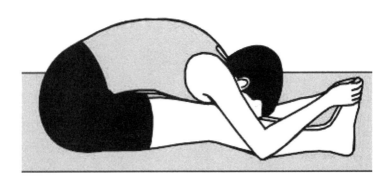

Awareness

✧ On the various bodily movements and breaths synchronized with them

✧ On the stretch of the back, lumbar region, and hamstrings

✧ On always recalling the sentient forms of "Radhey Krishna" flowing through your inhalations and exhalations

Benefits

✓ The advantages of Gatishil Pashchimottanasan are similar to that of Pashchimottanasan (See page 169). However, this is more dynamic as it naturally speeds up the blood circulation and metabolic processes throughout the body.

✓ It makes the body exceedingly flexible, strengthens the spine, and also supplies the body with both—physical and *prāṇic* energy.

✓ It massages all the visceral organs.

✓ It tones up both—the stomach and waist.

Contraindications

- People with slipped-disc, sciatica, and hernia should not practice this *asan*.

24. Stambhan Asan (Posture of Retention)

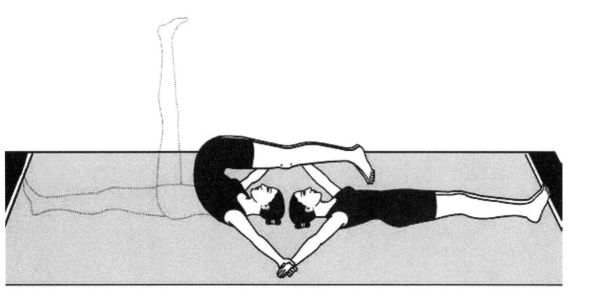

Procedure

i. For this posture, two people of similar height and size should lie in Simple Supine Posture (See page 227) with their crowns touching each other.

ii. Their bodies should be in a single line.

iii. Now, extend the arms sideways up, at the shoulder level, and catch hold of one another's hands firmly.

iv. Make sure the arms remain straight, touching the floor at all times.

v. Slowly inhaling (Radhey), the first person should raise the legs together without folding them until they gain vertical position.

vi. Now with an exhalation (Krishna), the same person raises the buttocks and again pushes them backward over the head, lowering the legs until they are exactly over the other person's navel.

vii. Stay in this pose for five seconds with normal breathing.

viii. Then, come back to the centre by reversing the process.

ix. In the same manner, the second person will perform the method.

x. This completes one round; repeat for 5-10 rounds in the same way.

xi. Finally, come to Shavasan (See page 227) and relax.

Awareness
- On the breaths synchronized with the downward, upward, and backward movements
- On always feeling relaxation in the stretched and contracted parts
- On the other person and the abdomen
- On feeling the presence of "Radhey Krishna" and psychic uttering of the Divine Names

Benefits
- ✓ Like Dynamic Plough Pose, Stambhan Asan also exercises the abdominal organs that helps remove constipation and flatulence.
- ✓ It brings a sense of physical and mental equipoise for it requires a great alertness while raising the legs vertically up and then lowering them over to the other person's navel.

25. Kandharasan (Shoulder Pose)

Procedure

i. Lie flat on your back with both your legs together and touch the outer sides of the thighs with your palms, i.e. Simple Supine Pose (See page 227).

ii. Gently fold your legs and place your heels near the buttocks.

iii. Now, grasp the ankles properly.

iv. Then, inhale (Radhey) and raise your back, abdomen, and buttocks.

v. Make sure the chest and navel are lifted as high as possible by pushing the chest up—toward the chin.

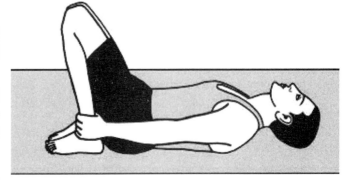

vi. Ensure the head, shoulders,

arms, and the soles of the feet remain on the floor.

vii. Stay in the final pose for 15-20 seconds with normal breathing.

viii. Exhaling (Krishna), come back to the floor by lowering the back, abdomen, and buttocks carefully.

ix. This finishes one round; try this pose for two more rounds.

x. Finally, come into Shavasan (See page 227) and relax.

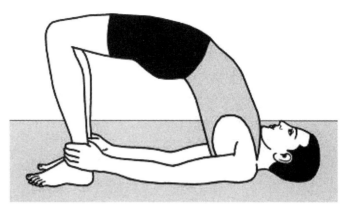

Awareness

✧ On the bodily movements and breaths synchronized with them
✧ On the pressure around your abdominal region, thyroid gland, and the back
✧ On spontaneously uttering the Holy Names "Radhey Krishna" in your mind

Benefits

✓ Kandharasan supports the prevention of menstrual disorders, asthma, bronchial, and thyroid conditions.
✓ It also heals backache and helps straighten the "rounded or arched shoulders."
✓ With a regular practice of this pose, there is improvement on the digestion as it stretches and massages the colon.
✓ It helps alleviate stomach and waist pain.

Contraindications

- People suffering from peptic or duodenal ulcer and abdominal hernia should not attempt it.
- Also, people with severe eye problems such as glaucoma should avoid it from their daily *Yogic* exercise(s).

26. Vipareet Karani Asan (Inverted Pose)

Procedure

i. Lie flat on your back with both your legs together and touch the outer sides of the thighs with your palms, i.e. Simple Supine Pose (See page 227).

ii. Inhaling (Radhey), taking support of your arms, gradually raise your legs together till they become perpendicular to the floor.

iii. While exhaling (Krishna), taking support of the arms—especially elbows, raise your lower back; ensure your legs stay perpendicular to the ground.

iv. In the final position, the weight of the body rests on the back of the upper arms, shoulders, and neck.

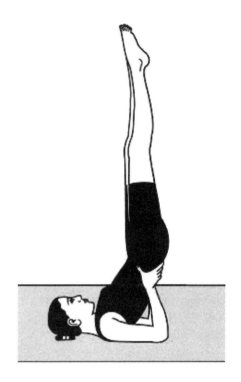

v. The trunk will be at an angle of 45 degrees to the floor. Also keep the elbows as much close to each other as possible.

vi. The eyes should be closed so that the whole body can be relaxed.

vii. Stay in this pose as long as possible with normal breathing.

viii. Now, come back to the initial position by following the steps in the reverse order.

ix. Finally, come into Shavasan (See page 227) and relax.

For Other Details: See Sarvangasan (Next *asan*).

27. Sarvangasan (Shoulder Stand Pose)

Procedure

i. Lie flat on your back with both your legs together and touch the outer sides of the thighs with your palms, i.e. Simple Supine Pose (See page 227).

ii. While inhaling (Radhey), gently raise both legs together.

iii. While exhaling (Krishna), taking support of the arms and elbows, raise your lower back; ensure your legs remain perpendicular to the ground at 90 degrees.

iv. Place your elbows firmly on the ground and support the back with both hands.

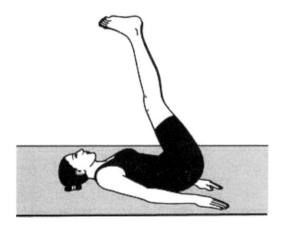

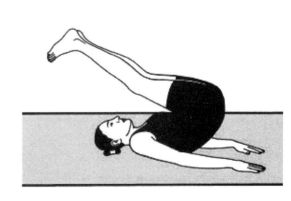

v. Now try to lower your feet towards your head until the legs get parallel to the floor; inhaling (Radhey), raise your back; then shift your supportive hands to the middle spine to support the back; then raise your legs and lower trunk vertically.

vi. As you exhale (Krishna), make both—the trunk and legs—erect by stretching your back, settling chin in the suprasternal hollow.

vii. In the final position, the body-weight is on the neck, head, and the arms.

viii. Stay effortlessly for as long as possible with normal breathing.

ix. Gradually reverse the order, and return to the initial phase.

x. Eventually, come into Shavasan (See page 227) and relax the whole body.

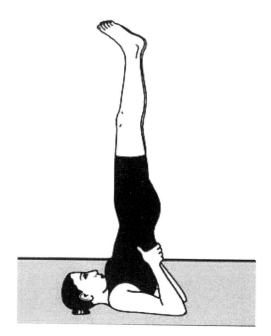

Awareness

✧ On your breaths and the bodily movements synchronized with them
✧ On mentally chanting the Revered Names "Radhey Krishna" along with your breathing and always realizing Their presence in front of you
✧ On the balance of your body in the final state

Benefits

✓ Sarvangasan develops our immune system by stimulating the thyroid gland.
✓ Similarly, it increases blood circulation in the brain area, which helps in relieving mental and emotional stress.
✓ It also cures many other diseases such as asthma, diabetes, thyroid disorders, menstrual troubles, cough, cold, and flu.
✓ This inverted pose works by reversing the effects of gravity on different parts of the body.
✓ It promotes proper blood circulation by directing the blood flow of the entire lower body toward the heart.
✓ It also prevents varicose veins by reducing the pressure on the legs and directing blood blocked in the veins/valves upwards to the heart.

Contraindications

- People with high blood pressure, glaucoma, hernia, cervical spondylitis, slipped-disc, heart problems, weak eye vessels, impure blood, thrombosis, kidney problems, active menstrual cycle, and pregnancy should not include this *asan* in their exercise. Also, people suffering from neck injuries should not do it without the counsel and guidelines of a *Yog* expert.

28. Urdhwa Mukh Pashchimottanasan (Posterior Stretch with Face Upward)

Procedure

i. Lie flat on your back with both your legs together and touch the outer sides of the thighs with your palms, i.e. Simple Supine Pose (See page 227).

ii. Inhale (Radhey); then exhaling (Krishna), gradually raise your legs and bring them over the head.

iii. Now raise your arms, hold both soles firmly by interlocking the fingers, and then lock the legs.

iv. Make sure your whole back lies on the floor in this state.

v. Again inhale (Radhey); while exhaling (Krishna), gently move your legs downward to the floor by widening the elbows.

vi. Attempt to keep the pelvis as much close to the floor as possible.

vii. Relax the chin on the knees and keep the legs locked at all times.

viii. Hold the position for almost 15-20 seconds with normal breathing.

ix. Now, comfortably come back to the central position.

x. This completes one round; repeat it for two more rounds.

xi. Lastly, come to Shavasan (See page 227) and relax.

Awareness

✧ On different physical movements and breaths synchronized with them

✧ On the stretch of your legs, knees, thighs, pelvic region, and the lumbar region

✧ On the unbroken feeling of the presence of "Radhey Krishna" standing in front of you and watching you

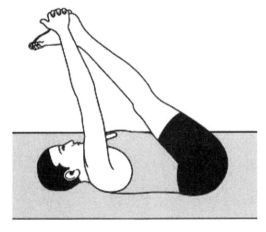 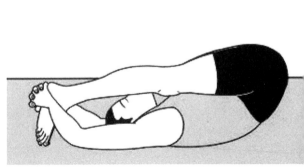

Benefits

- ✓ It tones up and massages the abdominal and pelvic regions including the pancreas, stomach, liver, adrenal gland, and spleen, etc.
- ✓ It helps alleviate disorders of the uro-genital system.
- ✓ It controls diabetes, menstrual problems, colitis, kidney troubles, bronchitis, and eosinophilia.
- ✓ The thighs and calves become slim; hernia is prevented and severe backaches are alleviated.
- ✓ It lengthens the leg muscles.
- ✓ It even helps relieve backaches.

Contraindications

- - People with slipped-disc and sciatica should not practice it. It should not be practiced before perfecting Halasan and Pashchimottansan.

29. Urdhwa Padmasan in Sarvangasan (High Lotus Pose in Shoulder Stand)

Procedure

i. Assume the final pose of Sarvangasan, steps i-vii (See pages 256-257), progressively.

ii. Fold your legs; cross them by first resting the right foot over the left thigh and then the left foot over the right thigh. Place your hands on knees to support them.

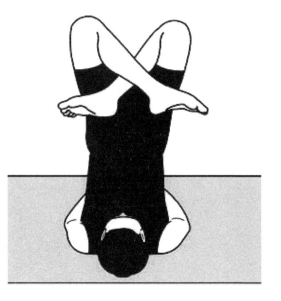

iii. While inhaling (Radhey), raise your thighs vertically up and also attempt to bring the knees closer to each other.

iv. Exhaling (Krishna), maintain balance on the neck and shoulders.

v. With normal breathing, remain in this pose for as long as comfortable without any strain.

vi. Slowly reversing the order, regain the starting position.

vii. Repeat with the alternate leg-position in Padmansan (See page 116).

viii. Finally, come to Shavasan (See page 227) and relax.

Awareness

- ✧ On the bodily movements and breaths synchronized with them
- ✧ On always feeling the presence of "Radhey Krishna" in front of you
- ✧ On the balance in the final position

For Other Details: See Sarvangasan (See page 256) and Padmasan (See page 116).

30. Pindasan (Embryo Pose)

Procedure

i. Come to the final position of Urdhwa Padmasan in Sarvangasan, steps i-iv (See page 259), progressively.

ii. Inhale (Radhey) in this position.

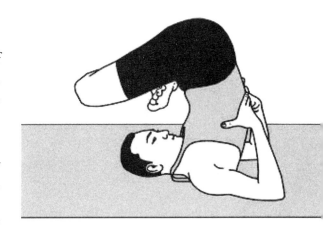

iii. While exhaling (Krishna), slowly lower the legs in Padmasan, bringing close to the forehead.

iv. Now, wrap both the arms around your knees and pull them as much close to the chest as possible.

v. Stay in this posture at your ease with normal breathing.

vi. Come back to the initial pose by following the reverse process.

vii. Repeat with the alternate leg-position in Padmansan (See page 116).

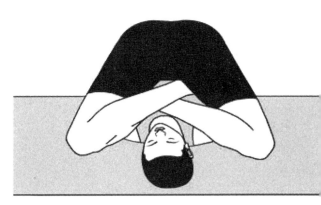

viii. Finally, come to Shavasan (See page 227) and relax.

Awareness

✧ On the pressure in your shoulders, neck, and lower abdomen

✧ On the balance

✧ On remembering the sentient and dynamic forms of "Radhey Krishna" in your breaths

Benefits

✓ Pindasan strengthens the skeletal muscles and purifies *nāḍīs*, *chakras*, blood vessels, and the neural network.

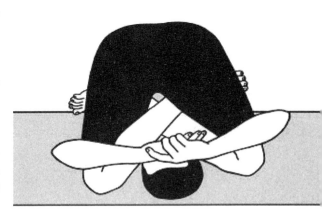

✓ It tones excellently up the lower abdomen, spinal column, liver, spleen, and stomach.

✓ It relieves constipation.

✓ It keeps the stomach slim and fat-free.

Contraindications

- Persons with high blood pressure, heart disease, thrombosis arteriosclerosis, chronic catarrh, acute constipation, kidney problems, impure blood, weak eye vessels, and also suffering from headaches or migraines should not attempt this *asan*.
- Women should not attempt this pose during pregnancy and menstrual cycle.

31. Drut Halasan (Dynamic Plough Pose)

Procedure

i. Lie flat on your back with both your legs together and touch the outer side of the thighs with your palms, i.e. Simple Supine Pose (See page 227).

ii. Now, bring your arms close to the body with the palms flat on the floor.

iii. Inhale (Radhey).

iv. Exhaling (Krishna), raise your legs over the head rapidly and touch the floor—behind the head—with the toes.

v. Ensure the legs remain outstretched and joined together throughout.

vi. Now inhaling (Radhey), revert the body rapidly, back to the initial position.

vii. Quickly return to sitting posture with an exhalation (Krishna); while continuing to exhale (Krishna), lean the whole body forward into Pashchimottanasan (See page 169), holding the big toes with the hands.

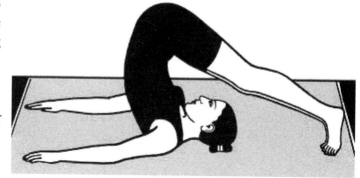

viii. Try to touch the knees with the forehead; your hands remaining on either side of the thighs.

ix. Again, with a regular inhalation (Radhey), without pausing, return to the seated position by rapidly raising the head and trunk until they become perpendicular to the floor.

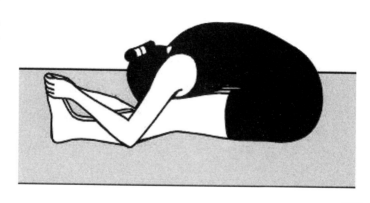

x. Now continuing to inhale (Radhey), go back to Supine Position.

xi. This completes one round; try this for 5-10 rounds with rapid but smooth movements.

xii. Lastly, come into Shavasan (See page 227) and relax.

Awareness

✧ On mentally chanting "Radhey Krishna" with your each breath
✧ On the back and forth movements synchronized with your breaths
✧ On the stretches and strains of the back

Benefits

✓ This Dynamic Halasan provides the double benefits of both—Halasan (See page 249) and Pashchimottanasan (See page 169).
✓ It stimulates the intestinal peristalsis, which helps in improving digestion and removing constipation.
✓ It is a boon for people with obesity as it helps in the breakdown of fats by exercising the liver and gall bladder.
✓ Besides, it gives relief to the pelvic region.

Contraindications

- Those with sciatica, back and neck pain, and high blood pressure should omit this *asan*.

32. Ardh Padma Halasan (Half Lotus Plough Pose)

Procedure

i. Lie flat on your back with both your legs together and touch the outer sides of the thighs with your palms, i.e. Simple Supine Pose (See page 227).

ii. Now, bend your left leg at the knee and place the left foot on the right thigh, just as in the Half Lotus Position (See page 111).

iii. Rest your arms on either side of the body, keeping the palms flat on the floor.

iv. Inhale (Radhey); taking support of your arms on the floor, slowly raise your right leg until

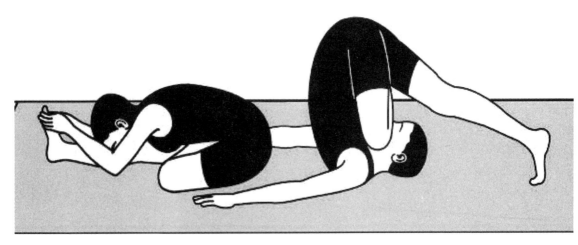

it becomes perpendicular to the floor.

v. Now raise your upper back as in Halasan (See page 249), supporting your middle-spine with the hands.

vi. Exhaling (Krishna), lower your right leg backward—over your head—to the floor.

vii. Attempt to move your forehead to the knee of the outstretched leg without any strain.

viii. Breathing normally, maintain this position for as long as you are comfortable.

ix. Then, come back to the initial lying position in the reverse order.

x. Now, repeat the process with the alternate leg.

xi. Finally, come into Shavasan (See page 227) and relax.

For Other Details: See Poorva Halasan.

33. Chakrasan / Urdhwa Dhanurasana (Wheel Pose)

Procedure

i. Lie flat on your back with both your legs together and touch the outer side of the thighs with your palms, i.e. Simple Supine Pose (See page 227).

ii. Gently bend your legs at the knees and touch the buttocks with your heels.

iii. Ensure your feet as well as knees remain at about one foot distance.

iv. Keep both hands by the sides of your head in such a way that the fingers point toward the shoulders.

v. Inhaling (Radhey), slowly and carefully raise the whole body with the support of the hands and shoulders.

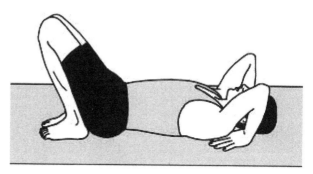

vi. Then, keeping the crown on the floor, shift the body-weight onto the head and arch the body upward.

vii. Continuing to inhale (Radhey), try to straighten the arms and legs, without any strain.

viii. Also, try to arch your back as much as possible in this condition.

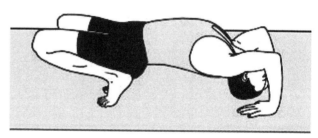

ix. Slowly try to bring the hands and the legs toward each other and maintain a proper balance.

x. Stay in this posture to your comfort

with normal breathing.

xi. Then, come back to the initial position by first slowly lowering the body so that your head touches the floor, and then bringing the remaining parts of the body down to the floor.

xii. Lastly, come to Shavasan (See page 227) and relax.

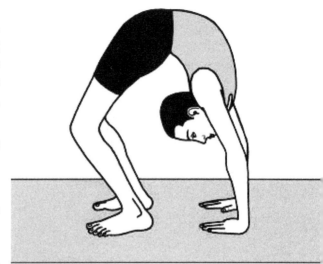

Awareness

✧ On the stretches and strains in the chest and abdomen

✧ On relaxing the spine

✧ On always remembering sentient and mobile forms of "Radhey Krishna" while breathing

✧ On the balance in the final position

Benefits

✓ By Chakrasan, there is an increase in the flexibility of the spine and stimulation in every part of the body.

✓ It makes the shoulders, arms, and legs very powerful.

✓ *Yog* therapists also consider it as a very effectual pose for the nervous, digestive, respiratory, cardiovascular, and glandular systems.

✓ Especially, women are given considerable relief as it helps cure several gynecological disorders.

✓ Mainly, it is excellent for the heart functions for it stretches the aorta.

✓ It is a must-do for diabetics.

Contraindications

- Those who have problems of the wrists and back should not do this *asan*.

34. Setu Bandh Asan (Bridge Constructing Pose)

Procedure

i. Lie flat on your back with both your legs together and touch the outer sides of the thighs with your palms, i.e. Simple Supine Pose (See page 227).

ii. Flex the legs and spreading your knees slightly, bring the heels toward the buttocks.

iii. The heels should be joined together with their outer sides touching the floor.

iv. Place your hands on either side of the head, keeping shoulder-width distance in between both hands; inhale (Radhey).

v. Now with the support of your hands, gently arch your upper body by raising the trunk so that the crown of the head rests on the floor.

vi. Try to draw your head backward, as far as possible, by stretching the neck.

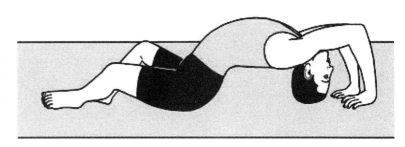

vii. Now exhale (Krishna) in this state, and then taking the support of your arms and head, raise your hips and inhale (Radhey).

viii. Continuing to inhale (Radhey), extend your legs straight and join them together with sufficient balance on the floor.

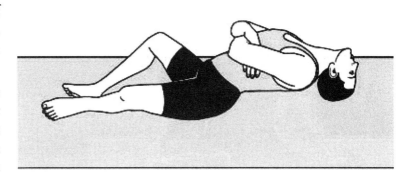

ix. Maintaining the balance, fold the arms across the chest, with the left elbow grapsed by the right hand and the right elbow by the left.

x. With the crown of the head and the legs as supports at the two ends, the whole body resembles a shape of an arch or a bridge.

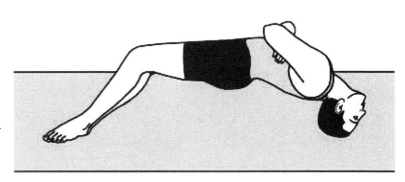

xi. Remain in this posture to your comfort with a normal breathing.

xii. Following the steps in the reverse order, come back to the central position.

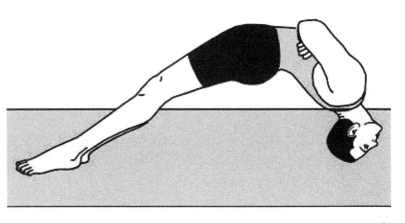

xiii. Lastly, come into Shavasan (See page

227) and relax.

Awareness
- ✧ On your bodily movements and the breaths synchronized with them
- ✧ On the stretch of the legs and back
- ✧ On the pressure of the neck
- ✧ On the balance
- ✧ On realizing the sentient forms of "Radhey Krishna" with your each breath

Benefits
- ✓ This difficult pose firms the neck and tones the cervical, dorsal, lumbar, and sacral regions of the spine.
- ✓ It strengthens the muscles of the back extremely and also exercises the hips perfectly.
- ✓ It also helps in monitoring the blood supply in the pineal, pituitary, and thyroid glands.
- ✓ It increases flexibility and elasticity of your body; it mainly strengthens the lower back and abdominal muscles.
- ✓ It relieves pain in the spine and the hip joints.
- ✓ It soothes the brain and helps reduce stress and mild depression.
- ✓ It relieves the female practitioners from the symptoms of menopause.
- ✓ Even the tired legs are rejuvenated if done regularly.

Contraindications
- Persons suffering from neck injury and lumbar spondylitis should get counsel of a *Yog* therapist. Only the persons with more suppleness and normal health should try this *asan*.

35. Urdhwa Padmasan (High Lotus Pose)

Procedure
i. Assume the final position of Sarvangasan, v-vii steps, (See pages 256-257) progressively.

ii. Slowly folding the right leg first and then the left leg, come into Padmasan (See page 216).

iii. Now, keeping the knees and thighs parallel to the floor, balalnce the whole body on the shoulders, neck, and the back portion of the head.

iv. Ensure your trunk remains erect on the floor and place your hands on the knees to support the bent legs.

v. Be in this posture for as long as possible with normal breathing.

vi. Come back into the base postion by reversing the whole process.

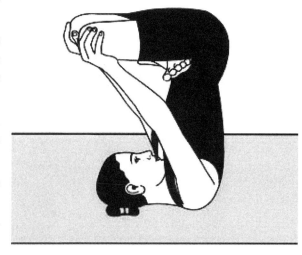

vii. Perform the posture again with the legs crossed the other way.

viii. Finally, come to Shavasan (See page 227) and rest.

Awareness

✧ On maintaining the balance

✧ On realizing the sentient forms of "Radhey Krishna" everywhere

Benefits

✓ This combined exercise of Sarvangasan and Padmasan purifies the colon and urinary tract.

✓ It strengthens the anterior part of the spinal column.

✓ It purifies the heart, lungs, and other parts of the body.

Contraindications

- People with high blood pressure, hernia, cervical spondylitis, slipped-disc, heart problems, weak eye vessels, impure blood, and women during active menstrual cycle and pregnancy should avoid it.

36. Setu Bandh Sarvangasan / Uttan Mayurasan (Bridge Formation in Shoulder Stand Pose / Intensely Stretched Peacock Pose)

Procedure

i. Assume the final pose of Vipareet Karani Asan, vii step (See page 255).

ii. Inhale (Radhey); while exhaling (Krishna), either bring your legs back, keeping them straight, or fold them at the knees and also let your feets go over the wrists and touch the floor.

iii. Without any strain, extend your legs and keep them together.

iv. Bearing the whole weight on the elbows and wrists, try to form the shape of a bridge.

v. Only the back of the head and neck, shoulders, elbows, and the feet will be in contact with the floor.

vi. Hold the posture to your comfort with normal breathing.

vii. Return to the initial position unhurriedly.

viii. Lastly, come to Shavasan (See page 227) and relax.

Awareness

✧ On the movements synchronized with the breaths

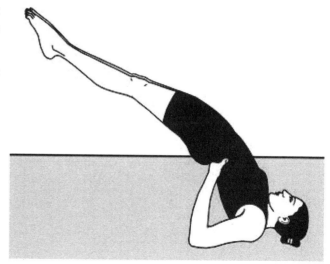

- On the stretch and strain of the spine
- On the pressure in your elbows and wrists
- On always feeling the presence of "Radhey Krishna" with your each breath

Benefits

- ✓ It provides movement to the spine—thus helps exercise the nerves and relieves the strain on the neck caused by the different movements of Sarvangasan.
- ✓ It increases blood circulation in the brain area, resulting in relieving mental and emotional stress.
- ✓ Like Sarvangasan, it is also versatile in healing several diseases such as asthma, diabetes, thyroid disorders, menstrual troubles, cough, cold, and flu.

Contraindications

- As in Sarvangasan, people with high blood pressure, hernia, cervical spondylitis, slipped-disc, heart problems, weak eye vessels, impure blood, active menstrual cycle, and pregnant women should not do this *asan*.

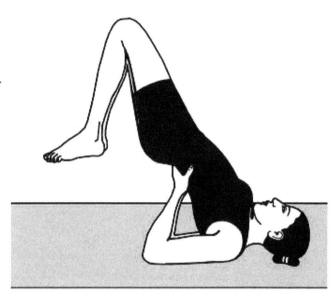

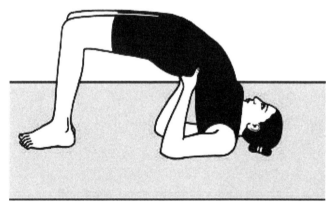

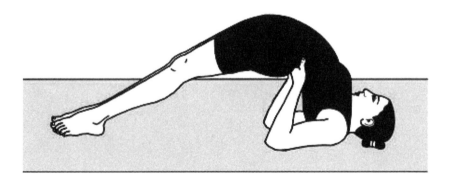

G. Topsy-Turvy Poses

1. Ardh Shirshasan (Half Head Stand Pose)

Procedure

i. Sit in Vajrasan (See page 113).

ii. Then, interlock all your fingers and inhale (Radhey).

iii. While exhaling (Krishna), gently bend your upper body and place your forehead on the floor; ensure your thighs remain perpeduicular to the floor; simultaneously taking support of your elbows rooted on the floor, support the crown with the interlocked fingers.

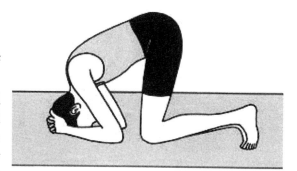

iv. Ensure the distance between your elbows is between 1-1.5 feet.

v. Now, place your crown between the interlocked fingers.

vi. Inhale (Radhey); as you exhale (Krishna), comfortably raise your buttocks and straighten the legs with the support of your feet and arms.

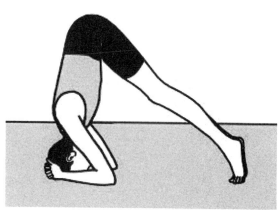

vii. Take a step forward and make a triangle with the body and the floor.

viii. Remain in this position at your ease with normal breathing.

ix. Then, with an inhalation (Radhey), slowly flex your legs and lower the knees to the floor.

x. Then exhale (Krishna); while inhaling (Radhey), come back into Vajrasan.

xi. Ultimately, come to Shashankasan (See page 117) and relax.

Awareness

✧ On breathing in and out along with various body movements
✧ On the balance
✧ On the stretch of the hamstrings
✧ On the pressure in the neck and head
✧ On always remembering the Divine Names "Radhey Krishna" flowing with your breaths

Benefits

✓ Practicing this *asan* fortifies the neck muscles and prepares one for Shirshasan—one of the most arduous postures.

- ✓ Its main benefit is to decrease anxiety and tension.
- ✓ It corrects the upper part of the spine.
- ✓ It develops concentration and memory power.
- ✓ It nourishes the facial skin and hair.
- ✓ It also improves blood circulation and empowers the immune system.

Contraindications

- People with high blood pressure, heart disease, swollen ears, acute asthma, vertebral problems, myopia (short-sightedness), and weak blood vessels should not perform this *asan*.

2. Shirshasan (Head Stand Pose)

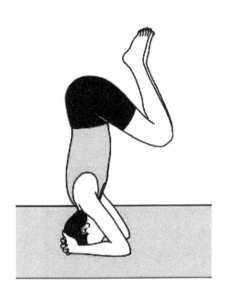

Procedure

i. Progressively assume the final position of Ardh Shirshasan, steps v-vii, (See page 269).

ii. Take 2-3 small steps forward; then while inhaling (Radhey), bend your legs at the knees and slowly raise them one by one—off the floor.

iii. Gently, straighten your legs; try to balance on the crown and forearms.

iv. In the final state, make sure your head rests at the bottom on the floor while the feet on the top.

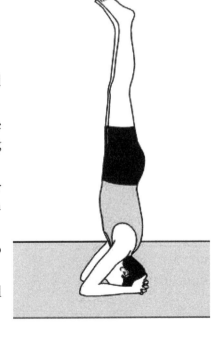

v. Stay in this position to your comfort with normal breathing.

vi. Exhaling (Krishna), gradually bend the legs at the knees and carefully lower them to the floor—returning to the final position of Ardh Shirshasan.

vii. Then inhaling (Radhey), drop your knees to the floor and raising your upper body to erect position, return to Vajrasan (See page 113).

viii. Perform all these steps unhurriedly and steadily; do not rush or make any rash movements.

ix. Finally, come into Shashankasan (See page 117) and relax for a while.

Note: Since this is one of the difficult *asans*, to begin with, you may take the support of a wall. This *asan* should be done only under the guidance of a trained *Yog* instructor. Sarvangasan (See page 256) is a safer *asan* to begin with.

Awareness

✧ On the balance in the last state

✧ On spontaneously remembering "Radhey Krishna" with your breaths and feeling Their presence everywhere

Benefits

✓ Shirshasan—one of the challenging poses—increases the blood circulation to the brain and pituitary glands, which boosts up the nervous system and memory power.

✓ It is considered as the king of the *asans* because of its immense benefits.

✓ As it corrects disorders related to the reproductive system, it produces a tremendous impact on women's health.

✓ The weight of the abdominal organs in the diaphragm during its practice causes rapid exhalation, resulting in the expulsion of carbon dioxide, toxins, and bacteria.

✓ Also, it rectifies asthma, hay fever, diabetes, and menopausal imbalances.

Contraindications

- Person with high blood pressure, heart disease, swollen ears, acute asthma, weak eye blood vessels, vertebral problems, myopia, and weak blood vessels in the body should avoid it.

3. Niralamb Shirshasan (Unsupported Headstand Pose)

Procedure

i. Come into Vajrasan (See page 113).

ii. Inhale (Radhey) and as you exhale (Krishna), slowly lean forward and place your palms on the floor, in front of the knees, with a distance of four inches between them.

iii. Slowly raising the buttocks, lean forward and rest the crown of your head between the two palms.

iv. Now, slide the hands backward and rest them flat on the floor, on the either side of the calves.

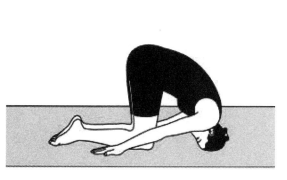
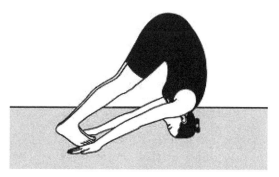

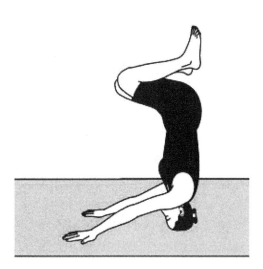

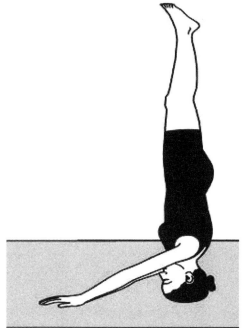

v. Inhale (Radhey); exhaling (Krishna), raise your buttocks and legs; balance on your toes, forming a triangle with the floor.

vi. Comfortably move toward your head, on your tiptoes till your torso is vertical; make sure your legs remain locked in this process.

vii. Balancing on your arms and crown, inhale (Radhey); then gradually fold the legs and raise the feet off the floor one by one by moving the knees toward the chest.

viii. Next, gently raise the thighs till they are almost parallel to the floor; relax with normal breathing for 4-5 seconds.

ix. Without any strain and carefully raise the legs vertically, pointing the sole upward.

x. Finally, make sure your whole body becomes perpendicular to the floor and the body-weight is shifted to the head, with a minimal support of the arms.

xi. Remain in this pose at your ease with normal breathing.

xii. Come back to the initial position by following the steps in the reverse order.

xiii. Lastly, come to Shashankasan (See page 217) and relax.

For Other Details: See Shirshasan (See page 270).

4. Mukt Hasta Shirshasan (Free Hands Head Stand)

Procedure

i. Assume the final position of Shirshasan, steps i-iv (See page 270), progressively.

ii. Ensure your wrists face upward and also the distance between them equals the shoulder width.

iii. Again inhale (Radhey).

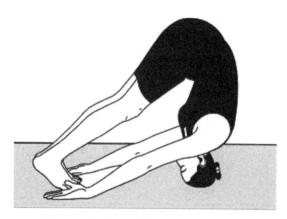

iv. Now while exhaling (Krishna), slowly raise your trunk until it becomes vertical.

v. And then, again with an inhalation (Radhey), raise your feet by the rooting the wrists on the floor.

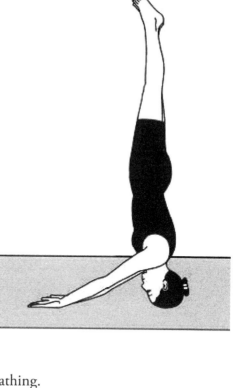

vi. Now make sure your legs stay vertical—in a single line with the head and the trunk.

vii. Also ensure your legs stay locked in this position.

viii. Hold the pose to your possibility with normal breathing.

ix. With an exhalation (Krishna), slowly bring your legs down to the floor; then come back to Vajrasan with an exhalation (Krishna).

x. Lastly, come to Shashankasan (See page 217) and relax.

For Other Details: See Shirshasan (See page 270).

5. Kapali Asan (Forehead Supported Pose)

Procedure

i. Come to the final position of Shirshasan, steps i-iv (See page 270), progressively.

ii. Maintain your balance for a few seconds; then comfortably transfer the body support from the crown to the forehead and relax.

iii. In the final step, slightly lean back the spine and legs so that there will be a perfect balance.

iv. Stay in the final position for as long as you are comfortable with normal breathing.

v. Gently, come back to Shirshasan; while inhaling

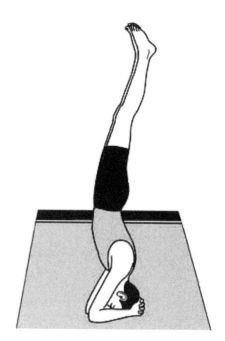

(Radhey), slowly lower the body to the floor.

vi. Now return to Vajrasan, and then come to Shashankasan (See page 217) for complete relaxation.

Variation - 1

i. Come to the final position of Kapali Asan, step iii (See page 273).

ii. Balancing your body, slowly fold the right leg at the knee and then rest the right sole on the front portion of the left thigh.

iii. Now, fold your left leg backward in such a way that the foot points toward the floor/sole—just behind the body.

iv. Stay in this posture to your comfort with normal breathing.

v. Again return back to Kapali Posture; then repeat with the other leg.

vi. Return to the initial position by following the steps in the reverse order.

vii. Finally, come back to Vajrasan and then to Shashankasan (See page 217) to relax the whole body completely.

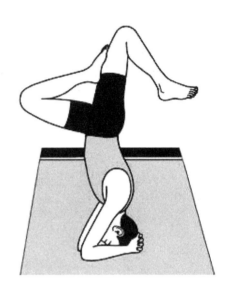

Variation - 2

i. Come to the final position of Kapali Asan, step iii (See page 273).

ii. Balancing your body, gradually fold the left leg at the knee and place the heel on the left buttock.

iii. Inclining the hips slightly forward, flex the right leg and then move the right knee to the chest.

iv. In the final position, ensure your left thigh rests on right sole and left folded-leg remains slanted, i.e. left knee points forward and the right knee downward.

v. Stay in this posture for as long as possible with normal breathing.

vi. Again, come back to Kapali Posture; repeat with the alternate leg.

vii. Return to the initial position by following the steps in the reverse order.

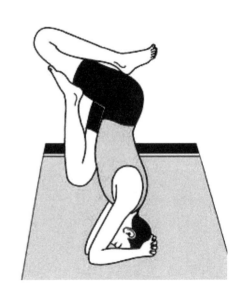

viii. Ultimately, come back to Vajrasan; then to Shashankasan (See page 217) and relax.

For Other Details: See Shirshasan (See page 270).

6. Padmasan in Shirshasan (Head Stand Lotus Pose)

Procedure

i. Come into the final position of Shirshasan, steps i-iv (See page 270).

ii. After maintaining the balance, gently and slowly fold the legs and cross them into Padmasan (See page 116).

iii. Remain in this pose to your capacity with normal breathing.

iv. While returning back to Shirshasan, carefully release the legs and straighten them.

v. Come back to the initial position by reversing the order of the Shirshasan.

vi. Repeat the method with alternate leg position in Padmasan.

vii. Lastly, come into Shashankasan (See page 217) and relax for a while.

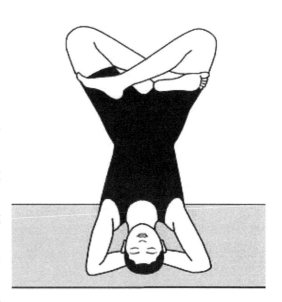

Note: This *asan* should be done only under the guidance of a trained *Yog* instructor. Sarvangasan is safer *asan* to begin with.

Awareness

✧ On the balance in the final position
✧ On spontaneously remembering "Radhey Krishna" with your breaths and feeling Their presence everywhere

Benefits

✓ Along with the benefits of Shirshasan, it helps expand the chest and entire back.
✓ It invigorates the whole body—enhancing plentiful blood circulation in the pelvic region.
✓ It also corrects disorders of the reproductive system.

Contraindications

- People with high blood pressure, heart disease, swollen ears, acute asthma, weak eye blood vessels, problems in the vertebrae, myopia, and weak blood vessels in the body, should not practice this *asan*.

7. Ek Pada Shirshasan (One Leg Head Stand)

Procedure

i. Come to the final position of Shirshasan steps i-iv (See page 270), gradually.

ii. Inhale (Radhey); while exhaling (Krishna), lower your right leg to the floor—just in front of the head.

iii. Make sure your left leg remains vertical, both—at the time of lowering the right leg to the floor and placing it there.

iv. Stretch out both legs and also firm the lower part of your abdomen.

v. Be in this pose for as long as possible with normal breathing.

vi. Now while exhaling (Krishna), raise the right leg up to Shirshasan and lower the left leg to the floor, just in front of the head.

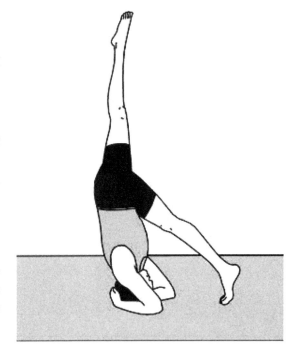

vii. Attempt to hold the pose for as long as possible with normal breathing.

viii. This completes one round; try one more round.

ix. After this, go back to Shirshasan slowly and then to the initial position in the reverse order.

x. Eventually, come to Shashankasan (See page 217) and relax for a while.

For Other Details: See Shirshasan (See page 270)

8. Vrishchikasan (Scorpion Pose)

Procedure

i. Assume the final position of Shirshasan, steps i-iv (See page 270), progressively.

ii. Keep the whole body relaxed; then as you inhale (Radhey), slowly fold the legs backward and arch the back like a bow.

iii. After acquiring a proper balance, move your forearms to the sides of the head with the palms lying on the floor.

iv. Gently, try to lower your feet downward—as much as you can.

v. Make sure your knees and ankles stay together and the toes point forward.

vi. Now, slowly raise your head upward and backward.

vii. Then, raise the upper arms so that they will be vertical.

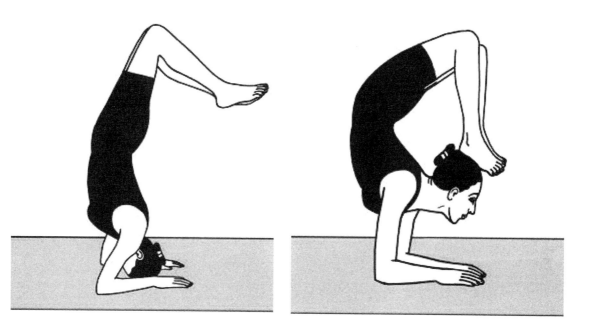

viii. Hold the pose to your capacity with normal breathing.

ix. Exhaling (Krishna), return to Shirshasan carefully and gently lower the feet to the floor.

x. Finally, come to Shashankasan (See page 217) so that you can relax.

Awareness

✧ On the balance

✧ On spontaneous remembrance "Radhey Krishna" along with your breathing act and feeling Their presence in front of you

Benefits

✓ This arduous *asan*—Vrishchikasan—expands the lungs completely by stretching the abdominal muscles and toning the whole spine.

✓ Chiefly, it refreshes the mind to a great extent by increasing the blood flow to the brain and pituitary glands. This significant function assists in revitalizing all the body's systems and rectifying nervous and glandular disorders.

✓ As the back has to be arched like a bow in the last position, it stretches the back so excellently that the nerves of the spine are firmed well.

✓ Besides, a sense of balance is developed as one has to balance carefully in the final position.

Contraindications

- Those who have problems like high blood pressure, vertigo, chronic catarrh, cerebral thrombosis, and any heart disease should not try it.

H. Hasyasans (Laughter Poses)

Hasyasan is formed by the two words "*Hasya*" meaning "to laugh" and "*asan*" meaning "a pose." Thus, the integrated sense of it is to laugh in different poses. Here are five types of Hasyasans that will really free you from your anxieties, stress, and unnecessary tensions.

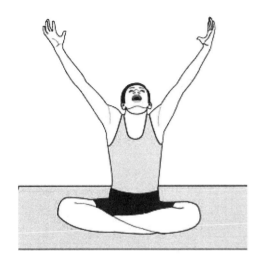

1. Attahas Hasyasan

Procedure

i. Sit in Sukhasan (See page 111).

ii. Raise your hands up and laugh boomingly.

2. Gur-Gur Hasysan

Procedure

i. Sit in Sukhasan (See page 111).

ii. Laugh with your mouth shut.

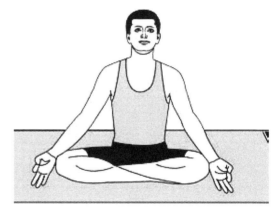

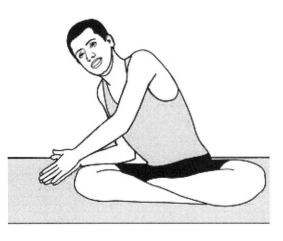

3. Dandiya Hasyasan

Procedure

i. Sit in Sukhasan (See page 111).

ii. Tilt leftward; clap your hands, and laugh loudly.

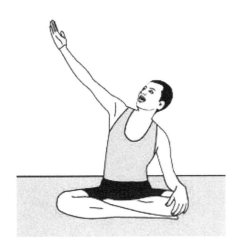

4. Anaram Hasyasan

Procedure

i. Sit in Sukhasan (See page 111).

ii. Raise your hands one by one and laugh enunciating the *swar varṇa* (vowels) of the *Devanāgarī* alphabet.

iii. You could also use vowels from the English alphabet—"a, e, i, o, u."

5. Gud-Gud Hasyasan

Procedure

i. Get another person to pair with you, and sit in Sukhasan, (See page 111) facing each other.

ii. Tickle each other and laugh.

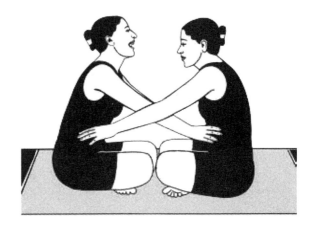

Benefits

✓ Hasyasans make your heart very healthy.

✓ They activate about 75 muscles in different parts of your body, thus resulting in the increase of blood level throughout the whole body.

✓ They release mental and emotional strains and help inducing zeal and vigor.

✓ You feel extremely released, vibrant, and fresh upon practicing the above mentioned of Laughter Poses.

✓ They strengthen your immune system.

✓ It helps growing the intellectual performance and boosting information retention.

✓ Laughter poses significantly help control diabetes by reducing blood sugar levels thus.

✓ These *asans* are cathartic exercises, which assist the practitioners in venting out their condensed emotions in systematic and organized way. Thus, they help develop positive emotions and reduce the negative ones, thereby ensuring a healthy life.

✓ According to Dr. Otto Warburg, a German scientist and Nobel Laureate, the main cause of our illness is due to the deficiency of oxygen in our body cells. Laughter poses bring adequate oxygen to both—the body and brain; adequate supply of oxygen is the basic factor for keeping a sound health. Thus, these *Yogic* exercises are equally significant for people suffering from cancer and different chronic respiratory diseases like bronchitis and so on.

✓ Everybody knows that immune system plays a crucial role in the causation and prognosis of cancer; the most probable trigger for the occurrence of cancer is the weak immune system of a person. Laughter poses increase the number of natural killer cells—the main factors of the immune system; thus these *Yogic asans* assist in both—overcoming and terminating cancer cells.

Contraindications

- People with the problems like depression, high blood pressure, and heart ailments; and also those who have undergone recent surgical operations of abdominal parts should not attempt any of these Hasyasans.

V. Surya Namaskār (Sun Salutation)

"*Surya*" is a Sanskrit word that means "the Sun" and "*Namaskār*" refers to "the act of paying Namaste with folded hands." Hence, "*Surya Namaskār*" means "Salute to the Sun." Symbolically, the act of prostration is a devotional one, representing the surrender of the self to the Supreme, Who is both—within and outside—of us. In the field of *Yog*, the Sun symbolizes the source of cosmic energy, represented by *piṅgalā* or Surya *nāḍī*, (*prāṇic* channel or life-giving force). This sequence consists of 12 poses, which are connected together by inhaling (Radhey) and exhaling (Krishna)—one pose flowing into the other. This can also be set as the "Synchronization of the Breaths with the Bodily Movements."

This is a dynamic exercise that loosens up, stretches, and tones all the joints and muscles in the body and also helps in massaging the internal organs of the body. It has the combined effect of both—the warm-up and relaxation. This is usually done both—at sunrise and sunset. But it can be practiced at other times of the day too, provided the stomach is empty. There are 12 levels of "Salute to the Sun." Together they set a wonderful warm-up routine, which limbers the spine, generates internal heat in your body, and prepares you for the rest of the sequences. These flowing series of 12 poses help improve strength and flexibility of the muscles and spinal column. In the practice, one should try to visualize the rising Sun, which is a symbol of love and enlightenment that annihilates both—ego and ignorance.

Although it is an indispensable warm-up exercise, readying the body for the different *asans*, it is in itself a complete exercise. Its versatility and application make it a distinct exercise among all. Here, both—postures and *pranayam*—are performed together. When you do it for the first time, try to follow the rhythm of performing one complete movement with each breath. Focus very carefully on the breath—inhaling (Radhey) while bending backward; exhaling (Krishna) while bending forward and/or sideward. By doing this, all 12 *asans* flow together progressively, one after other.

1. Namaskar Asan (Prayer Pose)

Procedure

i. Stand up straight—in an upright position—with both feet joined together and arms by your sides, i.e. Saral Tadasan (See page 25).

ii. Now close your eyes and join the palms together in front of your chest.

iii. Relax the whole body and visualize the shining Sun God (Surya Narayan) before you—emanating love, knowledge, and inspiration.

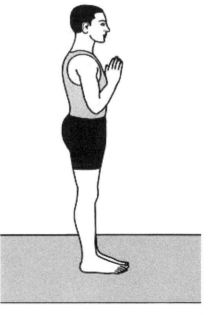

2. Hasta Utthanasan (Raised Arms Pose)

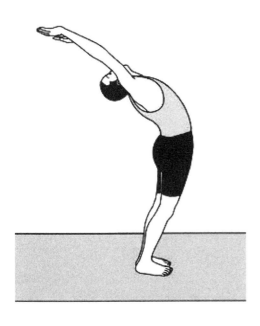

Procedure

i. While inhaling (Radhey), raise your arms up (next to the ears) above the head.

ii. Recline your trunk backward, with your head falling back.

iii. Stretch your arms and fingers fully.

iv. Make sure your spine forms a mild curve.

3. Pada Hastasan (Hand to Foot Pose)

Procedure

i. While exhaling (Krishna), bend forward from your waist to touch the knees with the forehead.

ii. Then, place your hands flat on the floor on either side of your feet, locking the knees.

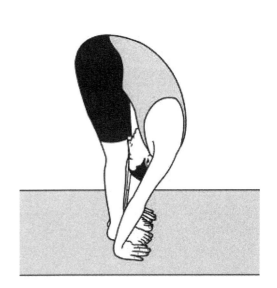

4. Ashwa Sanchalanasan (Equestrian Pose)

Procedure

i. As you inhale (Radhey), simultaneously bend your left leg at the knees between the arms, and stretch the right leg backward as far as possible; look up.

ii. Palms will be flat on the floor on either side of the left foot.

iii. Then, push the buttocks/pelvis forward.

iv. The right toe and right knee will touch the

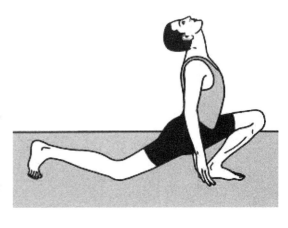

floor while the head should fall backward, forming a curve with the spine.

5. Parvatasan (Mountain Pose)

Procedure

i. Now, while exhaling (Krishna), move the left foot back—beside the right foot.

ii. Then, push your heels as far as possible into the floor, and simultaneously raise your buttocks.

iii. Also, push the palms against the floor and lower the head between the arms.

iv. Lastly, look at your feet.

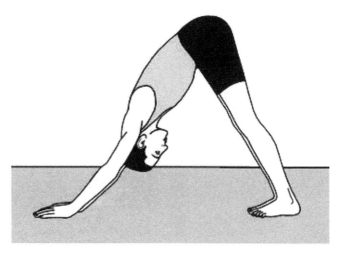

6. Ashtang Namaskar (Salute with Eight Parts/Points)

Procedure

i. Retaining the breath, fold your arms and then lower the knees, chest, and chin to the floor simultaneously so that the body come into a push-up position.

ii. You will look straight ahead in this state.

iii. Now, raise the buttocks off the floor.

iv. Ensure the toes, knees, chest, hands, and chin touch the floor in the final position.

v. The hands should be on either side of the chest.

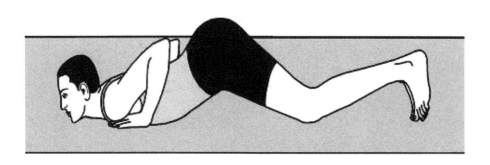

7. Bhujangasan (Cobra Pose)

Procedure

i.   As you inhale (Radhey), lower your buttocks to the floor and arch your back; straighten the elbows and raise the head, and simultaneously tilt the head backward.

ii. Unless the spine is very flexible, the arms will remain slightly bent.

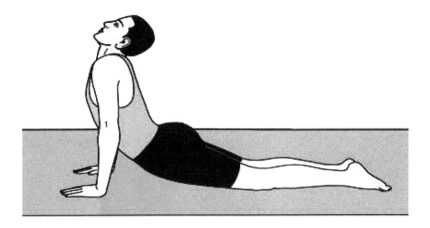

8. Parvatsan (Mountain Pose)

Procedure

i.   Now, raise your buttocks and lower your chest; tucking the head between both arms, regain the final position of Parvatasan (See page 285).

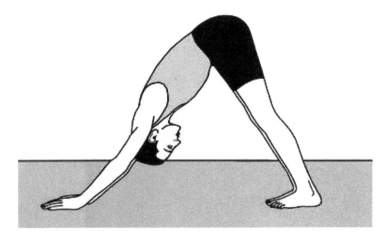

9. Ashwa Sanchalanasan (Equestrian Pose)

Procedure

i.   Inhaling (Radhey), bring the right foot forward between the hands.

ii. Then, lower the left knee to the floor, pushing the chest forward.

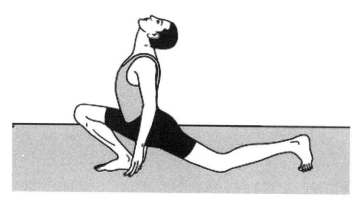

iii. Also, arch your spine and tilt the head backward.

10. Pada Hastasan (Hand to Foot Pose)

Procedure

i. Exhaling (Krishna), bring the left foot forward next to the right foot.

ii. Then, straighten both the legs as much as you can.

iii. Finally, try to touch the knees with your forehead.

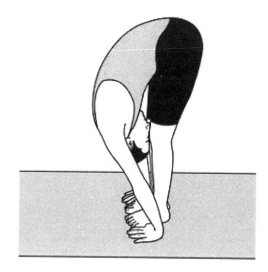

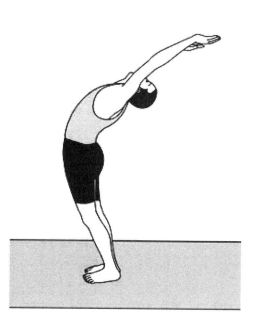

11. Hasta Utthanasan (Raised Arms Pose)

Procedure

i. As you inhale (Radhey), raise your upper body and come to the standing postion.

ii. Simultaneously, raise your arms upward and gradually recline backward.

12. Namaskarasan (Prayer Pose)

Procedure

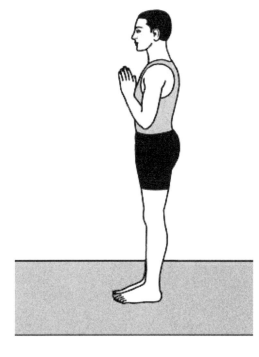

i. Inhaling (Radhey), lower your arms and form Namaste Mudra.
ii. This is one complete round.
iii. You can do 3-5 slow rounds of Surya Namaskār.
iv. Later on, you can increase the speed and number of rounds about 10-15.

Benefits

✓ The chief aim of Surya Namaskār is to balance the entire system of the body.
✓ The smooth alternation between forward-bending and backward-bending massages the solar plexus that promotes deep abdominal breathing. This kind of organized breathing improves the respiratory capacity of the lungs.
✓ The sequential movements in coherence with the breaths develop a state of relaxed attention and also develop the suppleness of the hips, pelvis, upper back, neck, and shoulders.
✓ As it consists of different *asans* combined as a package, it has multitudinous impacts on the entire body. The first is that it influences the pineal gland and hypothalamus. Next, it helps prevent pineal degeneration and calcification.
✓ Further, Surya Namaskār practiced with breath awareness helps cure pulmonary problems.
✓ The circulation of oxygenated blood in the brain contributes in the growth of mental peace and purity.
✓ The regular performance also tones up the body after 1-2 months of delivery.

Contraindications

- People with high blood pressure, hernia, heart problems, recent or chronic injury to the back, knees, hips, and intestinal tuberculosis should not practice Surya Namaskār. Also, do not practice it during menstruation; though it can be done in the first two months of pregnancy and even after two months of delivery.

VI. Radhey Krishna Pranayam

Secrets of *Pranayam*

Pranayam has been derived from two words "*pran*" and "*āyām*." In simple terms, it means to expand the *prānic* (vital) energy of the body. Normally, it is recognized as a respiration technique of inhalation and exhalation. But along with oxygen, we also take in vital *prānic* energy into our body. This *prānic* energy pervades the whole cosmos, and what we exhale is only a part of it. Therefore, only breathing in and breathing out cannot be termed as *pranayam*, rather it is a way to realize God by making an inner journey within ourselves, to develop cosmic consciousness. Although the level of oxygen increases in the body through *pranayam*, the meaning should not be confined to this physical aspect alone.

In general, *pran* is a life-giving energy that is subtler than oxygen and present everywhere. It is *pran* that sets other things in motion. In a broad sense, the whole universe is energized by *pran*. It is *pran* that gives life and vitality to all the creatures of this cosmos, and everything that happens in the body is energized by *pran*. Hence, it is also *pran* that gives energy to all the sense organs. It provides us with immunity that helps the body fight against various diseases. *Pran*, created by Brahma, has the inherent quality of being in motion. This quality is felt easily in *vāyu* (wind), which is also referred as a part of *pran*. According to the functions and locations in the body, *pran* is classified into five categories: *pran, apān, samān, udān, and vyān*. It enters the body through the nostrils. Through controlled breathing, our mind can look closely into the inner world and assist an aspirant in realizing God.

According to the Yog Darshan, as you sit in any convenient *asan* and regulate the act of breathing, it is regarded as *pranayam*. In this definition, "*pran*" refers to the breath or *prānic* energy, and "*āyām*" means to control. The process of taking air into the lungs is known as inspiration, and the process of taking out the same air is known as expiration. In typical terms, inhaling air into the body means *pūrak*, whereas exhaling air from the body means *rechak*. The Yog Darshan also states that the aspirant reaches a very high level in his or her *sādhanā* by sincerely performing *pranayam*.

The Upanishadic Seers and *Yog* Masters had a knowledge as to how the mind functions through *pran*, and by which it controls and governs various activities in the physical body. Just as an unseen magnetic force can move physical objects, so can the mind change the *prānic* distribution, and thereby impact various functions in whole body. Hence, the mind has a very subtle but strong connection with *pran*.

Undeniably, our lifestyle deeply affects the *prānic* forces. Our actions, sleep, diet, thought, senses, etc., have intense effects on our *pran*. An irregular and indiscriminate lifestyle depletes the *prānic* energy and eventually leads to *prānic* blockages. This is the reason why people feel loss of energy from time to time. The depletion of *prānic* forces leads to various ailments in the organs and muscles. The different *pranayam* practices largely contribute in the expansion of these forces and also in the balance of the five types of *pran* in the body. In *pranayam*, special breathing techniques are used to encourage that very vital force. One can achieve the full effects of *pranayam* only if it is done after some *yogasans*.

Prāṇ and the mind are closely related. When we are absorbed in deep thinking, our breathing slows down naturally. Whilst, when we are agitated and tensed, breathing moves faster than normal, quite unnaturally. When we are in deep sorrow, breathing becomes irregular and broken. This clearly proves that breathing process and the mind are deeply intertwined.

Importance of *Pranayam*

In physical terms, *pranayam* is a systematic and organized exercise of breathing that makes the lungs stronger, improves blood circulation along with making it pure, and relieves from almost all physical diseases. In this way, it makes us healthier from within. One should not forget the fact that the imbalances in breathing hinder the physiological functions, which later become psychological.

It is a known fact that most people use only 25% of the lungs' capacity in daily breathing. Due to this, all the remaining parts of the lungs remain inactive, which results in the emergence of multifarious ailments like asthma, tuberculosis, etc. Regularly performing *pranayam* helps curb all the maladies—including even psychic disturbances, like excitement, anxiety, fear, anger, disappointment, lasciviousness, and other mental perversions to vanish without any treatment from medical science. In addition, its daily performance also results in good memory power and improvement in the discrimination and observation tendency, resulting in the cultivation of spirituality in life.

Similarly, *prāṇ* and the mind are so much affiliated to each other that one cannot function in isolation of the other. The fluctuating mind is brought into a specific point of focus by controlling breathing through *pranayam*. The *Haṭha Yog Pradīpikā* mentions that *pranayam* helps in freeing the mind from untruthfulness, ignorance, and other sorrowful and painful experiences of both—the body and mind. Once in a state of *pranayam,* the aspirant can easily concentrate on the desired object or devotion to God.

Through a systematic exercise of breathing, the vital organs like the lungs become stronger, and thus it easily regulates blood circulation throughout the whole body. Most people do not breathe deeply in their daily life because either they do not know about the prominence of deep breathing, or they are always in a rush for worldly attainments. During normal breathing, only about 20 million pores in the lungs get oxygen, whereas the remaining 53 million pores remain deprived of fresh oxygen. As a result, they get affected by infectious diseases like tuberculosis, respiratory problems, and other manifold diseases like coughing, bronchitis, etc.

The continuous practice of *pranayam*, along with the practice of devotion, helps controlling mental abnormalities such as passion, lust, anxiety, despair, greed, etc., which have troubled everyone. Apart from that, the functions of cells improve in such a way that both—memory and rationality—grow wonderfully. An equally vital facet is that it increases our life span, for we learn to do very organized and systematic breathing, i.e. deep and slow breathing in our day to day life. Scientifically too, it is proven that impatient and short breathing triggers the appearance of innumerable maladies inside our body.

Thus, taking all the points into consideration, with the help of *pranayam* we can hone our life with both—sound body and sound mind, which is a must for the present generation. In addition, we can divert our nature from an extrovert (materialist) to an introvert (spiritualist), which is a key factor for spiritual life.

Guidelines for *Pranayam*

Generally speaking, one can find innumerable dos and don'ts mentioned in various books pertaining to *pranayam*. Nonetheless, the most significant factors are the guidance of an experienced *Yog* teacher; and moderation, balance, and the use of common sense. Additionally, it is also necessary to follow some basic rules of *pranayam* for deriving its benefits. If these rules are not followed, it can have manifold adverse effects on our health. So, a practitioner needs to be aware of the rules of performing *pranayam* which are as follows:

- *Pranayam* should be practiced on empty bowels or at least four hours after heavy meals and two hours after light meals.

- It should be practiced where adequate fresh air is available.

- The proper time for *pranayam* is in the morning, but it can be practiced even after sunset. It is advisable that the time and place of performing *pranayam* should be consistent.

- The sheet or cloth on which you sit must be a non-conductor of electricity. Loose and comfortable clothes made of fibre or cotton should be worn while practicing *pranayam*.

- *Pranayam* should be practiced after daily routines are completed like cleansing the mouth and relieving in the morning. If there is a problem of constipation, then mild laxatives (Ayurvedic medicines like *Triphalā*, etc.) can be taken before going to bed.

- Ways of performing *pranayam* may differ as per the season and also the mental attitude. Therefore, one should not forget that some *pranayams* may increase your body temperature while others may reduce or bring your body temperature to a moderate level.

- Pregnant women, hungry, or medically ill people should not practice *pranayam*. However, medically ill people can do it under the guidance of a *Yog* therapist.

- One should not be impatient; rather, one should practice *pranayam* slowly and cautiously—with confidence and vibrancy.

- One should not take bath for at least 20-30 minutes after practicing *pranayam*.

- One should always bear in mind that *pranayam* practiced without maintaining disciplines like timely eating, having a proper diet, regular working, etc., will not yield full benefits in spite of a daily practice of both—*Yog* and *pranayam*. There must be a disciplined life style as per the principles of the scriptures so that one would enjoy real peace and tranquility in life.

- The most essential point is the avoidance of strain and the use of unnecessary effort while doing *pranayam* because the lungs are such delicate organs that any misuse can easily injure them.

- It is not good for *pranayam* practitioners to either smoke or take tobacco of any kind.

- While practicing *pranayam* for the first time, myriad side-effects like sensation of itching, feelings of heat or cold, feelings of lightness or heaviness etc. may appear. Nevertheless, one should remember that these are due to the purification and the removal of unwanted products from our body, and these symptoms only persist temporarily.

- Remember God's Name along with *pranayam*. Mentally chant "Radhey" during inhalation and "Krishna" during exhalation. You can also remember any other Names of God as per your wish.

- Eyes should be totally closed so that the mind does not get diverted.

- Mild smile on your face while practicing *pranayam* brings a positive feel to the exercise. Let there be no sign of any tension or anxiety on the face.

- You should not over-exert yourself while practicing *pranayam* or else it may adversely affect your health.

- One can sit in any meditative position, such as Padmasan, Vajrasan, or Siddhasan, etc. but the spine and neck should be straight—without any stiffness in the body.

Advantages of *Pranayam*

It is quite natural that one can derive several benefits, both physical and mental, by the regular and organized practice of *pranayam*. However, if it is done with *Roop Dhyan* of God, i.e. meditation on the Forms of God, it will surely yield much better outcome. The person who practices *pranayam* in a routine and time-bound program of about 20-30 minutes, along with various *yogasans*, will certainly benefit from the following points that are mentioned briefly below:

- The three *doshas*, viz. *vāt*, *pitta*, and *kaph*, get adjusted in harmonious proportion and the abnormalities in them are removed, which helps uproot all the probable diseases that originate in the body.

- Digestive power gets toned and activated, and the various maladies pertaining to digestive organs are treated naturally.

- Ailments pertaining to the lungs, heart, and brain are cured.

- Other severe ailments like obesity, diabetes, cholesterol, constipation, flatulence, acidity, respiratory troubles, allergy, migraine, high blood pressure, diseases associated with the kidneys, sexual disorders of males and females, etc. are remarkably cured.

- Resistance power against different diseases increases, which is very essential for a sound body and mind.

- Even hereditary problems like diabetes and heart disease can be cured without any side effects.

- The problem of stress in the mind is solved as conditions like tension or depression are eliminated because there naturally emerges stability and tranquility in the mind. A sense of satiety and vigor, or enthusiasm, appears. Psychological conditions like depression, monotony, etc. are easily relieved.

- There is a redemption from negative thoughts, which assists the mind to develop the inclination of creative and constructive thinking.

- Immunity of the body increases immensely, resulting in the control of genetic diseases like diabetes and heart problems.

- Hair loss, facial wrinkle, poor eyesight, ageing, absent-mindedness, etc. are cured slowly and naturally without any side effects.

- There appears brilliance on practitioner's face that brings a peaceful attitude to him.

Radhey Krishna Pranayams

1. Vibhagiya Pranayam (Sectional Breathing)

Vibhagiya Pranayam is an introductory breathing practice for all kinds of *pranayams*. It rectifies the breathing pattern and increases lungs' capacity so that the practitioners can perform complete breathing. It soothes both—the body and mind—wonderfully. This breathing can be categorized into three kinds:

a. Diaphragmatic / Abdominal Breathing

Procedure

i. Sit in any meditative position with the spine and head erect.

ii. Inhale slowly (while chanting "Radhey" in the mind) and inflate your abdomen to your capacity, without any strain. In this position, the diaphragm at the base of the lungs will move down, and the lungs will expand.

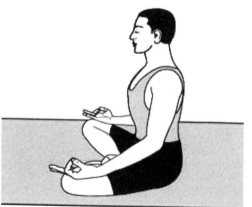

iii. Do not expand your chest or move the shoulders, rather just feel the expansion and contraction of the abdomen.

iv. Contract the abdominal muscles while exhaling slowly (while chanting "Krishna" in the mind).

v. In this position, the diaphragm will move upward and the lungs will contract.

vi. This is one round. Go up to 10 rounds of this *pranayam*.

b. Intercostal / Thoracic Breathing

Procedure

i. Sit in any meditative position with the spine and head erect.

ii. Inhale slowly (Radhey) and deeply, inflating your chest area to your ability.

iii. Feel the movement of your ribcage outward and upward along with the expansion of the lungs while breathing in air.

iv. Ensure there is no movement of the diaphragm and the abdomen in this breathing.

v. Exhale (Krishna) while relaxing the chest muscles.

vi. Be conscious of the contraction of the ribcage along with the air flowing out of the lungs.

vii. This completes one round. Repeat the process 10 times.

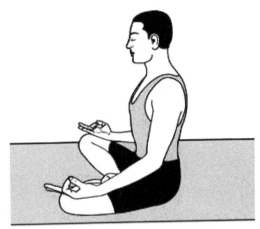

c. Clavicular / Upper Breathing

Procedure

i. Sit in any meditative position with the spine and head erect.

ii. Using the upper lobes of your lungs, inhale (Radhey) fully and let your shoulders and collarbones rise upward and backward.

iii. Do not move the chest and abdominal area.

iv. Now exhale (Krishna) slowly and come into the initial position.

v. Continue the process about 10 times.

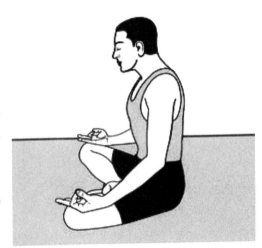

2. Jai Radhey Pranayam (Full Yogic Breathing)

Jai Radhey Pranayam is the integration of Abdominal, Thoracic, and Clavicular Breathing. It is also called Full Yogic Breathing. Full Yogic Breathing is a foundation to the advanced *pranayams* techniques. It is commenced with Abdominal breathing and continued with the Thoracic and Clavicular breathings.

Procedure

i. Sit in any meditative position, keeping the spine and head erect.

ii. Inhale (Radhey) slowly and deeply, using the bottom part of the lungs, let the abdomen swell; then use the middle part of the lungs to expand the chest and then finally using the upper portion of the lungs, allow your shoulders and collarbones to move up.

iii. Now exhale (Krishna) slowly, depressing the shoulders; then your chest and finally relax the abdomen.

iv. Breathe in and out equally and rhythmically.

v. Continue the process for 10-20 rounds.

Benefits

✓ As maximum portion of the lungs is used in this *pranayam*, it maximizes the intake of oxygen from the atmosphere and expel of carbon dioxide.

✓ Not only does it work as a tonic for the body, it also purifies the blood.

✓ It is a great boon for those who have high blood pressure.

✓ It tranquilizes and stabilizes the mind, and thus easily helps control anger.

✓ This *pranayam* can even be done when you feel tired, angry, or anxious so that you can easily overcome these anxieties.

✓ This Full *Yogic* Breathing defends us from the impacts of pollution.

✓ This *pranayam* also revitalizes the body against the physical fatigue and mental depression.

✓ It relaxes muscular restriction in and around the diaphragm, ribs, and chest, resultantly lets the breath flow freely and naturally.

3. Kapalbhati Pranayam

Kapalbhati has been derived from a Sanskrit word; "*Kapal*" means "forehead" and "*bhati*," "glow." Therefore, the practice of Kapalbhati enhances glow on the forehead.

This *pranayam* is most effective in Vajrasan. However, if you cannot conveniently adopt that posture, you may sit in any other meditative posture.

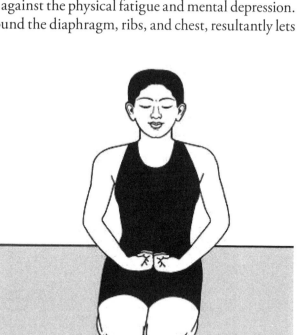

Procedure

i. Sit in any meditative pose, with the spine and head erect. Relax your shoulders.

ii. Bring your hands to Brahma Mudra (See page 312), i.e. clench your fists and place them side-by-side above the navel. The little finger side of the hands should be toward the navel. The folded fingers of both hands should be adjacent to each other.

iii. First inhale (Radhey) slowly and then exhale (Krishna) forcefully by contracting your

295

abdomen.

iv. Allow the abdominal muscles to relax; thereby, the breath will naturally flow into the lungs. In this *pranayam*, effort is not used for inhalation; it occurs naturally.

v. In Kapalbhati, it is important to note that the breathing should be performed with the use of the stomach; there should not be any use of the chest and the shoulders.

vi. While practicing this, one should be aware of the contraction and especially, the relaxing expansion of the abdominal muscles to allow the air in.

vii. This completes one cycle; practice 60 cycles. This makes one *chakra*. In the beginning you may get tired after 10 to 15 cycles. Over a few weeks, you will be able to reach one *chakra*.

viii. With a regular practice, you can go up to five *chakras*, with short breaks in between.

Timing

- The exhalation is done in $1/4^{th}$ of a second. The inhalation is done in $3/4^{th}$ of a second. So, one cycle of Kapalbhati Pranayam is completed in one second. In this way, one *chakra* takes 60 seconds.

- Beginners may find this strenuous. In that case, they may complete one cycle of Kapalbhati in two or three seconds.

Benefits

✓ With a regular practice of Kapalbhati Pranayam, the abdominal problems such as constipation, piles, etc. are alleviated and fat is removed from the abdominal area.

✓ Many *Yog* therapists consider it as a useful *pranayam* in diabetes, emphysema, gastric, hepatitis B, allergic problems, acidity, Parkinson's disease, liver cirrhosis, sinusitis, snoring, concentration, tuberculosis, cancer, and AIDS.

✓ It activates the kidneys tremendously, which are delicate but vital organs in our body.

✓ It also balances the *iḍā* (left psychic passage) and the *piṅgalā* (right psychic passage) nerves, which aid to increase concentration.

✓ It helps releive respiratory problems such as bronchitis, asthma, etc. and the elimination of various toxins to assist in the purification of blood in the body.

✓ It has other multitudinous effects such as balancing and vitalizing the nervous system, removal of lethargy, and healing diseases—thyroid, tonsils, and other ailments of the throat—without any side effects.

✓ It balances three *doṣhas* (*vāt*, *pitta*, and *kaph*) of the human body; the disorder of these elements triggers several diseases in the human body.

✓ Kapalbhati entirely eliminates blockages in arteries and controls cholesterol.

✓ Feminine diseases like uterus cysts, breast cysts, cancer cysts, or any type of cysts in the body are perfectly dissolved without any surgical operation.

✓ The daily practice of Kapalbhati Pranayam can even control excess hair loss.

✓ It increases oxygen supply and helps in purifying the blood.

✓ If this *pranayam* is practiced before *Roop Dhyan* Meditation, concentration increases and mind remains away from negative thoughts.

Contraindications

-   People with high blood pressure, heart problems, spinal problems, epilepsy, hernia, gastric ulcer, slipped-disc, and cervical spondylitis should not do this *pranayam*. It is also prohibited during menstrual periods and advanced stages of pregnancy.

4. Bhastrika Pranayam

Bhastrika has been derived from the Sanskrit word "*Bhastrika*" that refers to the bellows used by a blacksmith. Just as a bellow increases the flow of air into the fire producing more heat, similarly the forceful expansion and contraction of the lungs enhance the heat inside our body.

This *pranayam* can be done in three speeds—fast, medium, and slow. Beginners should do it in slow speed, and gradually—over months—should increase the speed, under the guidance of a *Yog* instructor.

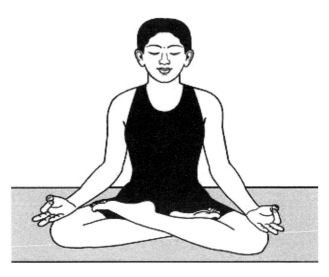

Procedure

i.   Sit in any meditative position with the spine and head erect.

ii. Now, relax the whole body and mind, and then close both eyes.

iii. Inhale deeply and forcefully (Radhey).

iv. Then, exhale (Krishna) with a forceful abdominal contraction.

v.   The length of time for inhalation and exhalation should be equal.

vi. Breathe in and out equally and rhythmically throughout the practice.

vii. This finishes one cycle; initially begin with 10 cycles, and afterwards this can be extended up to 50-100 cycles.

Note: As in Anulom Vilom, this *pranayam* can be practiced in either a medium, or fast pace. Nonetheless, in the initial stages, it should be practiced in a medium pace only. A healthy and physically fit person can do this *pranayam* in a fast pace. While practicing it, the facial expression should not be distorted and the body should be kept steady. Feeling giddiness and nauseated are the indications of doing the exercise incorrectly. During such a situation, consult a *Yog* therapist, or a doctor at the earliest.

Benefits

✓ One of the benefits of Bhastrika Pranayam is that it provides respiratory comfort to asthma patients.

- The rapid movements of the diaphragm massage the abdominal organs and help induce digestion.
- This practice burns up the toxins: *vāt* (wind), *pitta* (bile), and *kaph* (phlegm) due to the rapid exchange of oxygen and carbon dioxide in and out of the lungs.
- It balances and strengthens the nervous system, which tranquilizes the mind and builds up concentration to a great extent.
- It cures the diseases like cold, cough, allergy, and also respiratory diseases.
- It tones up the lungs by supplying adequate oxygen.
- With a regular practice of this *pranayam*, ailments related with the throat like thyroid, tonsils, and others are alleviated or even cured.
- It also balances three *doshas*—*vāt*, *pitta*, and *kaph*.
- It stabilizes *prāṇ* and calms the mind which is so supportive in performing *Roop Dhyan* Meditation.

Contraindications
- People with high blood pressure, heart problems, spine-related maladies, epilepsy, hernia, and gastric ulcer should not perform this *pranayam*. People with pulmonary ailments, such as chronic Bronchitis, Tuberculosis, etc. should also avoid it.

5. Surya Anulom Vilom Pranayam
Procedure
i. Sit in any meditative position with your spine and head well erect.

ii. Apply Nasagra Mudra as in Anulom Vilom Pranayam (See page 299) and close the left nostril with your ring finger.

iii. Now inhale (Radhey) and exhale (Krishna) through the right nostril only.

iv. Make sure the left nostril remains closed throughout the practice.

v. Comparatively, exhalation should be longer than inhalation.

vi. Continue the method for 10-20 times.

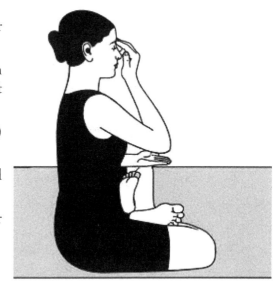

Benefits
- It is helpful in treating nose related allergies.
- This *pranayam* helps reduce weight if practiced daily before breakfast, lunch, dinner, and night sleep.

Contraindications
- People with high blood pressure, heart problems, and those who are underweight, should not practice this *pranayam*.

6. Chandra Anulom Vilom Pranayam

Procedure

i. Sit in any meditative position with the spine and head erect.

ii. Assume Nasagra Mudra like in Anulom Vilom Pranayam and close the right nostril with the thumb.

iii. Inhale (Radhey) and exhale (Krishna) through the left nostril.

iv. The right nostril will remain closed throughout.

v. Duration of exhalation should be longer than inhalation.

vi. Continue the process for 10-20 times.

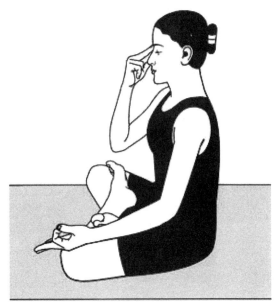

Benefits

✓ Chandra Anulom Vilom Pranayam is a blessing for treating the nose-related allergies.

✓ In contrast to Surya Anulom Vilom, this *pranayam* helps gain weight if practiced regularly prior to breakfast, lunch, dinner, and night sleep.

Contraindications

- This *pranayam* should not be practiced by people suffering from obesity and also by those with other allergies.

7. Anulom Vilom Pranayam (Nadi Shuddi Pranayam)

Procedure

i. Sit in any meditative position with your spine and head well erect.

ii. Keep the whole body relaxed and loose.

iii. Place the index and long fingers of the right hand (left hand in the case of left-handers) on the forehead.

iv. The little finger will remain a little curled.

v. Keep your elbow in front, with the upper arm parallel to the floor. This is called Nasagra Mudra.

vi. Now, close your right nostril with your thumb. Exhale (Krishna) completely through your left nostril.

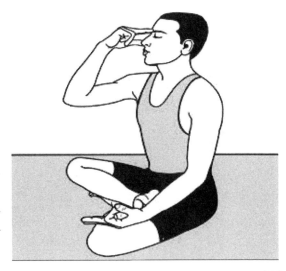

vii. Then, breathe in through the left nostril (Radhey) with the right nostril remaining closed.

viii. Next, close the left nostril with the ring finger and breathe out (Krishna) through the right nostril.

ix. Then, breath in (Radhey) through the right nostril.

x. Again, close your right nostril and breathe out (Krishna) through the left nostril.

xi. Make sure you breathe in and out equally and rhythmically.

xii. In this *pranayam*, always make use of the chest while breathing.

xiii. This completes one cycle; perform 10-20 cycles.

Note: Anulom Vilom Pranayam can be done in three ways—low, or medium, or fast pace. Initially, this *pranayam* should be practiced in a slow, or medium pace only.

Benefits
✓ It helps purify the 720 million *nāḍīs* of the body, making it lustrous and powerful by harmonizing the *prāṇ* at different parts of the body.

✓ Almost all kinds of diseases associated with *vāt* problems such as rheumatism, urinary and reproductive diseases are alleviated or even cured.

✓ The usual diseases like cold, cataract, sinus, mild fevers, eye and ear problems, cough, etc. get healed naturally.

✓ Most significantly, it relieves mental stress and decreases the level of cholesterol in the blood.

✓ It also cures different heart maladies like heart attack, etc. along with opening blockages in the heart arteries.

✓ It regulates pathogenic cholesterol, triglycerides, H.D.L., and L.D.L., which makes the arterial channels clear for effective blood flow in the heart.

✓ As it induces positive thoughts in the mind of the practitioners, the aspirant feels fearless and peaceful.

✓ It is quite beneficial in alleviating various ailments such as high blood pressure, arthritis, ligaments, Parkinson's disease, paralysis, migraine, depression, asthma, and allergy.

8. Ujjayi Pranayam
Procedure
i. Sit in any meditative position with the spine, neck, and head straight.

ii. Now, relax your shoulders and place the hands in any *mudra* on the knees.

iii. Then, close both eyes and relax the entire body.

iv. Concentrate on the nostrils, feel the air going in and coming out through the nostrils.

v. After 2-3 normal breaths, shift your concentration to the throat.

vi. Then, inhaling (Radhey) deeply and slowly through either of the two nostrils, contract the throat as if you are breathing through a narrow pipe (in the throat).

vii. Due to the constriction of the respiratory passage, the incoming breath will produce a soft sound like "urrmh," as if you are snorting. It may be a low sound, and though it should be audible to you, someone sitting a few feet away from you may not be able to hear it.

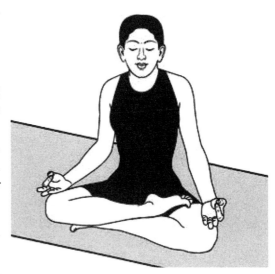

viii. Then close one of the nostrils with your thumb and exhale (Krishna) completely through the other. You may use either of the nostrils for exhalation, but alternatively.

ix. The time for inhalation and exhalation should always be the same.

x. This is one cycle of Ujjayi Pranayam; repeat up to 15-20 cycles.

Benefits

- ✓ Ujjayi Pranayam has a calming and soothing effect on the body.
- ✓ As it tranquilizes the nervous system, it has a positive influence on the mind, which helps relieve tension and other negative thoughts.
- ✓ Insomnia is healed totally if one performs it under the supervision of a *Yog* expert.
- ✓ It releases and enhances psychic energy, and hence it is preferred by many long-term *Yog* practitioners.
- ✓ Particularly, the disorders of the *dhātu* (semen), marrow, bone, blood, fat, flesh, and skin are removed naturally.
- ✓ In case of fluid retention too, it aids well.
- ✓ It is quite effectual in thyroid related problems.
- ✓ It greatly aids in strengthening the capacity of will-power.
- ✓ It is equally useful in curing heart diseases as well.
- ✓ It stimulates blood circulation, metabolism, and olfactory glands.
- ✓ It opens alveoli in the lungs, which helps the lungs absorb more oxygen.

Contraindications

- People who are introvert should not do this *pranayam*. Heart patients should not strain themselves and should practice one round of Jai Radhey Pranayam between two rounds of Ujjayi Pranayam.

9. Sheetali Pranayam

Procedure

i. Sit in any meditative position, with your spine and head erect.

ii. Now, relax your shoulders and place the hands on the knees in any *mudra*.

iii. Now, close both eyes and relax the whole body.

iv. Stick out your tongue and roll the sides of the tongue up, forming a tube shape.

v. Slowly and deeply, breathe in (Radhey) through this tube in such a way that the breath will produce a sound similar to rushing wind.

vi. At the end of the inhalation (Radhey), draw the tongue back, close your mouth and exhale (Krishna) deeply through your nose.

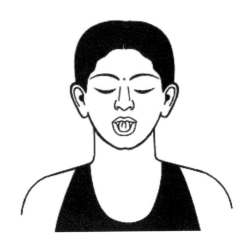

vii. This completes one cycle; perform up to 15-20 cycles.

Benefits
- ✓ Sheetali Pranayam benefits in purifying the blood.
- ✓ It also has a cooling effect on the body and the mind.
- ✓ Interestingly, it even quenches thirst and hunger, making one feel satisfied.
- ✓ It removes tension and anxiety and relaxes the mind.
- ✓ It helps alleviate allergies, as it soothes the nerves.
- ✓ Along with the improvement in digestion, Sheetali Pranayam also reduces acidity.
- ✓ High blood pressure gets alleviated if it is done regularly.
- ✓ It can even be done during the hot day to cool down the body.
- ✓ According to Swami Swatmarama in *Haṭha Yog Pradīpikā*—the practitioner becomes young and attractive by practicing this *pranayam*; it removes excess heat accumulated in the system, decreases the excess biles, rectifies the disorders of the spleen and works on fever.
- ✓ It soothes the entire nervous system; it stimulates the parasympathetic nervous system, thus inducing muscular relaxation and stress management.

Contraindications
- - People with low blood pressure should not practice it. This should not be done when a person has the common cold, throat-related problems, bronchitis, etc.
- - It should not be performed during winter and in cold places.

10. Sheetkari Pranayam

Sheetkari Pranayam is a breathing technique involving hissing act that causes a cooling effect on the entire body. People, who cannot roll the sides of the tongue due to genetic problem, can do Sheetkari Pranayam.

Procedure
i. Sit in any meditative position with the spine, neck, and head erect.

ii. Relax your shoulders and place the hands on the knees, forming any *mudra*.

iii. Now, close both eyes and relax the whole body.

iv. Clenching your teeth, flatten or fold your tongue against the soft palate.

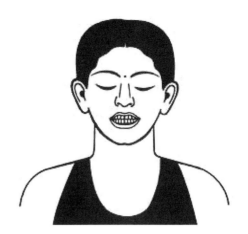

v. Then, breathe in (Radhey) slowly and deeply through the holes between the teeth.

vi. Shut your mouth and exhale (Krishna) through your nostrils.

vii. This completes one cycle; perform up to 15-20 cycles.

Benefits

✓ Its benefits are the same as those of Sheetali Pranayam (See page 301).

✓ Besides, Sheetkari is effectual for cooling the mouth; good for the teeth and gums; it even cures pyorrhea.

✓ It cools the body by decreasing the body temperature; thus it even helps endure very hot weather.

✓ It is highly recommended during a fasting.

Contraindications

- The limitations of it are the same as those of Sheetali Pranayam. Moreover, those with less teeth, no teeth, or artificial teeth should not practice this *pranayam*. They can, however, do Sheetali Pranayam.

11. Bhramari Pranayam

The word "*Bhramari*" has been derived from "*Bhramer*," which means "a humming bumblebee." In this *pranayam*, you shut your lips, and you gently and smoothly make a sound like a humming bumblebee in your throat. This *pranayam* gives a tingling sensation while performing it. It is done generally after performing Anulom Vilom Pranayam for its full effect.

Procedure

i. Sit in any meditative pose, keeping the spine and head erect.

ii. Now, close both eyes and relax the whole body.

iii. Then, fold your arms at elbows and shut the earlobes or close the ear holes with the index fingers.

iv. Make sure your elbows stay in a straight line with the shoulders so that air passes through the respiratory system without any intervention.

v. Now inhale deeply (Radhey) and while exhaling (Krishna), produce a humming sound like that of a bumblebee or an aeroplane.

vi. This is one cycle of Bhramari Pranayam; repeat it 5-10 times.

Note: One may feel cold and tingling sensation, so it advisable that breathing should never be stopped under any circumstances. Ensure that there is no strain involved while you are humming. Do not inhale or exhale any deeper or longer than you are comfortable. Always breathe through your nose as it not only warms the air to your body temperature, but it also helps you to breathe deeply and longer.

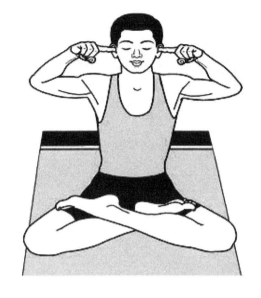

Meditation

While doing Bhramari Pranayam, with your eyes closed, you may imagine yourself to be a bee creating a humming sound. Just as a bumblebee hums around and drinks nectar from a flower, visualize yourself moving around the lotus feet of your *Ishta Dev* (the form of God that you worship).

Benefits

✓ Bhramari Pranayam is a very special *pranayam* for servicing the parts of the brain.
✓ The problems of insomnia and high blood pressure are easily treated.
✓ It is advantageous in heart diseases, thyroid problems, respiratory ailments such as asthma and diabetes.
✓ It also helps reduce depression and release mental stress and anxiety.

Contraindications

- People suffering from severe ear infections should not perform it until the infection clears up.

12. Shyam Uchcharan (Shyam Chanting)

"Shyam" is one of the Names among Shree Krishna's infinite Names. Like the sound "*Oṁ*" is used for chanting by different *Yog* practitioners, we will use the Divine Name "Shyam" for chanting in our JKYog. Repetition of the Divine Name "Shyam" dissolves the mind in its Divine source and helps largely to connect our minds with Shree Krishna, His Names, His Qualities, His Pastimes, His Abode, and His Associates (Saints). Thus, the chanting of "Shyam" several times loudly and rhythmically purifies the body, mind, and atmosphere.

Procedure

i. Sit in any meditative position, keeping the spine and head erect.

ii. Now close both eyes; relax the whole body entirely and place the hands on the knees, forming any *mudra*.

iii. Then, concentrate on the respiration process and meditate on one of the Divinely Forms of Shyam.

iv. Now, breathe in (Radhey) slowly and deeply through the nostrils.

v. After that, open your mouth and with a slow exhalation, start chanting the Divine word "Shya……am" very slowly—with a rhythm—till your lungs are fully contracted.

vi. While chanting the Divine Name "Shyam," feel the Divine vibrations produced in the heart area. Also, meditate on one of His sentient and dynamic Forms in your mind.

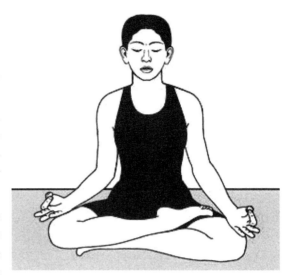

vii. There should not be any pause in chanting until you have exhaled completely.

viii. This is one cycle of Shyam Uchcharan; repeat it up to 5-10 times.

Benefits

✓ The power of concentration increases amazingly if Shyam Uchcharan is done regularly.

✓ The problems of insomnia and blood pressure are easily cured.

✓ It has a healthy effect on the heart diseases and diabetes.

✓ Shyam Uchcharan also contributes in alleviating depression and releasing mental stress and anxiety by cleansing the mind and controlling emotions that help divert the mind naturally—from material aspects to the spiritual world of ever increasing Bliss.

✓ It not only relaxes the practitioner physically, mentally, and emotionally, but also charges the surrounding atmosphere with positive thoughts and Divinely vibrations.

13. Jagadguru Kripaluji Pranayam

Procedure

i. Stand up straight—in an upright position, with both feet joined together and arms by your sides—i.e. Saral Tadasan (See page 25).

ii. Then, spread your feet about a foot apart.

iii. Either close the eyes completely or fix them on a certain point in front of you.

iv. Now with a deep inhalation (Radhey), slightly move the arms backward at first; then rotate both hands forward—through 360 degrees—so that the arms make a complete vertical circle.

v. Make sure your arms are stretched and straight while rotating.

vi. There should be continuous inhalation (Radhey) in the course of rotational movement of the arms.

vii. After finishing one cycle of rotation, when the arms reach the shoulder level, with the palms facing upward, make fists with the thumb inside and fold the arms at the elbows.

viii. Now without losing momentum, exhale (Krishna) forcefully and pull the forearms backward—jerking the whole arm—bringing them by the sides of the chest.

ix. Make sure forming the fists and pulling the forearms backward along with folding the elbows are done simultaneously while exhaling (Krishna).

x. For ease and effectiveness, one can even stand on tiptoes while exhaling (Krishna).

xi. This completes one cycle.

xii. At the beginning, you can start with 10 cycles and then gradually go upto 30-40 cycles.

Benefits
✓ Its benefits are similar to that of general Bhastrika Pranayam (See page 297).
✓ Moreover, it is more effective and intensive than general Bhastrika because the rotation of your arms aids more expansion and contraction of the lungs.

Contraindications
- The contraindications of Jagadguru Kripaluji Pranayam are the same as those of Bhastrika (See page 297).
- Besides, persons with defects in the shoulder joints, high blood pressure, or respiratory ailments like asthma, etc. should not perform this *pranayam*.

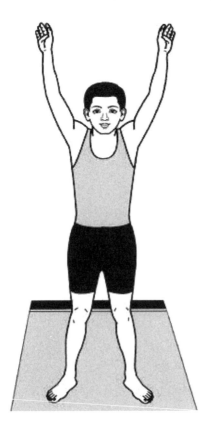
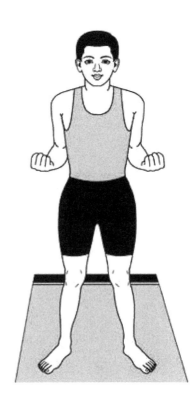

VII. Selected *Mudras* (Symbolic Gestures)

Introduction to *Mudras* (Symbolic Gestures)

The word "*Mudra*" is derived from the root word "*Mud,*" meaning "to be glad or to have a delight in." *Mudras* are postures that bring delight to the deities and also to the performers, and cause the *drava* (dissolution) of the mind. However, the term *mudra* also denotes "seal" because the hand gestures seal the body, thus aiding to fetch joyousness to a large extent. A *mudra* also represents a spiritual gesture and an energetic seal of validity, which are used in the iconography and spiritual practice of Indian religions. They are the means of controlling the energy in the body and also the symbolic representations of our inner state. Persons who are even a bit sensitive to the body's vibrations or energies can easily feel that a change of mood can be experienced by the movement of one's hands. They begin to feel mentally more aware of our inner vibrations and energies. With a slight alertness, the multifarious inner states induced by the *mudras* become clearly noticeable. It is generally said that there are nearly 108 hand gestures, quite popular as sacred symbols among Hindus. Most *mudras* are performed with the hands and fingers and some involve the whole body.

Generally speaking, *mudras*, which are considered as the developed form of *asans*, have significant influences on our body. Basically, they are techniques to stimulate the glandular functions and the dormant psychic power centres with two facets of uses—physical and mental. In *asans*, sensory organs are major and *prāṇ* is minor, whilst in *mudras*, the sensory organs are minor, and *prāṇ* is the major one. To highlight the prominence of *mudras*, the scriptures clearly state:

नास्ति मुद्रा समं किञ्चित् सिद्धिदं क्षिति मण्डले।

nāsti mudrā samaṁ kiñchit siddhidam kṣhiti maṇḍale

"There are no other actions in this planet that can yield benefits like *mudras*." From the above mantra, one can easily realize the paramount importance of *mudrās* in both—mental and physical respects.

In *mudras* of the hand, the five fingers are used. Our body is built up of five elements. The five fingers represent and are directly linked to these five elements. The thumb, index finger, middle finger, ring finger, and little finger are the symbols of fire, air, space, earth, and water respectively. Moreover, such *mudras* are also the way to control the involuntary organs, which are associated with the different nerves of the body. In reality, they help one become conscious and closer to the inner energy. Aspirants can improve their *sādhanā* if they know the secret of *mudras* perfectly. They also enhance the consequences of *pranayam*, and nowadays it has become so common that while any *pranayam* is performed, at least one of the *mudras* is selected—to have additional effects.

There are many types of *mudras*, and amongst them, in Jagadguru Kripaluji Yog, we have chosen the most effective *mudras*. Most of these *mudras* are so natural that they can be practiced at any place, at any time, and under any circumstance. One also should not forget that they produce more advantages if done along with the meditative *asans* such as Padmasan, Vajrasan, Sukhasan, etc.

Mudras with Radhey Krishna Pranayams

In a simple sense, *mudra* is a physical attitude. We can send different messages to the brain by adopting a physical arrangement of the fingers and hands for carrying out a *mudra*.

The *Yogīs* take recourse to the various *mudras* in the practice of *pranayam* as well as meditation, and undeniably, this empowers *pranayam* with more beneficial results. The *Yogīs* have developed *mudras* that speed up various attitudes of the body and relate to the specific attitudes of the mind. Thereby, both—the psyche and the body—get involved. For Radhey Krishna Pranayams, where the involvement of the body and psyche are equally vital, these *mudras* help immensely.

These *mudras* can be performed at any time and any place. When these are practiced alone, one should breathe normally so that the mind becomes focused on perfoming the *mudras*.

1. Gyan Mudra / Dhyan Mudra

Procedure

i. Sit in any meditative pose.

ii. Join the tip of the thumb and the index finger.

iii. Make sure the remaining fingers remain straight.

iv. Palms should face downward.

v. Place your palms on the knees and relax the hands.

Benefits

✓ Gyan Mudra / Dhyan Mudra helps focus the mind.
✓ Its regular practice strengthens the nerves of the brain, which helps to control the psychological disorders like tension, insomnia, hysteria, headache, and agitation.
✓ It helps in sharpening your brain and improving the memory power.

2. Chin Mudra

Procedure

i. Sit in any meditative pose.

ii. Join the tip of the thumb and the index finger.

iii. Make sure the remaining fingers remain straight.

iv. Contrary to Gyan Mudra, the palms should face

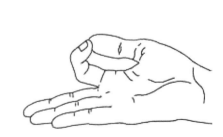

upward.

v. Now, rest the palms on the knees and then relax the hands.

Benefits

✓ The benefits of Chin Mudra are same as those of Gyan Mudra (See page 308).

✓ Besides, it creates a *prāṇic* circuit that helps in maintaining and redirecting *prāṇ* within the body.

✓ It also prevents insomnia.

3. Vayu Mudra

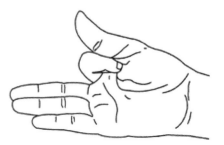

Procedure

i. Sit in any meditative pose.

ii. Place the tip of the index finger at the root of the thumb.

iii. Press the index finger with your thumb.

iv. Make sure the remaining fingers remain straight.

v. Place the palms on the knees and relax the hands completely.

Benefits

✓ Vayu Mudra is useful in treating wind-related problems such as arthritis, sciatica, gout, pain in the knees, gas, and even Parkisnson's disease.

✓ It also alleviates backache, neck problems, and blood circulation disorders.

✓ It gives relief in the neck and spinal pain.

4. Shunya Mudra (Akash Mudra)

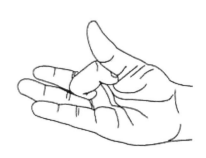

Procedure

i. Sit in any meditative pose.

ii. Place your middle finger at the root of the thumb.

iii. Press the middle finger with your thumb.

iv. Make sure the remaining fingers remain straight.

v. Place your palms on the knees and relax the hands.

vi. You may perform it as necessary, or perform thrice daily, for 15 minutes, as a course of treatment.

Benefits

✓ Shunya Mudra is immensely supportive in healing bone and heart-related problems.

✓ It alleviates throat and thyroid-related ailments.

✓ If practiced regularly, it assists in treating impaired hearing and other aural problems.

✓ It even cures numbness in any part of the body.

✓ Even the problems like nausea and vertigo can be overcome with a regular practice of Shunya Mudra.

Contraindications

- This *mudra* should be performed regularly until the disease is totally healed. It should be avoided while eating food or walking.

5. Prithvi Mudra

Procedure

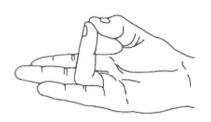

i. Sit in any meditative pose.

ii. Now join the tip of your ring finger with your thumb.

iii. Make sure the remaining fingers remain straight.

iv. Place your palms on the knees and then relax the hands.

v. You may do this *mudra* half an hour a day or thrice a day for fifteen minutes.

Benefits

✓ The regular performance of Prithvi Mudra helps to get rid of physical weakness.

✓ It assists in correcting poor digestion.

✓ It also increases *sattva guṇa*, develops the *prāṇ* (life-force), and replenishes the inadequacy of different vitamins.

6. Pran Mudra

Procedure

i. Sit in any meditative pose.

ii. Now join the tips of your little finger, ring finger, and thumb.

iii. Make sure the remaining fingers remain straight.

iv. Place your palms on the knees and then relax the hands.

Benefits

✓ Pran Mudra generates vitality and energy in the body.

✓ It alleviates various eye diseases.

✓ It removes tiredness from the body.

✓ Like Prithvi Mudra, it replenishes the deficiency of different vitamins too.

✓ It even unfolds the dormant *prāṇic* forces.

✓ If performed daily and sincerely, it increases immunity.

✓ Interestingly, it helps tolerate hunger and thirst during the period of *sādhanā*.

7. Apan Mudra

Procedure

i. Sit in any meditative pose.

ii. Now join the tips of the middle finger, ring finger, and thumb.

iii. Make sure the remaining fingers remain straight.

iv. Place your palms on the knees and then relax the hands.

Benefits

✓ Apan Mudra is most advantageous to diabetics.

✓ It helps in curing the heart-related problems.

✓ It even corrects the disorders of the brain, kidneys, teeth, and abdomen.

✓ Its long-term practice also normalizes urine problems, expels the toxins from the body, and purifies it.

✓ It transfers energy to the peripheral body.

✓ It also helps in constipation and urinary problems.

✓ It provides energy and makes the practitioners more self-confident.

8. Apan Vayu Mudra

Procedure

i. Sit in any meditative pose.

ii. Now combine the procedures of both—Apan Mudra (See page 311) and Vayu Mudra (See page 309), i.e. join the tips of the middle finger, ring finger, and thumb and place index finger-tip at the thumb-root, by pressing thumb with index finger.

iii. Only the little finger will remain straight.

iv. Lastly, place your palms on the knees and relax the hands.

v. You may do this *mudra* thrice a day for fifteen minutes.

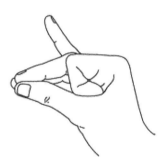

Benefits

✓ Problems like heart ailments, gas formation, insomnia, anxiety, asthma, high blood pressure, headache, rheumatism, and physical weakness are naturally alleviated by the daily performance of Apan Vayu Mudra.

✓ Those who feel difficulty in climbing up the stairs may perform this *mudra* while climbing to avoid exhaustion.

✓ It is also called "Lifesaver" and is the first aid for heart attacks.

9. Adi Mudra

Procedure

i. Sit in any meditative pose.

ii. Now, make fists with your thumbs covered by your fingers as shown in the figure.

iii. Place both the fists on your thighs and relax the arms.

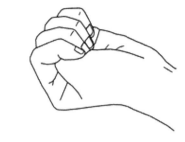

Benefits

✓ The upper parts of the lungs get fully utilized in Adi Mudra, thereby enhancing the effects of *pranayam*.

10. Brahma Mudra

Procedure

i. Sit in any meditative pose.

ii. Now, make two fists with your thumbs covered by your fingers.

iii. Then, place both fists on either side of the navel with the knuckles placed against each other.

iv. Ensure your palms face upward.

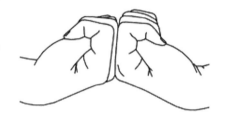

Benefits

✓ The entire chest and lungs are brought into play if this *mudra* is practiced along with the *pranayams*.

11. Varun Mudra

Procedure

i. Sit in any meditative pose.

ii. Now, join the tips of the little finger and the thumb.

iii. Make sure the remaining fingers remain straight.

iv. Place your palms on the knees and relax the hands.

v. You may do this *mudra* thrice a day for fifteen minutes.

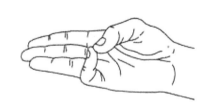

Benefits

✓ Varun Mudra plays a great role in retaining body moisture, which makes the skin supple and glowing.

✓ The main purpose of doing this *mudra* is the healing of skin diseases, blood impurities, acne, pimples, and other ailments caused by water deficiency in the body.

✓ It is also effective in the following disorders—dryness of the eyes, dryness of the digestive tract (especially mouth, throat, and intestines), indigestion, degeneration of the joint-cartilage, osteo-arthritis, anaemia, cramps, deficiency of hormones, oliguria (scanty urination), scanty semen (oligospermia), and tongue disorders.

Contraindications

- Those who have cough problems should avoid it.

12. Surya Mudra

Procedure

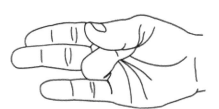

i. Sit in any meditative pose.

ii. Now, place your ring finger at the root of the thumb.

iii. Make sure the remaining fingers remain straight.

iv. Lastly, place your palms on the knees and relax the hands.

v. You may practice it daily twice, for 5 to 15 minutes.

Benefits

✓ Surya Mudra helps reduce weight, increase the moisture in the body, and induce digestion wonderfully.

✓ It reduces depression and cholesterol levels in the blood, and induces vitality.

✓ Many *Yog* therapists consider it highly useful in the treatment of diabetes, liver problems, and the enhancement of the digestion power.

✓ This *mudra* helps reduce fat, thus helps in weight loss.

✓ It releases the practitioners from anxiety and mental burden.

Contraindications

- Surya Mudra should not be practiced by feeble persons, or during the hot season. Also, it becomes ineffective if done for a long time.

13. Khechari Mudra

Procedure

i. Sit in any meditative pose, with both—the head and spine—erect, and the hands in Dhyan / Chin Mudra (See page 308).

ii. Before closing your eyes, relax the whole body and then roll your tongue backward and raise upward in such a way that the lower part of the tongue touches the upper palate.

iii. Without any strain, roll the tip of the tongue as far back as possible.

iv. Now breathing slowly and deeply, practice Ujjayi Pranayam for as long as possible.

v. If the tongue gets tired, relax for a few seconds.

vi. This ends one round; repeat this *mudra* for up to five rounds.

Benefits

✓ It activates various pressure points located at the back of the mouth and the nasal cavity, which affect the whole body.
✓ It massages different glands by activating the secretion of hormones and saliva.
✓ It assists in remaining calm and patient by decreasing the feeling of hunger and thirst.
✓ Besides, it is tremendously effectual for inner healing as it helps store energy in the body.

Contraindications

- Persons suffering from tongue ulcers, or other mouth problems should not practice this *mudra*.

14. Bhoochari Mudra

Procedure

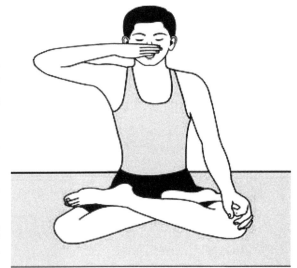

i. Come into any meditative pose.

ii. While keeping both—the head and spine—erect, form either Dhyan or Chin Mudra (See page 308) with the left hand.

iii. Place the left hand with Dhyan or Chin Mudra on the left knee.

iv. Slowly, raise your right hand exactly in front of the face.

v. Keep your right elbow pointing sideward, making it parallel to the floor.

vi. In this pose, your palm faces downward, with all fingers joined together and the side of the thumb touches the top part of the upper lip.

vii. Fix your eyes on the tip of the little finger for 30-40 seconds, without blinking.

viii. Then, remove your hand and focus into a blank space at the same location of the little finger.

ix. Ensure your mind remains clear of any thoughts; do not distract your mind from the space in front of your face.

x. Stay in this state for as long as possible with normal breathing.

xi. This is one round; practice this *mudra* for about 3-5 rounds.

Benefits

✓ Bhoochari Mudra's benefits are the same as those of Nasikagra Drishti (See page 318) and Shambhavi Mudras (See page 319).

- ✓ Additionally, this *mudra* helps in improving concentration power and tranquility of the mind.

Contraindication
- Those with eye diseases should not perform this *mudra*.

15. Akashi Mudra (Concentration into the Inner Space)

Procedure
i. Sit in any meditative pose.

ii. Keep the head and spine erect and the hands in either Dhyan / Chin Mudra (See page 308).

iii. Close both eyes for 30-40 seconds and relax the whole body.

iv. Assuming Khechari Mudra (See page 313), roll your tongue backward against the palate.

v. Focus the eyes at the *Āgyā Chakra* (centre between the eyebrows) as you would do in Shambhavi Mudra (See page 319) and perform Ujjayi Pranayam (See page 300).

vi. Simultaneously, move your head back at an angle of 45 degrees.

vii. Now lock your arms, pushing hands on the knees.

viii. Perform it with ease with very slow and deep breathing in this position.

ix. To return back to the initial state, loosen your arms freely; free yourself from the Khechari and Shambhavi Mudras and stop Ujjayi Pranayam.

x. Take a few breaths with alertness into the inner space and then repeat it again.

xi. Repeat the steps above for 3-5 times.

Benefits
- ✓ As Akashi Mudra is the combination of Khechari Mudra (See page 313), Shambhavi Mudra (See page 319), and Ujjayi Pranayam (See page 300), it increases mental peace and helps develop control over the senses.
- ✓ It even helps in controlling the thoughts and indirectly increasing the level of consciousness.

Contraindications
- Those with high blood pressure and mental disorders should not perform this *mudra*.

16. Bhairav Mudra (Fierce Attitude)

Procedure
i. Sit in any meditative pose.

ii. Keep your head and spine erect.

iii. Now, relax the whole body.

iv. Then, bring your cupped right hand on top of the left cupped hand in such a way that both

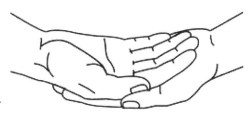

palms face upward, with elbows facing sideward.

v. Now, place both hands on the lap below the navel.

vi. Keep your hands steady.

vii. Lastly, close the eyes and relax the whole body.

Note: When your right hand is placed on top, it is the Shiv aspect—Bhairav Mudra. When the left is on top it is Bhairavi Mudra, the Shakti aspect—consciousness and manifestation.

Benefits
✓ It enhances the benefits of *pranayams* and meditation.
✓ Its regular practice alleviates the feeling of fear or anxiety.

Contraindications
- People with low blood pressure should not attempt this *mudra*.

17. Shankh Mudra

Procedure
i. Place your left thumb inside the right fist by closing all the fingers of the right hand.

ii. Then, join the tip of the left index finger with that of the right thumb.

iii. This makes a shape of a conch, which is Shankh Mudra.

iv. Give pressure to the right fingers, by pressing the remaining left fingers.

v. Likewise, it can be done by alternate set of hands.

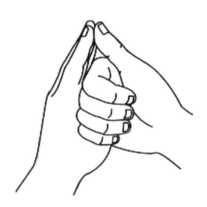

Benefits
✓ Shankh Mudra helps alleviate all disorders related to the stomach.
✓ It increases appetite by correcting the digestive system.
✓ The nervous system gets activated to perfection.
✓ Additionally, disorders in the vocal system, throat, and thyroid glands are completely cured by regular and systematic practice.

18. Shaktisanchalini Mudra

Procedure
i. Comfortably sit in Vajrasan (See page 113).

ii. Now pull the genital muscles inward strongly as if trying to stop urine, and then release it.

iii. Repeat the process about 20-30 times.

Benefits

✓ Shaktisanchalini Mudra has great effect on the reproductive organs as they are toned by regular movement.

✓ Additionally, exhaustion in the body is removed easily by regular practice of this *mudra*.

19. Yoni Mudra (Attitude of the Womb)

Procedure

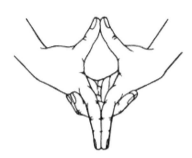

i. Sit in any meditative pose.

ii. Keep your head and spine erect.

iii. Now, relaxing the whole body, bring your palms together in such a way that the fingers and thumbs remain straight and point opposite to the body.

iv. Joining the pads of the index fingers together, interlock your little, ring, and middle fingers.

v. Join pads of your thumbs together and bring them toward the body.

vi. Slowly place the hands on the lap below the navel so that the thumbs come closer to the navel.

vii. Keeping your hands steady, close the eyes and relax the whole body.

Benefits

✓ As the fingers are interlocked, there is a flow of energy from the right hand to the left.

✓ It also aids in harmonizing the activities of both the hemispheres of the brain—the right and the left.

✓ The most significant point is that it gives stability to the mind and the body during meditation.

20. Ling Mudra

Procedure

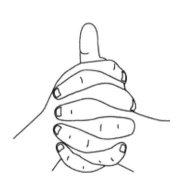

i. Sit in any meditative pose.

ii. Make a fist by interlocking your fingers of the two hands together.

iii. Keep your left thumb erect, pointing upward.

iv. Make sure the remaining fingers remain interlocked.

v. Place the fist just below the navel, on the lap.

vi. You may practice this *mudra* thrice a day for 15 minutes.

Benefits

- ✓ Ling Mudra increases heat in the body.
- ✓ It is highly supportive for cold, asthma, cough, sinus, and low blood pressure.
- ✓ By this method, one can even stop disorders due to the seasonal changes.
- ✓ It increases the body's immune system.
- ✓ It loosens the mucous accumulated in the lungs and also makes the body more resistant to colds and chest infections.

Contraindications

- After Ling Mudra is performed, either eatable or potable things such as water, fruits, juice, ghee, and milk should not be taken in a large amount for an extended period of time.

21. Kaki Mudra

Procedure

i.   Sit in any meditative pose.

ii. With both, the head and spine erect, place the hands on the knees in either Dhyan or Chin Mudra.

iii. Close your eyes for 30-40 seconds so that you can relax the whole body.

iv. Open your eyes and focus on the nose tip.

v.   Do not blink the eyes throughout the whole process.

vi. Open your mouth in a round shape (like a beak of a crow), without straining the tongue.

vii. Now inhale (Radhey) slowly and deeply through your mouth; close the mouth and exhale (Krishna) slowly through the nostrils.

viii. This finishes one round; do Kaki Mudra for up to five rounds.

Benefits

- ✓ Kaki Mudra increases concentration power as one has to continuously focus on the tip of the nose.
- ✓ The most significant factor is that it pacifies both the mind and the body, which aids to root out maladies such as high blood pressure.
- ✓ Additionally, the air taken inside stimulates the membranes of the mouth, which considerably benefits the digestion process.

Contraindications

- Patients of low blood pressure, depression, and acute constipation should avoid this *mudra*.

22. Nasikagra Drishti Mudra

Procedure

i. Sit in any meditative pose with the hands in either Chin / Gyan Mudra (See page 308).

ii. Now, look at the tip of your nose.

iii. Be in this position for a while, and then close your eyes.

iv. There should not be any strain; if you feel a burning sensation in the eyes, then close them immediately.

v. Now rub your palms and place them over your eyes.

vi. Try to feel the warmth and relax the eyes for some time.

vii. This is one round; practice up to five rounds.

For Other Details: See Shambhavi Mudra (See page 319).

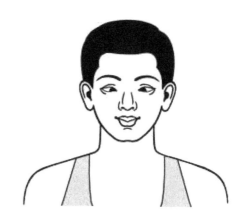

23. Shambhavi Mudra

Procedure

i. Sit in any meditative pose with your hands in either Chin / Gyan Mudra (See page 308).

ii. Look at the space between the eyebrows, just above the nose.

iii. Remain in this position for a while, and then close your eyes.

iv. Ensure that you do not feel any strain, and if you feel a burning sensation in the eyes, close them immediately.

v. Now, rub your palms and place them over the eyes.

vi. Feel the warmth of the palms and relax the eyes.

vii. This completes one round; practice up to five rounds.

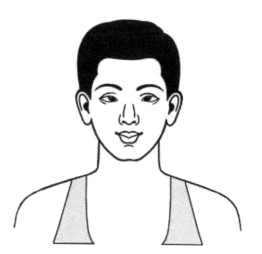

Benefits

✓ Shambhavi Mudra strengthens the eye muscles.
✓ It also soothes the mind and builds up one's mental concentration.

Contraindications

- Those with any kind of eye ailments should not try this *mudra*.

24. Pashinee Mudra (Noose Bound Attitude)

Procedure

i. Come into Karnapidasan (See page 251) progressively.

ii. Keeping a distance of nearly 1.5 feet between your two feet, wrap both arms tightly around the back of the knees.

iii. You may close the eyes while relaxing the whole body.

iv. Breathe (Radhey and Krishna) slowly and deeply in this state.

v. Stay in this position for as long as you are comfortable.

vi. Release the arms and come into Halasan (See page 249).

vii. Lastly, come into Shavasan (See page 227) so that you can relax for a while.

Benefits

✓ The benefits of Pashinee Mudra are similar to those of Akashi Mudra (See page 315).

✓ Besides, it yields benefits of Halasan and Karnapidasan, such as toning the spinal nerves and massaging all the abdominal organs.

Contraindication

- Those who have got spinal problems should not perform this *mudra*.

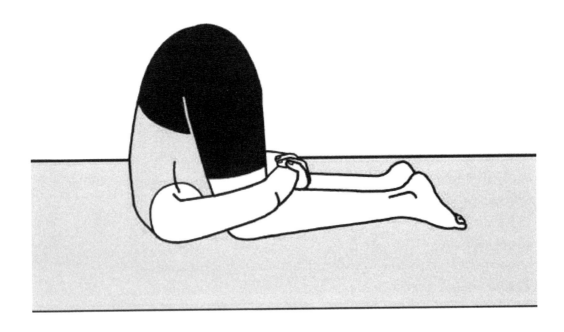

IX. *Ṣhaṭkarmas* (Cleansing Practices)

What is *Ṣhaṭkarm*?

Generally speaking, the compound word "*Ṣhaṭkarm*" is formed by "*Ṣhaṭ*" meaning "six" and "*karma*" meaning "action,"consisting of six purification processes developed by the ancient *Yogīs* for the purpose of removing unwanted substances accumulated inside the human body. These consist of certain techniques used in cleansing the inner channels of the body and also certain hygiene related techniques involving both—bathing and cleaning—of the eyes, ears, and mouth. The cleansing of the inner channels involves—cleansing the gastrointestinal tract, nasal passages, and sinuses. They are also used to balance the three *doṣhas* (humours) in the body: *kaph*, i.e. mucus; *pitta,* i.e. bile and *vāt,* i.e. wind.

Our body constantly throws different useless matters like perspiration, urine, stool, and carbon dioxide through different mechanisms. In case they do not come out properly and entirely, it is very difficult to maintain normal health. Consequently, to keep ourselves healthy and fit, we can practice *Ṣhaṭkarm*. These practices are also used before *pranayam* and other advanced *Yogic* practices to eliminate the toxins from the body so that we could attain an excellent health. Following are the details of the *Ṣhaṭkarmas*:

Ṣhaṭkarmas

1. *Neti* (Washing)

Neti is a process of cleansing the nasal passage (sometimes known as *Ṣhaṭkriyā*). Jal Neti and Sutra Neti are the two main variants of *Neti* practice.

a. Jal Neti

For this technique, tepid salt water is poured into one nostril, so that it comes out through the other. The process is then repeated on the other side. At last, the nose is dried by leaning forward and finally by forceful exhalation to remove any residue in the nasal passage.

Items

- *Neti* pot
- Half a litre tepid water
- One teaspoonful of salt

Procedure

i. Dissolve the salt into lukewarm water and fill the *Neti* pot.

ii. Now, stand with your feet slightly apart and hold the *Neti* pot with the left hand.

iii. Lean a little forward from your waist and tilt your head to the right side.

iv. Keep the mouth slightly open and breathe through the mouth.

v. Then, insert the nozzle of the *Neti* pot inside the left nostril and let the salty water pass through it; water will flow from the right nostril.

vi. Continue the process till the pot is empty; then take the pot away from the nose and place it aside.

vii. Wait until the water stops dripping through right nostril; then straighten the neck and look frontward.

viii. Shutting your left nostril, blow out from the right nostril.

ix. Repeat the method with the right nostril.

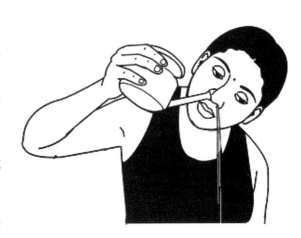

Benefits

✓ Jal Neti is a sterling procedure to remove mucus and other unwanted objects from the nasal passages and sinuses.

✓ It helps prevent the respiratory tract diseases like asthma, pneumonia, bronchitis, etc.

✓ With a regular practice, the various defects of the ears, eyes, and throat are easily cured.

✓ It produces a very soothing effect on the mind, which is extremely beneficial for the treatment of epilepsy and migraine, and for the elimination of anxiety, anger, depression, etc. as well.

✓ In addition, it helps stop hair loss and untimely graying, which is a common problem nowadays.

Contraindications

- Those infected with ear infection, or have undergone a nasal septum operation, or with bleeding problems of the nose should not practice it.

b. Sutra Neti

For this technique, a wet string or thin rubber catheter (36-40 cm) is carefully inserted through one of the nostrils so that one of its ends can be pulled out of the mouth. Holding both ends, the string or catheter is alternately pulled in and out of the nostrils and sinuses.

Item

- A thin rubber catheter (width 4-6 mm and length 36-40 cm) lubricated with butter.

Procedure

i. Either stand in Tadasan (See page 25) or squat down.

ii. Spread your feet about one foot apart and relax the whole body.

iii. Then, tilt your head slightly backward and insert the narrow end of the rubber catheter into one of the nostrils.

iv. When the catheter reaches the back of the throat, insert your index and middle fingers inside the mouth so that the catheter can be pulled out of the mouth.

v. Now, hold the two ends of the catheter and gently pull it back and forth.

vi. Then, remove the catheter carefully, pulling it out through the nostril.

vii. Repeat the same steps above with the opposite nostril.

viii. Breathe in (Radhey) and out (Krishna) through your mouth during the practice.

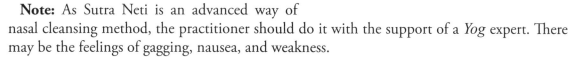

Note: As Sutra Neti is an advanced way of nasal cleansing method, the practitioner should do it with the support of a *Yog* expert. There may be the feelings of gagging, nausea, and weakness.

Benefits
✓ The effects of Sutra Neti are the same as Jal Neti (See page 321).
✓ It corrects the problem of deviated nasal septum.
✓ It clears the nasal passages and eliminates cold, hypersensitivity, headache, sinusitis, bronchitis, etc.
✓ The regular practice of Sutra Neti also helps clear the obstructions due to deformed bone or fleshy outgrowth in the free movement of breath.

Contraindications
- People with a nasal ulcer, severe malformation of nasal bone, or chronic bleeding problems should not practice Sutra Neti. Those with asthma and other breathing problems should breathe in and out several times with the opposite nostril, before practicing this *Neti*.

2. *Dhauti* (Intestinal Wash)

Dhauti (sometimes known as *Ṣhaṭkriyā*) is the *Yogic* method of cleansing the digestive tract in its full length. However, it also affects the respiratory tract, external ears, and eyes.

a. Mukh Dhauti

See page 19

b. Vaman Dhauti (Kunjal/Gaja Karani)

Vaman Dhauti is the *Yogic* method of cleansing the upper digestive tract that regurgitates the solid food contents of the stomach. As the action here is like that of an elephant's water drinking process, it is also known as Kunjal or Gaja Karani.

Items

- Two litres of lukewarm water.
- Three tablespoon of salt.
- A glass of 200 ml.

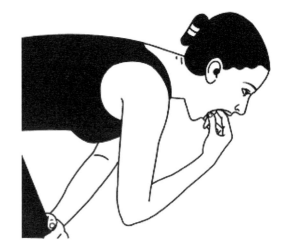

Procedure

i. First dissolve the salt into the water properly.

ii. Either stand in Tadasan (See page 34) or squat down.

iii. Spread your feet about one foot apart and relax the whole body.

iv. Start drinking salty lukewarm water, as fast as you can till you feel that your stomach cannot hold any more.

v. When the stomach is full, the urge to vomit is automatic.

vi. Now, bend slightly forward from the waist, keeping the trunk as horizontal as possible.

vii. Open your mouth; insert the middle and index fingers of the right hand to the back of the tongue, and press it.

viii. The water will flow out from the stomach.

ix. Repeat it until all the water comes out.

x. After sufficient practice, vomiting can be done even without using the fingers.

Benefits

✓ Like other *Ṣhaṭkarmas*, it tones and stimulates the abdominal organs by inducing strong muscular contraction.

✓ It also alleviates indigestion, acidity, and gas problems.

✓ Mucus is easily and effortlessly removed from the body and cold, cough, bronchitis, asthma, and other respiratory ailments are cured as well.

✓ The problem of bad-breath is also rooted out naturally.

Contraindications

- People suffering from hernia, heart problems, peptic ulcer, and diabetes with eye problems should not perform it. Also, those who suffer from high blood pressure should use lime water instead of salty water.

c. Vastra Dhauti

Vastra Dhauti is cleaning the stomach by swallowing a long thin strip of cloth (preferably muslin) in a squatting position and then retiring it after some time.

Items

- A fine piece of white thin and soft cotton (preferably muslin) cloth, 5-6 cms wide and 7-8

meters long without stitched borders.
- A mug of tepid water to keep the cloth wet.

Procedure

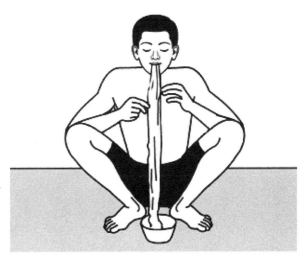

i. First put the cloth into the water.

ii. Then, come into squatting position with your heels on the ground.

iii. Comfortably, put one end of the cloth into the mouth, and start swallowing it slowly and carefully—like the act of swallowing food.

iv. Sip water along with the cloth if it does not pass smoothly.

v. In the starting phase, swallow only one foot of the cloth, and after keeping in the mouth for a few seconds, take it out very slowly and carefully.

vi. You may increase the capacity of swallowing more on the next day.

vii. As the cloth may stick in the lowest part of the throat a feeling of vomiting occurs, pause for a few seconds till the cloth passes downward.

viii. Never swallow it quickly, and also leave at least 30 cms cloth to protrude from the mouth.

ix. After completion, contract and relax the abdomen for a few seconds; then leaning slightly forward, start pulling the cloth out of the mouth gradually.

x. If it does not come out easily, take a few breaths, drink some water, and continue again.

Benefits

✓ Quite distinctively, it cleans the throat and chest region well by expelling the mucus; the muscles of the bronchial tubes relax, eliminating the problem of asthma.

✓ The excessive *kaph* is controlled and the *pitta doṣh* is balanced, which helps in alleviating biliary disorders.

✓ The function of the upper gastro-intestinal tract is also improved.

✓ It is also good for curing headache, cold, leprosy, etc.

Contraindications

- This practice should be done only under the supervision of a *Yog* expert. Also, those with hypertension, hair-related problems, or general illnesses should not include this in their daily *Yog* practice.

d. Vahnisara Dhauti / Agnisar Kriyā (Stimulation of the Digestive Fire)

The word "*Agni*" means "fire," "*sār* " means "essence," and "*kriyā*" means "action." The essence or nature of fire is attributed to the digestion process. If the abdominal organs are not working properly, the digestive fire smolders and needs to be stoked or fanned to increase its power. Agnisar Kriyā not only fans the digestion power but, also purifies the digestion system and the organs related with it, and allows assimilating maximum nutrients from food ingested.

Beginners may find it difficult and get tired due to no voluntary control over their abdominal muscles. The control has to be developed slowly and gradually over an extended period of time. Three rounds of 10 abdominal contractions and expansions is sufficient in the beginning phase. With a daily practice, its frequency can be increased. Also, gradually the time of breath-retention should be increased.

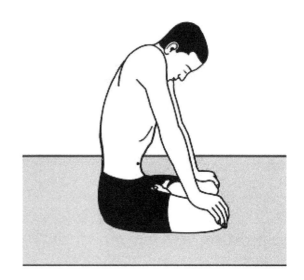

Timing

- On empty stomach, preferably in the early morning.

- After the completion of *asans* and *pranayams*.

Procedure

i. Sit in Padmasan / Vajrasan and separate your knees as far as possible, keeping the big toes in contact with each other.

ii. Rest your hands on the knees and relax your abdomen for a few minutes.

iii. First inhale (Radhey) deeply; as you exhale (Krishna), empty the lungs as much as possible.

iv. Lock your arms and lean a bit forward.

v. Push down on the knees with your both hands and do Jalandhar Bandh (See Page 340).

vi. Start contracting and expanding the abdominal muscles rapidly for as long as possible in order to hold the breath outside easily; do not strain.

vii. Release Jalandhar Bandh; straightening your neck, take a slow and deep inhalation (Radhey).

viii. This completes one round.

ix. Relax yourself till the breathing normalizes and only then start the next round.

x. You can do this *kriyā* for 5-6 rounds.

Awareness

✧ On the breaths synchronized with the rhythmic movement of the abdomen
✧ On mentally chanting the Divine Names "Radhey Krishna" along with each breath, and always realizing Their presence

Benefits

✓ Agnisar Kriya arouses the appetite and alleviates various digestional problems like indigestion, hyperacidity, hypoacidity, flatulence, constipation, and sluggishness of the liver and kidneys.

✓ It massages the abdomen by stimulating the associated nerves and muscles, and different abdominal organs.

✓ It also stimulates the five *prāns*, especially *samān*, and increases the energy levels.

✓ If practiced regularly, other problems like depression, dullness, and lethargy are rooted out completely.

Contraindications

- Those suffering from high blood pressure, heart ailments, acute duodenal or peptic ulcers, overactive thyroid gland, or chronic diarrhea should omit this *kriyā* .

- Women at the pregnancy stage should not perform it.

Precautions

- It should be performed very carefully in the summer season because it may increase the body heat and blood pressure excessively.

- It is better to do the cooling *pranayams* like Sheetkari or Sheetali to lower the body temperature along with this practice.

e. Ganesh Kriyā / Mool Shodhan (Rectal Cleansing)

It is one of the types *Dhauti* for cleaning the rectum with the index or middle finger, or a turmeric root.

Timing

- Morning or any time after emptying the bowels.

Item

- *Araṇḍī* oil, viz. castor oil (or other natural oil such as coconut, peanut, etc.), or natural ghee.

Procedure

i. Apply *Araṇḍī* oil (castor oil) or any other natural oil or ghee on your left index or middle finger.

ii. Insert the index or middle finger about one inch into the rectum and start rotating it slowly and carefully around the inner side of the rectum.

iii. Rotate the finger around the rectum and draw the stool from its inner side.

iv. Then, wash your hands, and repeat the method until all the stool comes out.

Benefits

✓ Ganesh Kriyā tones the external and internal muscles of the anus by massaging them well; thus it helps in removing the problems like constipation and flatulence.

✓ As it helps removing the remaining stool after relieving, even the chronic pile gets eradicated easily. For this reason, people suffering from piles are recommended to do it regularly.

Precautions

- As the nail in the index finger can make wound in the rectum, one should trim the finger-nails prior to practicing this *kriyā*.

- Hands should be washed prior to this *kriyā* in order to remove harmful germs from your hand.

f. Shankh Prakshalan (Varisara Dhautī)

It is the *Yogic* process of cleansing, especially, the lower digestive track by evacuating a large quantity of water through the bowels. It can be further categorized into Laghu Shankh Prakshalan and Purna Shankh Prakshalan.

i. Laghu Shankh Prakshalan

Laghu Shankh Prakshalan is a short way of cleansing the lower digestive tract in which plenty of clean and salty tepid water is taken and expelled through the rectum.

Time

- Morning, after shower and emptying the bowels.

- During winter, practice only when the Sun rises, and the temperature becomes normal.

- Do not practice when the weather is cloudy, or when it is raining.

Item

- Plenty of clean, salty tepid water and extra hot water in case the tepid water's temperature drops down.

Preparation

- Start doing Tadasan, Tiryak Tadasan, Kati Chakrasan, Tiryak Bhujangasan, and Udarkarshanasan one week before doing Shankh Prakshalan.

- Take a light dinner on the night before the practice.

- People with high blood pressure and skin diseases should use tepid water with lemon, without salt. But those with cervical spondylitis, slipped-disc, joint and body pain, and phlegm problems should use tepid water with salt but without lemon.

- Special food like *khichaḍī* of *mūṅg* and rice, is to be prepared. It must be semi-liquid. And finally, mix a good amount of ghee with the *khichaḍī*.

Procedure

i. Drink two glasses of salty lukewarm water.

ii. Perform each of the following *asans* about eight rounds dynamically.

iii. While doing each *asan*, retain your breath for about five seconds in the final position.

1. Tadasan

See page 34.

2. Tiryak Tadasan

See page 36.

3. Kati Chakrasan

See page 28.

4. Tiryak Bhujangasan

See page 215.

5. Udarkarshanasan

See page 127.

After one cycle of the five *asans*, do the following:

- Drink two more glasses of water, and again perform the set of five *asans* mentioned above.

- Repeat the same for the third time.

- After completing this, go to the toilet but do not strain. Even if you cannot empty your bowels, do not worry, you will be able to clean your bowels after a while.

- Sometimes the bowel movement does not take place after three cycles. In such a case, you may go up to four or even five cycles, and then you will feel the pressure building up.

- After emptying the bowels, come into Shavasan (See page 227) and relax for half an hour. Do not sleep or the activated digestive fire will diminish. If you feel sleepy in Shavasan (See page 227), you can relax in any of the other relaxing poses too.

- After taking a rest, take light food, *mūṅg* dal *khichaḍī* (rice and lentils boiled together) with one or two teaspoons of clarified butter (ghee).

- You can have your lunch and dinner as usual, but avoid spicy, fried, and oily food.

Benefits

✓ As Laghu Shankh Prakshalan activates the whole digestion system, it is recommended for curing digestive disorders like constipation, flatulence, acidity, and indigestion, etc.

✓ It also corrects urinary dysfunctions, and thus the formation of stones in the kidneys is prevented.

ii. Purna Shankh Prakshalan

Purna Shankh Prakshalan is the surest way of cleansing the lower digestive tract in which plenty of salty tepid water (even lemon mixed) is taken and expelled through the rectum.

Procedure

i.   Drink two glasses of salty tepid water as fast as possible.
ii. Practice one round of the following *asans*: Tadasan, Tiryak Tadasan, Kati Chakrasan, Tiryak Bhujangasan, and Udarkarshanasan.
iii. Again, drink two glasses of water and perform the set of *asans*, second time.
iv. Repeat the process for the third time, and then go to the toilet but do not strain.

v. Come back again and repeat the process above.

vi. Generally this process is recommended to be repeated eight times.

vii. After completing each process, go to the toilet and remain there for a minute even if you do not feel like evacuating.

viii. Evacuation starts after completing the process for three times. First solid stool will appear, then a mixture of stool and water. Then, brownish, cloudy, and then plain water will drain out.

ix. It is advisable to stop when the cloudy water appears, but one should not exceed the point when plain water appears.

x. After completion of the process, lie down in Shavasan (See page 227) for 30-45 minutes. Mainly, Subtle Body Relaxation is preferable for this process.

xi. After relaxation, eat semi-liquid food such as *khichaḍī* to your feel. You should eat at proper time and in proper amount as it is necessary for the digestive system to regularize its function.

xii. Three components in *khichaḍī* help the restoration of correct digestive function. Ghee coats the intestinal walls until the new linings are produced. The rice is an easily digestible carbohydrate for energy, which also protects the inner lining of the alimentary canal. The *mūñg* (lentil) provides an easily digestible protein, which is necessary for nutrition.

xiii. *Khichaḍī* should be eaten in sufficient quantity as it stretches the gut; it is necessary to prevent the gut from cramping. It is also important to resume peristalsis, which prevents indigestion, diarrhea, and constipation.

xiv. One should rest for the whole day and one should sleep at least for three hours after having the first meal.

xv. One should not drink water or any liquid at least 2 to 3 hours after having the first meal. Any cold items should not be taken for the whole day. Body should be kept warm and no fans, cooler, and air-conditioner should be used. Sitting in the hot Sun or fire, having a cold bath, and doing any physical exercise is strictly prohibited.

Benefits

✓ One of the main reasons behind illness is abdominal disorder. This stomach cleansing process, Purna Shankh Prakshalan, strengthens the entire digestive system, thus helps in overcoming all the abdominal maladies.

✓ It is used to cure diabetes, obesity, high cholesterol, and high lipid levels.

✓ It is a boon for arthritis.

✓ It empowers the immune system in such a way that the external germs cannot attack the body easily.

✓ The blood is purified so well that almost all kinds of skin diseases are eliminated naturally without any side effects.

✓ Many *Yog* therapists even say that it has got the capacity to harmonize the *prāṇ* at five different places, especially by removing blockages.

Precautions

- Salty water induces thirst; so do not drink cold water as it results in weakness; only drink tepid water the whole day.

- Pregnant women, children, and feeble persons should not attempt to perform Shankh Prakshalan.

- Perform Laghu Shankh Prakshalan once in two months, and Purna Shankh Prakshalan only once in a year.

- Do not eat spicy or heavy food for a week and avoid all acidic foods for a month.

3. *Basti* (Colon Cleansing / Enema)

Basti/Enema is the method of introducing liquids like plain water or saline water into the rectum and colon. The lower intestinal tract expands rapidly due to the excess volume of the liquid and results in uncomfortable bloating, cramping, strong peristalsis, and an urgent feeling of evacuation of the lower intestinal tract.

Procedure

i. This is a process in which water is sucked into the large intestine through the rectum and then thrown out.

ii. Before it was performed by dipping half of the body into water with a tube inserted into the rectum. But nowadays enema is easily available, which has the same effect.

Benefits

✓ *Basti*/Enema cleanses the colon fully and eradicates maladies like abnormal growth in the abdomen, spleen, and liver.
✓ It helps in alleviating various eye diseases.
✓ It also assists in removing different urethral irregularities, dyspepsia, constipation, piles, fistula, pimples, boils, acidity, irregularities of the bowels, etc.

4. *Nauli* (Churning the Abdomen)

Nauli is one of the *Yogic* processes to cleanse the abdominal region, especially digestive organs and small intestine, by massaging the internal belly organs. As *Nauli* is a difficult *Yogic* method, it should be performed only under the guidance of a *Yog* expert.

Nauli is generally prescribed for the treatment of constipation. It is usually done in standing pose but it may be practiced in the positions like Padmasan, Sukhasan, Vajrasan, etc. Exhaling completely, the whole belly is strongly pulled in and then the middle belly muscle is contracted and rotated in a circle. It has four different types:

a. Madhya Nauli (Central Abdominal Contraction)

It is the isolated contraction of the central abdominal muscles—making a concave shape in front of the abdomen.

Procedure

i. Stand with the feet spread about two feet apart.

ii. Bend your knees a bit and lean forward—resting both palms on the thighs—just above the knees.

iii. Look at your abdomen.

iv. First breathe in (Radhey); then breathe out (Krishna) completely, and loosen the stomach muscles.

v. Now, lower your neck a little forward so that it touches the pit nearby the chest; raise your chest a bit upward and push the stomach back as far as possible, trying to draw the inner stomach toward the spine.

vi. Comfortably, press the thighs with the arms and pull up the lower abdominal muscles in such a way that they make a concave shape in front of the abdomen.

vii. While contracting the rectus abdominal muscles, there should not be any strain.

viii. After contracting to your comfort, release it gradually and return to an upright position.

ix. Relax fully by inhaling (Radhey) slowly and deeply so that the abdomen will expand freely.

x. This is one round; try the next round after maintaining a normal heartbeat.

Note: Madhya Nauli should be mastered before attempting Vama Nauli and Dakshini Nauli.

b. Vama Nauli (Left Abdominal Contraction)

It is the isolated contraction of the left part of the central abdominal muscles.

Procedure

i. First assume the final position of Madhya Nauli (steps vi-vii).

ii. Now, isolate the rectus abdominal muscles to the left side.

iii. Contract the muscles to the left as much as you can without any strain.

iv. After contracting to your comfort, return to Madhya Nauli; then release it, and return to an upright position.

v. Now, relax by inhaling (Radhey) slowly and deeply so that the rate of your heartbeat slows down.

vi. This finishes one round; repeat it for five rounds.

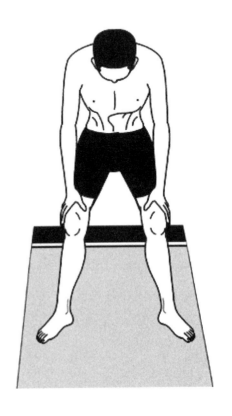

c. Dakshini Nauli (Right Abdominal Contraction)

Dakshini Nauli is the isolated contraction of the right part of the central abdominal muscles.

Procedure

i. Come into the final position of Madhya Nauli (steps vi-vii).

ii. Then, isolate the rectus abdominal muscles to the right side.

iii. Gently contract the muscles to the right as far as possible, without giving any unnecessary effort.

iv. Maintain the contraction to your comfort, and then return to Madhya Nauli.

v. Now, release it and return to normal standing position.

vi. Relax fully by inhaling (Radhey) slowly and deeply so that the heartbeat rate slows down.

vii. This is one round; do it for five rounds.

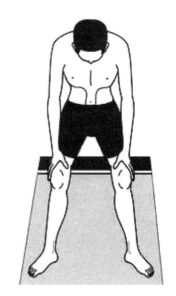

d. Purna Nauli (Abdominal Churning)

It is the *Yogic* process of making a circular movement of the central abdominal muscles.

Procedure

i. Assume the final position of Vama Nauli, steps ii-iii (See page 332).

ii. Then, start rotating the muscles to the right—Dakshini Nauli—and finally back to the left.

iii. Keep rotating the muscles from side to side, so that it appears like churning.

iv. Practice three successive rotations, and then release the abdominal contraction, and relax the abdominal muscles.

v. Then, assume the final position of Dakshin Nauli (steps ii-iii), and rotate the abdominal muscles from the right to the left, and then again to the right.

vi. After doing this for three successive rotations, come back to the final position of Madhya Nauli (steps vi-vii), and then to the standing position.

vii. Relax fully by inhaling (Radhey) slowly and deeply so that your abdomen expands naturally.

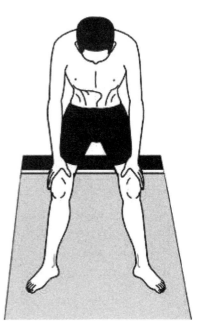

viii. This ends one round; try the next round after returning to a normal heartbeat rate.

ix. Repeat the above process for 5-10 rounds.

Note: Purna Nauli is done only after perfecting the Madhya Nauli, Vama Nauli, and Dakshini Nauli (Right Abdominal Contraction).

Benefits
✓ Purna Nauli cleanses all kinds of impurities stuck inside the intestines and thus helps remove all abdominal diseases like constipation, indigestion, flatulence, etc.
✓ It helps rooting out obesity, dyspepsia, depression, and hormonal imbalances.
✓ It helps in controlling urinal and different sexual problems.
✓ Naturally, the three *doshas* (humours)—*vāt*, *pitta*, and *kaph* are balanced, which makes the stomach so light that it develops a good appetite.
✓ Another purpose of doing Purna Nauli is also to rectify emotional imbalances, and restore sufficient energy in the body.

Contraindications
- Those with a swelling of the intestines, heart disease, high blood pressure, hernia, gall stones, or acute peptic ulcer should not perform Nauli. Also, pregnant women and those who have undergone recent abdominal surgery should avoid it.

5. *Kapālbhāti*

Kapālbhāti is one of the *Ṣhatkriyās* to cleanse the body especially—the cranial sinuses but with many other effects too. In *Kapālabhāti*, a practitioner has to do an act of short and rapid forceful exhalation, however, inhalation occurs naturally.

For Other Details: See page 295.

6. *Bhagwad Swaroop Darśhan* (*Trāṭak* / Fixed Gazing)

Bhagwad Swaroop Darśhan (*Trāṭak*) is a way to meditate by fixed gazing on a single point such as an idol of God, a black dot, or candle flame. The main intention of practicing this is to aide the practitioner to halt the restlessness of his eyes, pursuing something every moment; by concentrating his eyes, he can halt the restlessness of his mind too.

Procedure
i. Sit in any meditative *asan*.

ii. Place either an idol of Radha Krishna, or your favorite form of any God such as Ram, Shivji, etc. on the table or wall, in front of your eyes.

iii. The distance between you and the idol must be about 3-5 feet (the distance depends more on the size of the picture).

iv. The bigger the idol, the greater the distance one should sit away from the idol for proper Bhagwad Swaroop Darshan.

v. Perform each of the eye exercises five times successively:

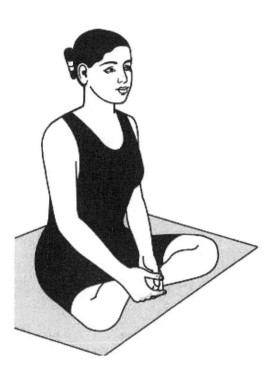
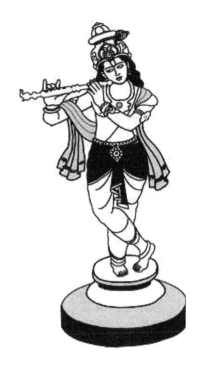

a. Sideways Viewing

See page 104.

b. Front and Sideways Viewing

See page 105.

c. Up and Down Viewing

See page 106.

d. Scattered Viewing (defocusing)

See page 107.

e. Rotational Viewing

See page 105.

Stage - 1

Procedure

i.   Gently open your eyes and look at the place below the idol.

ii. Slowly move your eyes to look at the picture, and start gazing at the whole idol effortlessly.

iii. Although in the beginning, you may feel an irritating sensation in the eyes, do not leave the performance.

iv. Using your will-power, do not blink; if tears come, let tears flow from your eyes.

v. Maintain this for about one minute.

vi. Then, close your eyes totally and rub the hands together, and place them over your eyes (Palming process).

vii. After 15-20 seconds, release your hands; then open your eyes with a few blinks.

viii. This is one round; do this for five rounds.

ix. End the final round with palming for a bit longer period (about 30 seconds).

x. Finally, release the hands but do not open your eyes instantly.

Stage - 2

Procedure

i. Slowly open your eyes, and look at the place below the idol and then carefully move the eyes to look at the idol.

ii. This time, just stare at one part of the picture like the eyes, nose, etc.—intensively.

iii. Your eyes may feel a burning like sensation at first, but control your eyes with will-power so that the eyes do not blink.

iv. If tears come, let them flow out freely as they purify the eye muscles.

v. Remain in this position for about one minute without straining the eyes.

vi. Then, close your eyes for a few seconds; rub your hands together, and perform palming.

vii. After 15-20 seconds, release your hands and open the eyes with a few blinks.

viii. This completes one round; repeat for five rounds.

ix. End the final round with palming for a bit longer period (about 30 seconds).

x. Finally, release your hands, but do not open your eyes immediately.

Stage - 3

Procedure

i. Slowly open your eyes and look at the place below the idol.

ii. Slowly, move your eyes from the place below the idol, to the idol.

iii. This time defocusing will be practiced; expanding your awareness, collect the details of the idol such as the colorful clothes, the posture, facial expression, the beautiful eyes, etc., in your mind.

iv. Now, while expanding your awareness more and more, observe the aura around the Lord.

v. Maintain the process for one minute, again close your eyes and try to visualize the image in your mind, remembering all the details you have collected. But try to visualize the sentient and dynamic Lord, as if He is smiling or playing on a flute or dancing with His pals in Vrindavan.

vi. When the image disappears, perform Palming process.

vii. Now, Bhramari (See page 303) can be practiced with palming; giving a gentle press over the eyes, breathe in and produce "Mm…" sound and feel the vibrations throughout the body.

viii. Perform Bhramari for five times.

ix. Then, release your hands; sit peacefully for some time and feel the changes in the body.

x. Realize that your mind has now become tranquil and your concentration, will-power, and eyesight have improved as well.

Benefits

✓ This meditative process, *Bhagwad Swaroop Darśhan* (*Trāṭak*), purifies the mind, maintains good eyesight by cleansing the eyes, and also relieves the practitioners from tension, insomnia, restlessness, depression, etc.

✓ It also stimulates the nervous system, which helps enhance the ability to concentrate.

✓ It increases memory and mental power.

✓ It also decreases the rate of breathing.

✓ This method exercises the centres—olfactive and optical; it also controls ciliary's reflex and helps in stimulating the pineal gland.

Precautions

- It is preferable to practice in the dark, especially in the evening time.

- One should sit comfortably in one of the meditative *asans* with the head, neck, and spine erect; for this reason, it is better to remove wrist watches, eye glasses, belts, shawls, chains, etc.

- While performing the palming process, the palms should not touch the eye balls.

- At the time of palming, breathe slowly.

- Palming should be done in such a way that there should be complete darkness.

- The face should remain relaxed—preferably keeping a gentle smile.

- One should not strain the eyes.

- Persons with insomnia should not go to bed for at least an hour after doing it as it awakens the mind, and it is really difficult to sleep just after practicing.

- In case of tension or headache, it is better to avoid this tyepe of *ṣhaṭkarm*.

IX. *Bandhas* (Locks)

Introduction to *Bandhas*

The term "*Bandh*" means "an act of binding, locking, arresting, capturing, or bondage that may be either internal or external to our body." All kinds of *bandhas* involve the contraction or squeezing of different muscles. There are three muscular locks—Jalandhar Bandh, Uddiyan Bandh, and Mool Bandh. They are applied in the throat, abdomen, and perineum respectively. When we apply these three *bandhas* together, it becomes—Maha Bandh—The Great Lock. The three *bandhas* are traditionally practiced to lock the *prāṇic* energy, and thereby enhancing the impacts of the accompanying pose or *pranayam*. Mostly *bandhas* are practiced after exhalation and on completion of inhalation. Practicing *bandhas* helps in regulating physical, emotional, and mental functions.

As there are three *bandhas*, there are three muscles groups involved—cervical (neck) muscles, abdominal muscles, and perineal muscles. Contraction of these muscles impacts the nervous, circulatory, respiratory, endocrine, and energy systems. As endocrine glands are intimately associated with the *chakras* located at different parts of the body, *bandhas* affect these *chakras* too. On all the *chakras*, the bandhas are directly associated with the active stimulation of three *chakras*—Mool Bandh (*Mūlādhār Chakra*), Uddiyan Bandh (*Maṇipūr Chakra*), and Jalandhar Bandh (*Viśhuddhi Chakra*). Each of these physical locations is co-related neurologically to a specific counterpart in the spinal cord, brain, and the mind. In *Yog*, bandhas are both—studied and practiced—with *pranayams* and *mudras*.

Various *bandhas* have been explicated in different *Yogic* texts and discourses. *Bandhas* have been described in *Haṭh Yog Pradīpikā*, especially, in the chapter relating to *mudras*. *Haṭha Yog* has mentioned four types of *bandhas*—Jalandhar Bandh, Uddiyan Bandh, Mool Bandh, and Maha Bandh. The fourth kind of *bandh*, viz. Maha Bandh, is the integration of the three classic *bandhas*. They are practiced together or separately at particular times during *kriyā*, *asan*, *pranayam*, *mudra*, and *dhyan*.

These internal energy locks direct the *prāṇ* upward—toward the spine rather than allowing it to go downward, because it has got normal tendency of converting it into spiritual energy. Jalandhar Bandh prevents *prāṇ* from crossing the upper body; Uddiyan Bandh forces *prāṇ* up the *suṣhūmṇa nāḍī*; and Mool Bandh prevents *apān* escaping from the lower body.

Bandhas withold back the dissipative energy as in *pratyāhār*, one of the eight fold ways of the *Yog Sūtras*. *Pratyāhār* is the process of restraining the scattering outward flow of *prāṇ* while bringing it back from the periphery, toward the centre. The fifth limb of the *Aṣhṭāṅg Yog*, *pratyāhār*, in turn acts similarly as a dominant vehicle for *tapas*. Even though generally known as locks, *bandhas* act as valves as they direct the internal energy flow to irrigate the *nāḍīs* and activate the energy body. When integrated with *yogasans*, *pranayams*, *mudra*, and *dhyan*, *bandhas* provide excellent benefits.

The three *bandhas*—Jalandhar Bandh, Uddiyan Bandh, and Mool Bandh—are associated with the three *granthis* and as such provide the motivational power to unlock higher dimensions (*Brahma Lok*, *Vishnu Lok*, and *Rudra Lok* which also refer to *Nirmāṇ Kāyā*, *Sambhog Kāyā*, and *Dharma Kāyā* respectively). Thus, the three classic *bandhas* and the Maha Bandh provide the keys to unlock these three *granthis* respectively.

Concept of *Bandhas* (Locks)

In most modern *Yogic* literature, *bandh* is defined simply as a "lock." Nevertheless, the correct meaning of *bandh* is essentially contradictory, for it is said that by locking or contracting certain muscles at the physical level, a subtle process of "unlocking" begins simultaneously at the mental and *prāṇic* levels. Most modern muscle relaxing therapies advocate that by the total, systematic contraction and relaxation of muscles all over the body, one can have both— physical and mental relaxation.

Bandhas work in a similar way, simultaneously impacting the physical, *prāṇic*, mental, psychic, and causal bodies. They have far reaching effects because they are associated with energy centres in the spine and brain. So effectively, *bandhas* are more dynamic and instant than simple contractions and relaxations of the different muscles in different parts of our body.

How do *Bandhas* Benefit us?

Bandhas direct the *prāṇ* inside the body so that blockages of jammed and repressed energy are released; areas without or less amount of *prāṇ* are nourished, and the life force energy (*prāṇ*)—which leaks out because of dissipative nature—is brought into coherence, activation, and integratation. In this way, *bandhas* bind back the dissipative energy.

Bandhas are the internal energy valves, which allow *prāṇ* to flow through various parts of the body, activating the dormant potential of spirit. *Bandhas*, *pranayam*, and *pratyāhār* possess the potentiality of availing the pathway for the spiritual reconnection.

Bandhas can only be perfected by full awareness on their practice while practicing them. This awareness is achieved through the practice of alertness and *vairāgya* applied concurrently. When the *bandhas* are perfected, progress in *asans*, *pranayams*, *mudras*, and *dhyan* are greatly enhanced and an aspirant can easily uplift himself/herself in the spiritual path.

1. Jalandhar Bandh (The Throat Lock)

The Sanskrit word "*Jaal*" refers to the net and "*Dhar*" means stream or flow. The next meaning of Jalandhar Bandh is the lock that controls the network of *nāḍīs* in the neck or throat. So Jalandhar Bandh is the throat lock that blocks the *prāṇic* energy moving down the *Viśhuddi* from *bindu* and prevents it from falling into the digestive fire, resulting in the conservation of *prāṇ*.

Procedure

i. Sit erect either in Padmasan (See page 116) or Siddhasan (See page 115).

ii. Keep your head and spine erect.

iii. Ensure your knees do not touch the floor properly.

iv. Make sure you press the perineum with the left heel and place the right heel on the left thigh, or sit in any other comfortable posture.

v. Place the palms on the knees; keep the neck and the spine erect. Close the eyes, and relax the whole body.

vi. Now inhale (Radhey) slowly and deeply; at the end of inhalation and the beginning of retention of breath, press the chin firmly against the chest so that your chin touches the pit on your neck.

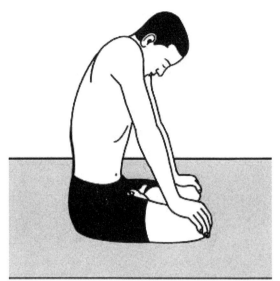

vii. Straighten your arms by pressing the knees down with the palms.

viii. Be in this final position for as long as the breath can be retained comfortably; do not strain.

ix. Then, bring the chin up and exhale (Krishna).

x. This is one round; repeat when the respiration has returned to normal; this practice may be repeated up to five times.

Note: This *bandh* is ideally performed together with *pranayams* and *mudras*. It can also be practiced on its own, or prior to meditation. Do not inhale or exhale until the chin lock and arm lock have been released and the head is fully upright. If you feel suffocated, you should immediately stop the practice.

Awareness
✧ On the throat pit
✧ On the breaths synchronized with the physical movements
✧ On feeling the presence of "Radhey Krishna" in your each breath

Benefits
✓ Jalandhar Bandh stretches the neck excellently.
✓ It stimulates the parasympathetic spinal area, located at the bottom of the brain and the top of the spinal cord, resulting in the regulation of heart rate, respiration, blood pressure, etc.
✓ It also compresses the carotid sinuses that are located in the neck. These sinuses help regulate the circulatory and respiratory systems.
✓ As it reduces depression, stress, anxiety, and anger, the practitioner attains a sense of rest, relaxation, and vibrancy.
✓ The stimulus on the throat also helps balance thyroid function and regulate the metabolism.

✓ Those who like to make their voice pleasant and appealing would better practice this *bandh* regularly.

Contraindications

- People suffering from cervical spondylitis, high intracranial pressure, respiratory problems, vertigo, high and low blood pressure, and heart disease should not attempt Jalandhar Bandh on their own, as long retention of the breath may cause some strain on the heart.

2. Uddiyan Bandh (The Abdominal Lock)

The Sanskrit word "*Uddiyan*" means to "rise up or to fly upward" because the physical lock applied to the body causes the diaphragm to rise toward the chest. "Uddiyan" is therefore often translated as the stomach lift. The physical lock helps *prāṇ* flow into *suṣhumṇā nāḍī* and from where it flows upward to *Sahasrār chakra*. Uddiyana Bandh can be combined with Nauli Shatkarm. It can be practiced either by standing or in sitting posture.

a. Standing Abdominal Contraction

Procedure

i. Stand up erect, in an upright position, with both feet joined together and arms by your sides, i.e. Saral Tadasan (See page 25).

ii. Separate your feet about 1.5-2 feet apart.

iii. Inhaling (Radhey), bend on the knees slightly, lean forward from the waist and place your palms just above your knees.

iv. Make sure your arms remain locked.

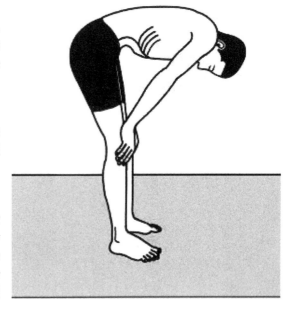

v. While exhaling (Krishna), contract your abdomen and place the chin on the hollow of the throat—pit. By the end of the exhalation, your abdomen should be fully contracted, drawn up and back, toward the spine—by pressing on the knees with your palms.

vi. With this contraction, the diaphragm expands and creates a cavity on the front side of the abdomen, under the rib cage. Your back curves slightly inward.

vii. Hold the position as long as possible without any strain and then release.

viii. This is one round; repeat when your breath returns to normal state.

ix. Repeat it up to five times.

x. When this *bandh* is mastered, the navel moves toward the spine, and the rectal and back muscles contract inside the abdomen.

b. Sitting Abdominal Contraction

Procedure

i. Sit in Siddhasan (See page 115) or Padmasan (See page 116), with your spine erect and the knees touching the floor.

ii. Rest the palms on top of the knees.

iii. Close your eyes and relax the whole body.

iv. Inhale (Radhey) deeply through the nostrils.

v. Exhale (Krishna) through the mouth with a whoosh, trying to empty the lungs to your capacity.

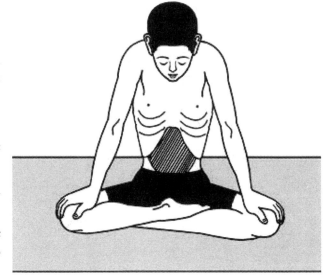

vi. Retaining the breath outside, bend forward and press down on the knees with your palms; also lock your elbows and raise the shoulders, letting further extension of the spinal cord.

vii. Do spontaneous Jalandhar Bandh—pressing your chin against the chest.

viii. Contract your abdominal muscles inward and upward; hold the abdominal lock and breathe outside for as long as you can without uneasy effort.

ix. Lift your head and then slowly inhale (Radhey).

x. Be in this state until the respiration returns to normal; then begin the next round.

Awareness

✧ On the abdomen
✧ On the breaths synchronized with the bodily movements
✧ On always feeling the presence of "Radhey Krishna" with your each breath

Benefits

✓ Sitting Abdominal Contraction compresses the digestive organs, adrenal glands, kidneys, and the most important—the solar plexus.
✓ It tones up the sympathetic nervous system, thus avoiding the effects of stress and anxiety in psychosomatic diseases.
✓ This *bandh* relieves for many abdominal and stomach ailments like constipation, indigestion, worms, diabetes, etc.
✓ The adrenal glands are balanced—which helps in alleviating lethargy, anxiety, and tension.
✓ It improves blood circulation throughout the torso area and empowers all the internal organs.

✓ It activates and peps up the whole body as the extra fat of the stomach is reduced considerably.

Note: During *pranayams*, this *bandh* is to be practiced only in the sitting position. It must be always practiced on an empty stomach. Never force the abdominal muscles outward; use force only in pulling the muscles in and upward.

Contraindications

- Avoid this exercise if there is any problem of high blood pressure, hiatal hernia, ulcers, or heart disorders. Women should omit it during menstruation or pregnancy period.

3. Mool Bandh (The Perineum Contraction)

"*Mool*" is a Sanskrit word that means "the root, or firmly fixed, or the source, or the cause." Together, the words "*Mool*" and "*Bandh*" refer to "the contraction of *Mūlādhār Chakra*." This contraction is triggered at the root of the spine—the perineum (or cervix in case of female). Mool Bandh is also known as the Perineal Lock. On the physical level, it is the physical contraction of muscles. However, when refined, Mool Bandh is the contraction of *Mūlādhār Chakra*.

Procedure

i. Sit in Padmasan or Siddhasan.

ii. Keep your palms on the knees and slightly press them.

iii. Close your eyes and relax yourself; also watch the natural rhythm of breaths for a while.

iv. Shift your awareness on to the anal area.

v. As you exhale (Krishna), contract the anal area by squeezing the muscles inward.

vi. Hold the contraction for some time, with normal breathing; however, do not hold the breath.

vii. Slowly releasing Mool Bandh, lift your head to the upright position.

viii. Repeat 10 times—with maximum contraction and relaxation.

ix. With further practice, the duration can be extended to 3-5 minutes.

Note: Mool Bandh is the contraction of certain muscles in the pelvic region. Nevertheless, it does not contract the whole perineum. In the male body, the area of contraction is located between the anus and the testes. In female body, the area of contraction is behind the cervix, where the uterus projects into the vagina.

Awareness

✧ On mentally chanting the Divine Names "Radhey Krishna" with each breath
✧ On the perineal (males) or crevical (females) contraction in the final position

Benefits

✓ Mool Bandh has got many physical, mental, and psychic benefits that help in the preparation of spiritual awakening.

✓ Mool Bandh stimulates both—the sensory-motor and the autonomic nervous systems—in the pelvic region. Sympathetic nervous stimulation also occurs in Mool Bandh, but at a subdued level.

✓ Intestinal peristalsis is also stimulated—thus relieving constipation and piles.

✓ If done sincerely and regularly, it helps alleviate anal fissures, ulcers, prostatitis (inflammation of the prostate gland), some cases of prostatic hypertrophy, and chronic pelvic infections.

Contraindications

- It should be performed under the supervision of a *Yog* therapist. If practiced wrongly, it may increase the energies very fast, and can even suddenly trigger symptoms of hyperactivity.

4. Maha Bandh (The Great Lock)

"*Maha*" refers to "the great." Maha Bandh is called the Great Lock, because it is the integration of all three classic *bandhas*.

Procedure

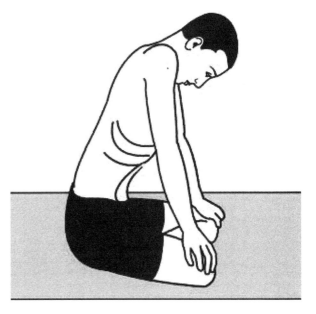

i. Sit in Padmasan (See page 116) or Siddhasan (See page 115).

ii. Keeping palms on the knees, slightly press them.

iii. Gently close your eyes and relax the whole body; also watch the natural breath for a while.

iv. Exhale (Krishna) forcefully and completely through your mouth.

v. Hold the breath outside.

vi. Do Jalandhar, Uddiyan, and Mool Bandh—serially.

vii. Hold the *bandhas* and the breath as long as possible for you, without straining. Then, release Mool, Uddiyan, and Jalandhar Bandhas consecutively.

viii. After releasing the *bandhas*, inhale (Radhey) slowly.

ix. This is one round; relax and let your breath return to normal state before starting the next round.

x. Repeat about 3-5 rounds.

Awareness

✧ After performing three classic *bandhas*, move your awareness through the perineal, abdominal, and throat regions consecutively

✧ Remain aware of each region for a few seconds and then move to the next

Benefits

✓ Maha Bandh gives the benefits of all three classic *bandhas*.
✓ It has positive effects on the hormonal secretions of the pineal gland and regulation of the entire endocrine system.
✓ The decaying, degenerative, and ageing processes are checked, and each cell of the body is revitalized.
✓ It reduces anger; keeps the mind peaceful and alert, and thus prepares the mind for meditation.
✓ When perfected, it can fully awaken *prāṇ* in the main *chakras*.

Note: One should not try Maha Bandh until other three classic *bandhas* have been perfected.

Contraindications:

- People who are suffering from high or low blood pressure, heart conditions, hernia, stomach or intestinal ulcer, physical weakness, and those recovering from visceral ailments should omit it.
- Also, women should not do it during menstrual or pregnancy period.

X. Subtle Body Relaxation

An uncontrolled mind is our worst enemy and a controlled mind is our best friend. An unbridled and overworked mind is the cause of stress, anxiety, tension, depression, ulcers, and innumerable other ailments. Often, mental activity reaches a state where one keeps thinking while eating, sitting, standing, walking, etc. If the mind could be taught to relax, one can find relief from most ailments.

Cause of Disease as Described in *Yog Vāsiṣṭh*

Yog Vāsiṣṭh describes a discussion between Shree Ram and the Sage Vasishth. When Lord Ram saw disease afflicting the people of His kingdom, He was moved by compassion, and asked His teacher about the cause of disease. Sage Vasishth explained that firstly the mind becomes disturbed due to negative thoughts, such as thoughts of anxiety, hatred, tension, regret, remorse, lamentation, etc. This causes a disturbance at the level of the *prāṇas*, or the "life giving forces." This manifests in the next stage, i.e. in the physical body, as disease. Hence, if we wish to cure disease from the root, we must address the mind.

Subtle Body Relaxation is a powerful mind management technique, and is one of the most important parts of Jagadguru Kripaluji Yog. It not only provides ultimate relaxation to the gross and subtle bodies, but also revitalizes them. Since the mind is applied to the Divine realm, it gets purified by mediating on God. From a physical viewpoint, the Subtle Body Relaxation technique is as beneficial as all the *yogasans* and *pranayams* put together. From the spiritual viewpoint, it brings about true "*Yog*" or union with God.

This relaxation technique is practiced in stages. First you have to lie down in Shavasan (See page 227). Then, you have to relax your body, not moving any part of thereof. The next stage is to develop sensations within your body. Then, you will make a firm resolve to meet God in the manner of your choice. In the final stage, you proceed to take out subtle body to the Divine realm.

Stages

There are three stages in every Subtle Body Relaxation.
1. Preparation
2. Meditation
3. Conclusion

Stage 1 – Preparation

Lie down in Shavasan (See page 227), keeping your hands on the ground with the palms facing upward, toward the sky. A gap of about 1/2-1 foot should be maintained between your feet. Keep your eyes closed; preferably, an eyeshade, handkerchief, or a piece of cloth should be used to cover your eyes completely. This is to avoid disturbing factors such as light, insects, etc. from disturbing your concentration.

Place your neck, hands, torso, waist, and other limbs in a comfortable position so that you will not need to adjust them later due to any discomfort or pain. Keep your eyes closed till the end; use a piece cloth if needed. Your breathing should be normal and rhythmic. Stop all movements in your body.

Relax your entire body. There should be no tension or tightness in any part of the body. Relax the toes of your feet. Let them free and loose. Relax your ankles and your lower limbs. Relax your knees and your thighs. Relax your waist or hips. Relax your stomach muscles and then your chest. Completely relax your fingers and your arms. Free your shoulders as much as you can. Relax your neck and finally your face. Relax all the muscles of your face and forehead. Thus, make your whole body totally relaxed.

You will now experience various sensations in the body. Develop the feeling that your body is getting heavier. Develop the feeling that the weight of every part of your body is increasing, and your body is slowly sinking into the ground. Be aware of the contact between your body and the ground.

Now, develop the opposite sensation. Feel that your body is becoming light. It is slowly becoming weightless and soon you can see yourself levitating in the air! You have now lost all your heaviness; now feel lighter than a dry leaf. Enjoy this feeling for a while.

Now, leave your body on the ground. Watch it from a few feet above; observe it lying calm and still. It is such a strange feeling! You are awake but your body is lying down below. It is like looking in the mirror. Look at your own body from head to toe. Look at your head. Look at your face. Observe your neck. Observe your shoulders. Watch your arms. Watch your hands. Watch your chest. Look at your stomach. Look at your hips. See your thighs. See your knees. Watch your feet. Observe your entire body—from the toes to the head.

Your body has now become transparent. Look within your body. You are able to see the various organs functioning within your body. You can see your heart pumping blood. The blood is running in the veins and arteries throughout your body. Your lungs are breathing in and out, their muscles are expanding and contracting.

Your body is in perfect health, glowing with light and positive energy rays. Physically and spiritually, you are feeling rejuvenated.

Stage – 2 : Mediation

1. Meditation – Meeting with God

Now, resolve firmly that you want to meet God today. Pray to your Spiritual Master for His grace, to enable you to fulfil this resolution. Also, resolve strongly that you will stay attentive and not fall asleep. Imagine that your body is beginning to fly. You are experiencing this in your subconscious mind. Miraculously, you are lifted off your feet and you are now rising up in the air. Look down and see the people lying in Shavasan on the floor. Soar up, watch the clouds roll by and you roll with them. Keep climbing higher and enjoy the silence.

The vast expanse of mother earth, the never-ending sheet of clouds, and the surreal horizon! Your city now resembles a matchbox from above. The glowing Sun washes your face with its gleaming rays. Your flight intercepts the path of birds, who are amused to see a unique creature emulate the flight of Icarus. Smile at the birds and continue to fly. It is such a perfect day and it is now imminent that you are going to meet your beloved and revered Guru.

High up in the sky, your Guru appears from a cloud ahead. Your heart leaps with joy at His gracious presence and you prostrate at His lotus feet. Place your head softly on His feet and pray to Him, Oh! My beloved and revered *Gurudev*! Please take me to God's abode as I yearn to meet Him today. All I want is a fleeting glance. Your Guru blesses you with His hands on your head. He is now leading you further into the skies. The turquoise blue skies seem to reach beyond the heavens, and there is not a speck in the skyline.

You are now breaking the forces of gravity and zooming past the stratosphere. A great event awaits you as your Guruji takes you beyond the outer edges of the galaxy. You are now seeing hundreds of other galaxies flashing before you. Are these Star Wars! How strange they all look to the naked eye. You are now headed for Golok, Shree Krishna's Divine abode and your heart races in anticipation of the Divine rendezvous. As you draw closer, you can see a glow up ahead in a distance. This must be Golok Dham. You slow down and come to a stop.

Imagine that you have now reached the Divine abode of Golok. Like a beacon on a moonless night. Golok illuminates everything in all directions. You enter inside, anxious to see the sights. As you step inside, a surreal world greets you. It is completely different to what you saw a while ago—on the celestial journey till here. The Divine Yamuna flows majestically through lush greenery and thick forests. Serene ponds dot the place. Everything you see is an eternal part of Radha Rani. Even the leaves seem to chant the Name, "Radhey" with every breath.

Remember your oath. You had prayed to your *Gurudev* to help you meet God today. Now too far away, you can hear the melodic sound of a flute being played and it is undoubtedly Shree Krishna's. The bewitching melody increases your anxiety to meet Shyam Sundar. Your *Gurudev* is now leading you toward your soul-Beloved, past the Divine trees. Every tree chants the Name—"Radhey Radhey."

As you walk eagerly, you arrive at an open area. On the other side, Tribhangilal Shyam Sundar, Murali Manohar is standing under the *Kadamb* tree. You heart skips many beats at His very sight and you are now seeing His wonderful Divine form. Your eyes begin to admire His bluish color and beautiful crown made of peacock feathers, perched so perfectly on His tender head. He is also looking at you. Desiring to get closer to Him, you leave your *Gurudev*'s hands and rush toward Shyam Sundar's feet and prostrate. Embrace His feet and hold them in your arms, as this is the moment you have been waiting for, since eternity!

Overwhelmed with love for Shree Krishna, tears of joy run down your face. They seem to trickle down gently and cleanse the feet of Lord Krishna. All this while, you are holding the Lord's feet close to your chest. Pray to Him fervently, "Oh Lord! Please make me a speck of dust that sticks to Your feet all the time. I am an eternal part of You and my sins have led me astray in this materialistic world. I have now realized that Your love and service is my only goal. Oh Shyam Sundar! Please have mercy on me and grace me so that I will be Yours forever in Your abode."

Shree Krishna is holding you in His arms, as He helps you stand up. You are now looking at Him closer than ever, and your eyes fall prey to His mesmerizing gaze, melting your heart in an instant. You have never felt this way before and your heart races for your Beloved. Every inch of Shree Krishna's presence overflows with love for His devotees and realizing this fact, you feel closer to Him. You are now admiring everything about Shree Krishna. His beautiful blue skin, the peacock feather crown, the little earrings dancing at His slightest movement.

Unable to resist the temptation, you embrace Shree Krishna. This is the greatest and the finest moment of your entire existence! Tears run down your face, as Shree Krishna consoles you. You feel the biggest of the burdens being taken off your chest. The love of your life is in your arms, what else can you ask for? You are now weeping uncontrollably and Shyam Sundar is pacifying you. An eternal journey has now come to fruition with this Divine meeting with God. A lost and wandering soul has now met its true source and eternal companion.

Lost in love, you have not noticed time racing by. Your insatiable thirst for His love keeps you stuck to His shoulders, nestled in His arms and craving for more. Shree Krishna smiles at you and whispers into your ears, "Do not worry my dear child. Continue to increase your surrender and devotion, and you will one day reach a stage where you will be with Me forever. To get there, you will have to practice sincere devotion and listen to your *Gurudev*'s instructions. Surrender to Him and you shall come to Me. I promise." With these blessings, you return home, brimming with sweet memories of a meeting that will linger in your mind forever.

You now walk toward your *Gurudev*, who had been watching this scene from the distance. A great sense of satisfaction fills the heart of your *Gurudev* to see his disciple being greeted by the Lord Himself. This is also a day of great joy for your *Gurudev*. You prostrate at his feet and thank Him profusely for His grace without which this meeting would be impossible.

You are now returning back from Golok, and swoop across the skies in a flash. You are descending toward the solar system and you can see the nine planets revolving around the Sun. You have now reached the point where you can see planet Earth just as you left it some time ago. Descending further, you are now entering the earth's atmosphere and rapidly losing altitude. You can now sight your city, and soon, you can see the spot where your body is lying unmoved. You can also see others lying next to you, as still and calm as you are.

Slowly, enter your physical body.

Conclude the practice as explained in Stage – 3 (See page 356)

2. Meditation – Welcoming God to your Home

Today, you shall extend an invitation to Shree Krishna and request Him to grace your home. You have to take care not to lose concentration during your meditation, else you may fall asleep.

Stay determined that you shall not be careless, so that you can host God at your house today. Imagine you are leaving your gross body on the ground. Visualize with your mind that you are getting up from the floor and walking out from this place.

You are now at your home. Start the grand arrangements for the auspicious arrival of Lord Shree Krishna. You begin cleaning your house and no corner is spared. Your family members are helping you in the task to ensure that house is most presentable. The complete household is engaged in the cleaning, and all the dirt is slowly being washed away. You are cleaning the hall, the rooms, the stairs, the kitchen, the dining hall, and the washrooms.

You pay special attention to the *pūjā* room (altar at home) and decorate it with special, fragrant flowers. You are now sweeping, brushing, and polishing every visible surface. Hand plucked mango leaves adorn the doors and the supple trunks of young plantain trees are tied outside the entrance to the house. Exotic sandal perfume is selectively sprayed to elevate the senses. The doors are thrown open, a carpet of the choicest margosa and jasmine flowers and along with rose petals are laid down along the path up to your door. You are now checking every detail at home to ensure that all arrangements are made. The excitement grows for the impending Divine visit.

Step outside your house and begin to sing the Lord's Name and *kīrtans* along with your family members. You are all eagerly waiting for Radha Krishna to arrive. Suddenly, a flash of light in the distance draws your attention and you watch it with abated breath. The brilliant white light draws slowly toward the crowd of people gathered around. Your heart is on tenterhooks and is beating anxiously faster. The brilliant light has disappeared abruptly to reveal the breath taking Divine Forms of Radha Krishna.

Behold the magnificent splendour of Yugal Sarkar (the Divine Couple), right in front of your eyes! You and your family are overjoyed at the sight of Radha Krishna, and the chanting of Their Names is filling the air around. The sacred conch is being blown to announce the arrival of the revered Guests. People are showering flowers as your entire family welcomes Radha Krishna to enter and grace your home. Amidst the fervor, your roving eyes steal a few glances at the Divine couple. Shree Krishna's body has a blue tinge, His peacock-feathered crown sits so perfectly on His head, the rarest of pearl necklaces decorate His neckline and He wears the softest of silky saffron clothes.

Radha Rani is standing close to Him and She oozes grace. She is extremely fair and is wearing a blue silk saree. She is wearing a majestic-looking diamond studded crown. Her eyes are filled with love and compassion. Her very presence radiates Divine love and grace. A soft halo is surrounding Them both. Every member of your family prostrates in front of Radha Krishna. It is your turn to pay obeisance to Shree Radha Krishna. You are now prostrating at Their feet and thanking Them for gracing your house and granting your wish. Welcome Them home and request Them to come inside.

As They begin to walk, you shower more flowers at Their feet. The conch is again blowing and people chant the glory of Their Names continuously. Feel Their causeless grace as They have personally accepted your invitation and sanctified your place.

Yugal Sarkar are now being seated in your drawing room. The sofa is draped in silk and decked with flowers. The *Ārati* (ceremonial offering of lamps) is being prepared and *diyā* (the symbolic flame) is lighted. Exotic flower garlands were prepared for Shree Radha Krishna and you are now placing them on Shree Krishna and Radha Ji. Both are now seated comfortably on your sofa and feeling at home. Now, begin to wash Shree Krishna's feet gently. Realize how lucky and gifted you are because you are now washing the very same Divine feet, that are the source of the mighty Bhagirathi River. What a priceless opportunity! You are now wiping Shree Krishna's feet. Proceed to clean Shree Radha Rani's feet. These are the very same feet that even the greatest of *Ṛiṣhis* and *Munis* (Sages) meditate upon, to gain Her grace and cross the ocean of ignorance. Collecting the Divine water, that has the power to grant *Bhakti*, you drink a part of it as *Charaṇāmṛit*, and distribute the rest to all the family members.

Start to perform the *Ārati* of Yugal Sarkar. Sing the *Ārati* song as written and taught by your *Gurudev*.

आरति प्रीतम प्यारी की, कि बनवारी, नथवारी की।
ārati prītama pyārī kī, ki banavārī, nathavārī kī

The *ḍholak* is being played along with other instruments in the background. The Creator and Protector of countless galaxies, the Soul of all souls is now seated in your living room and showering His causeless grace upon you. You are immensely gifted with the good fortune of having God as your esteemed guest today. Petals are being showed from the heavens above by the *devatas* (celestial gods and goddesses). Everyone in the family is taking their turns to perform the *Ārati*. Continue to sing the *Ārati* prayer. Everyone is enjoying the occasion and their hearts are filled with love and affection for God.

You have now completed the *Ārati* and everyone is seated on the ground, in front of Shree Radha Krishna. Thank God for accepting your invitation and for coming home today. Request Him to make this home His temple.

It is now time for you to serve food to the most Esteemed Guests. Request Radha Krishna to taste some of the food prepared for Them. Help wash Shree Krishna's hands in a bowl of water. Wipe His hands gently with a towel. Wash Radha Rani's hands and wipe Them gently with a cloth. You are now preparing to serve Radha Krishna on silver plates and you place them in front. Freshly prepared food is brought to the table and served. They are now enjoying the food prepared with love and affection and are relishing every dish served. Everybody at home is overjoyed to see God Himself at their dining table and eating food like mere mortals!

Radha Krishna have finished eating and are sitting back in a relaxed pose. You had prepared special *pāns* (beetle nut and leaves) for both of Them. Placing the *pāns* on the plate, you are now presenting it to Radha Krishna. Shree Krishna takes one and places it in His mouth. Radha Rani takes the other. You now request Radha Krishna to grace every room of your house. Radha Krishna accept your invitation and proceed to visit every room.

They are now looking at the temple in your house and smile when They see Their own photographs. Your Guru's photograph is also placed beside Them. Radha Krishna are very impressed to see your Guru's photographs. You thank Them once again for gracing your house.

It is now time for Radha Krishna to leave. They advise you to continue to do *Bhakti* (devotion), and assure you that They will be back again. With these words, They proceed toward the door and walk outside. A flash of brilliant white light is seen where They stood; in a moment Radha Krishna disappear, just the way they came. The Divine perfume and Their sweet memories still linger in your mind and you sit down near the sofa to recollect every moment of this Divine event.

Now, come out of your house, and return to where your body is. Watch all the people lying on the floor. See your body lying in exactly the same position as you had left it. Slowly, enter your physical body.

Conclude the practice as explained in Stage 3 (See page 356)

3. Meditation – Visiting Vrindavan Dham

Today, resolve that you will visit Vrindavan, Mathura—the Land of Shree Krishna on this earth. Decide firmly that you will visit in your subtle body, all the places in Braj where Shree Krishna performed His Divine pastimes. Also, resolve that you will not fall asleep due to carelessness.

Leave your gross body on the floor. In your mind, get up from the floor and go back to your home. Prepare for your journey to Vrindavan. Pack your bag with clothes, toiletries, and other items required for the journey. You are now proceeding toward the railway station, eager to get on the train. At the station, there are many of your fellow devotees waiting to go to Vrindavan on the same tour as yours. The train arrives and excited devotes board the carriage.

You spend the journey singing and listening to *kīrtans*. At times, look out of the window and see the green fields, farmers working hard and tilling their lands. You are now anxious to reach Vrindavan at the earliest and visit all the places of Shree Krishna's pastimes. With these thoughts, go to sleep in the train. At dawn, all devotees are waking up early and you are also ready to leave. Soon, the train pulls into Mathura Junction. You are now getting down hurriedly and realizing that you are in the Divine Land of Shree Krishna! As a mark of deep respect, collect a pinch of mud and place it on your forehead. Pray to Shree Krishna for His grace and for His priceless Divine love. Pray to Him that you may be able to see all the places of His Divine *leelas* and receive His Divine vision.

Leaving Mathura by a van, you approach Vrindavan where you proceed toward your *Gurudev*'s *āshram*. Inside, you are greeted by other devotees. You rush toward the prayer hall. *Kīrtans* resound the hall with thousands of inspired voices singing in unison. The songs reach a feverish pitch with the grand entrance of your revered and beloved *Gurudev*. A feeling of great satisfaction and relief descends on you at the very sight of your Guru. The hall reverberates with cries of "Glory to *Gurudev*! Glory to our beloved *Gurudev*!" He is now seated on his ceremonial seat, as the devotees get in line to pay their obeisances and respects to Him.

It is now your turn to pay your respects to your Guru. Fall at His feet, to take His blessings. Everybody is in a very cheerful mood. Your *Gurudev* is inquiring from everyone about their well-being and current affairs. Ask his permission to take a tour of Vrindavan. He agrees immediately and advices that you should tour the Divine Land whilst singing the *kīrtans* of

Shree Krishna. Devotees now retire for the night.

Early next day, everybody gets ready to leave for the tour of Vrindavan. You leave bare-footed along with other devotees. Starting to sing the *kīrtans*, you are now walking in the lanes of Vrindavan. You now begin to think about the greatness of Vrindavan. This is the same place where Shree Krishna manifested His Divine pastimes nearly 5000 years ago. These are the very lanes where He played with His Divine associates, and the dust touched His Divine feet. You place some of the dust on your forehead and proceed further. You have now reached the banks of the Divine River, Yamuna, that looks blue in colour from a distance. This is the same Yamuna where Shree Krishna enacted His Divine *leelas* with the *Gopīs*.

Looking at the gently flowing water, try to remember Shree Krishna's Divine form. This is the same Divine Yamuna that has descended from Golok, the Divne abode of Shree Krishna. You are now walking along the banks of the river and have reached the place where Lord Krishna killed and liberated Kalia, a fearsome serpent. A temple stands at the place where this Divine act took place. Bow your head in reverence to Shree Krishna, the slayer of the serpent, viz. Kalia. Visualize the Divine *leela*, in which Kalia is half-submerged in the Yamuna, with his hoods raised outside the water, and Shree Krishna dancing on those hoods. What an awe-inspiring sight! Shree Krishna's cowherd friends are frightened and very concerned for their dearest pal. Mother Yashoda and Nand Baba arrive at the scene and are aghast to find their beloved young child in the grasp of this gruesome serpent. His dancing on the heads of the serpent soon subdues the serpent as it starts to bleed profusely. A subdued Kalia is now surrendering to Shree Krishna. Finally, Shree Krishna slays the serpent to redeem the village from the grip of the fearful serpent. What a Divine sight! This holy land of Braj has appeared on earth only due to the grace of Radha Rani and every particle in this holy land is filled with devotion for Shree Krishna. Think about the greatness of this land and continue to tour Vrindavan.

You have now reached Chir Ghat, the place where Shree Krishna enacted the *Chīr Haraṇ leela*. Try and visualize the situation. All the *Gopīs* are bathing in the water whilst Shree Krishna is sitting atop a tree, holding all the clothes with Him. The *Gopīs* plead with Him to return their clothes but the Lord refuses and asks them to pick it up on their own. This Divine pastime symbolizing surrender to the Lord is very unique, and you now pay your respect to Shree Krishna at the Chir Ghat Mandir and continue on your tour across Vrindavan.

Walking the streets of Vrindavan, you reach a place called Vamshivat, a place with great Divine significance. Vamshivat is a tree on the banks of river Yamuna. It is here that nearly 5000 years ago, Shree Krishna played the mesmerizing tunes on His flute that drew all the *Gopīs* from their homes into the Divine *Mahārās leela*. Though the tree does not exist any more, locals have placed another tree to signify the spot where it all happened. You are now paying your respects to *Raseshwar* Shree Krishna.

You are now seated near the banks of the river with other devotees and start singing *kīrtans* in remembrance of the Divine *Mahārās leela*. Try and visualize the picture in your mind. It is a full moon night, auspiciously known as *Śharat Pūrṇimā* and Shree Krishna is standing under the tree, playing melodious tunes with His flute, late in the night. The sound of His flute echoes across Braj and hearing them, the *Gopīs* get impatient. They yearn to meet Shree Krishna the very next moment and run toward Him. Imagine this scene from the Divine *leela* and continue to walk.

As you continue to tour Vrindavan, take a right turn from Vamshivat. You are now in Nidhivan where Radha Krishna would rest at night after Their pastimes with the *Gopīs*, in the forest groves. Here, the *Gopīs* would serve their Lord in different ways to ensure His happiness. Radha Krishna would make them sleep comfortably, and before dawn, would ensure that they reached home safely before Mother Yashoda or Kirti could find out. Visualize this intimate *leela* of Shree Radha Krishna resting in beautifully decorated hut, on a cot. The *Gopīs* are serving Them with all their attention. They are surrounded by pristine trees everywhere.

After some more walking, you come to Seva Kunj. This is the same Seva Kunj where Shree Krishna performed the famous *Rās leela*. Pay your respects at the temple of Shree Krishna in Seva Kunj. Imagine the *Rās leela* in your mind now. Thousands of *Gopīs* are dancing in a circle and Radha Krishna are dancing in the middle. The *Gopīs* are clapping their hands in appreciation as Radha Krishna dance gracefully. Shree Krishna has now expanded Himself into innumerable forms, and is dancing individually with each *Gopī*. Celestial gods and goddesses shower flowers from up above and pay obeisances to Radha Krishna in this Divine *leela*.

Think of this in your mind and continue to walk further. You have now reached the temple of Bankey Bihari where a crowd has gathered to get a glimpse of Lord Krishna's deity in the temple. The unique feature in this temple is that people are allowed to see the deity of Shree Krishna for a short while, and then the curtain is drawn in front of it. People sing the glories of the Lord and are overcome with love for Him. You are now standing in line to see the black idol of Shree Krishna. Soon, some devotees begin to distribute *prasād*. The priest throws a garland into the crowd that happens to fall on you and around your neck. Think of this as the Lord's grace on you and a good sign. With these thoughts in your mind, you are slowly leaving the Bankey Bihari temple.

A lot of time has passed since you left this morning. You have not noticed that dusk is approaching fast. Soon, you reach the *āshram* of your Guruji where you do *sādhanā* (devotional practice) for a short duration since you have to go back home. Hurriedly, you take your *Gurudev*'s blessing and leave Vrindavan for Mathura. You are now waiting for the train to take you back to your city. Inside the train, you and your fellow devotees recollect the wonderful experiences you all have had and sing *kīrtans* all along, in glorious remembrance of Shree Radha Krishna. The train has taken you to your home city and you bid adieu to all your fellow devotees.

You have now reached the home and are fully satisfied with the trip. From home, come back to the where your physical body is lying presently. See all the people lying on the floor. Recognize your body amongst them. Now, come back into your physical body.

Stage 3 – Conclusion

Once you have completed the meditation, you will have to come back to your normal state. For this, you have to slowly bring consciousness and movement in your gross body.

Start feeling the weight of your own body, lying on the ground. Move the fingers and toes. Move your feet and arms. Bend your arms and feet. Lock the fingers of your hands and place them above your head. This is similar to Tadasan posture in *yogasan*. Keep your feet straight and stretch your arms above your head, keeping your fingers interlocked. Now, turn sideways and get up from either right or left side slowly. Sit in Sukhasan posture. Rub your palms and place them on your eyes. Open your eyes slowly with a few blinks.

XII. *Roop Dhyan* Meditation

The mind is a subtle machine that constantly generates thoughts. These thoughts create our personality. You look at someone and say, "He seems to be a very aggresive person," or "He appears to be a very simple, straightforward person," or "He seems to be very merciful," etc. The nature of thoughts that resides in the mind shapes both—personality and physical appearance.

The Latent Powers of the Mind

Modern scientists estimate that we only use three per cent of the potential of our mind. At present, our mind is scattered. Just as, if the channel button of a television set is spoilt, the channels keep changing sporadically. Similarly, our mind too keeps flipping from topic to topic. But if we can learn to concentrate our mind, we can increase the extent to which we are able to utilize its potential.

Concentration increases the effectiveness. Water vapor keeps rising from lakes, and ineffectively drifting in the sky. But the same water vapour, when concentrated in the form of steam and focused on the piston of the railway engine, becomes so powerful that it is able to push the engine along a railway track, with thousands of tonnes of carriages at high speeds. Similarly, an unwavering mind has tremendous powers. This is the reason why different people in different cultures around the world use a variety of meditation techniques to improve their concentration. Some mediate on the breath, others on the eyebrow centre, others on the psychic centres in the spinal cord, others on a tranquil lake, and others on light, etc. These different meditation techniques do improve the focus of the mind; however, their benefits are incomplete and impermanent. The reason is that they do not address the issue of purification of the mind. As long as lust, anger, greed, envy, illusion, etc. reside in the mind, these forces destroy whatever concentration was gained. It thus becomes vitally important to understand how to purify the mind.

Purification of the Mind

To cleanse the mind, we must fix it on an object of meditation that is itself pure. The material realm is dominated by the three modes of material nature—*sattva*, *rajas*, and *tamas* (modes of goodness, passion, and ignorance). If the object of meditation is material, it cannot purify the mind. Beyond this material realm, is the Divine realm of God, His Names, Forms, Virtues, Abodes, Pastimes, and Saints. If we fix our mind anywhere in this area, it will become pure. Shree Krishna told Arjun in the Bhagavad Geeta:

मां च योऽव्यभिचारेण भक्तियोगेन सेवते।
स गुणान्समतीत्यैतान् ब्रह्मभूयाय कल्पते॥ (भगवद् गीता १४.२६)

māṁ cha yo 'vyabhichāreṇa bhaktiyogena sevate
sa guṇānsamatītyaitān brahmabhūyāya kalpate (Bhagavad Geeta 14.26)

"I am Divine. If you fix your mind on Me, it will rise above the three modes of material nature." Jagadguru Shankaracharya says:

शुद्धयति हि नान्तरात्मा कृष्णपदाम्भोज भक्तिमृते।

shuddhayati hi nāntarātmā krishṇapadāmbhoja bhaktimrite

"The inner self, the mind, cannot be cleansed without fixing it in devotion on God." Jagadguru Shree Kripaluji Maharaj says:

सर्व शास्त्र सार यह गोविन्द राधे।

आठों याम मन हरि गुरु में लगा दे॥ (जगद्गुरु श्री कृपालुजी महाराज)

sarva śhāstra sāra yaha govinda rādhey

āṭhoñ yāma mana hari guru meñ lagā de (Jagadguru Shree Kripaluji Maharaj)

Hence in Jagadguru Kripaluji Yog, we learn to meditate on the Names, Forms, Virtues, Pastimes, Abodes, and Associates of God. Meditation on God can be of endless varieties, of which a few sample meditations are described below.

Types of *Roop Dhyan* Meditations

This section describes various meditation techniques with a sample meditation.

1. Meditation with Every Breath

In order to cleanse the mind, we need to fix our mind on God. To do that, we need to take the help of Divine entities like God's Names, Forms, Pastimes (*leelas*), Qualities, Abodes, and His Saints (Associates). In this mediation, we will use the Names of God to focus our mind on Him. The Scriptures say:

नाम्नामकारि बहुधा निज सर्व शक्तिस्। (चैतन्य शिक्षाष्टकम्)

namnāmakāri bahudhā nija sarva śhaktis (*Chaitanya Śhikṣhāṣhṭakam*)

कहहुँ नाम बढ़ ब्रह्म राम ते।

kahahuñ nāma baḍha brahma rāma te

कलियुग केवल नाम आधारा।

kaliyuga kevala nāma ādhārā

ब्रह्म राम ते नाम बढ़, बढ़ दायक बढ़ दानी।

brahma rāma te nāma baḍha, baḍha dāyaka baḍha dānī

The Vedas declare that God is fully present in His Name itself. He has put all His powers in His Name. So, He is present in the same form in His Name as He is in Vrindavan! This is another example of the causeless grace of God. The great Saints of India have given us a very easy and powerful way of remembering God. Recite and remember God with every breath you take in. This is the big secret. You do not need any *mālā* (beads); there is nothing else to show to the outside world nor do you have to remember the count.

Let us now practice this form of Meditation. We will take the help of God's sweet Names, Radhey Krishna. The reader is free to take the help of any Name of God like Seeta-Ram, *Oṁ Namaḥ* Shivaya, Wahey Guru, *Jai* Hanuman, Mother Mary, glory to Christ, Allah, and so on. There is no restriction on the Name of God.

Close your eyes and relax your body. Keep your eyes closed till the end of this meditation exercise. As you read on or listen to a *dhyan* (meditation) lecture, create the same type of feeling in your mind. Slowly and steadily breathe in and breathe out. Concentrate on your breathing rhythm. Take a slightly deeper breath and let it out. Practice this three times. Keep your eyes closed and body relaxed.

Now, we shall go to the next level. Imagine that there are two pipes in your nasal cavity— all through to the stomach. You are breathing in with one pipe and out with the other. Keep breathing steadily and visualize the same picture.

Let us now move ahead and add one more aspect to the meditation, the Name of God. As you breathe in, say the Name "Radhey," or your chosen Name, in your mind. Feel the sound travel from your nose to your navel through the pipe. Now, slowly breathe out and say the Name "Krishna," or your chosen Name in your mind. Feel the sound travel from the navel back to your nose, through the pipe.

Now, discard idea of the pipes from your mind and just concentrate on the Names of God, "Radhey Krishna, Radhey Krishna, Radhey Krishna." Just feel the Name and the sound within yourself with every breath.

God is present with all His powers in His Divine Name. Bring this fact to your mind, and experience the presence of God as the vibrations of the Names travel within you. Shree Radha Krishna are traversing your body, purifying you by Their presence and grace.

2. Meditation on Noble Thoughts

In this meditation, we work on bringing the noble thoughts and emotions in our mind. This helps us calm the mind and brings a sense of tranquillity that we have not experienced before. Let us learn to create thoughts of forgiveness, mercy, compassion, understanding, tolerance, friendship, devotion, servitude, and so on. This is generally called as "Positive Thinking" and quite commonly known to us. These thoughts strengthen the mind and at the same time, help us get rid of impure thoughts that plague us continuously and weaken our minds.

Think that God is standing right in front of you. He is the ocean of eternal happiness. Try to feel the peace and calm emanating from God. Feel the tranquillity slowly overtake your senses and fill your inner self. Your body is completely relaxed and free of stress. Now think about God and how tolerant He is. He is the protector of countless souls and knows each soul's every problem. Yet, He does not get angry or tense. His whole presence emanates peace, tranquillity, and calmness. Now, try and absorb the same feeling within you. Feel the calm presence of Shree Krishna in front of you and relax your body and mind.

Stop thinking of matters related to the outside world. Think of yourself to be a tolerant person and try to increase this feeling. People are disturbing and creating problems for you but you remain calm in front of any difficulty. You do not lose your mind or balance. You are now becoming as tolerant and humble as a tree.

God has all the noble characteristics we admire. He has the best characteristics and is the noblest of them all. Feel that all these good qualities are flowing from God toward you, into your body and your mind. As the goodness of God enters your system, you feel more peaceful and calm. Now, all the negative feelings are flowing out of your body. Out of them, the one that hurts you the most, your ego, is leaving you. You feel more humble in the presence of the almighty God, Who is the humblest of all. Humility is one of the best qualities one can possess and you are now learning to be humble and gentle with everyone. You take great pleasure in honouring others but not seeking fame for yourself.

All the negative thoughts and feelings in your body have gone away. You are now surrounded and filled with all the good qualities that belong to God. Your mind is as clear as a mountain stream and perfectly balanced. It has given up all the bad thoughts and is now thinking only of the Lord. Slowly, you begin feeling the Lord's grace and a feeling of gratefulness starts to flow through your body. It is due to the Lord's grace that all your negative feelings have gone away and you feel so good and positive. You have never felt this good before. Feel humble before God and see Him smile back at you. Look at the people around you, many of them leading a sad and dejected life. Just like you, they are children of God but they do not realize it. Pray to the Lord that He brings them on the right path and graces them so that they can follow Him truthfully and sincerely.

It gives immense pleasure to the Lord when He sees you as a changed person with all the Divine qualities taking seed in your thoughts. Continue to feel positive and pray to the Lord for the well-being of this whole world.

3. Meditation on the Greatness of God

Our next meditation is the practice of remembering the greatness and the grace of God. We have been gifted with the five senses, hearing, sight, touch, taste, and smell that we use in our daily lives. These five senses also reside within the mind in a subtle form. When we are asleep, all our organs also go to rest. We are unable to see or hear anything. However, when we dream, we perform all sorts of activities like seeing, walking, talking, hearing, and eating. How is this possible? It is due to the presence of the five senses in their subtle form that we continue to perform the same activities even in our dreams. We all know that we cannot dream at will. It happens by chance and takes its own course; our conscious mind has no control over it. In this meditation, we will utilize the five subtle senses within the mind to meditate. The world is full of God's magical creation and glimpses of His innumerable virtues. We all get to see, smell, hear, and touch the many objects that He has created for us. Every cell has some unique characteristic or the other. We perceive beauty, art, colour, melody, and many such innumerable aspects around us that are nearly impossible to be explained in words. Keeping this in mind, just think how great and immeasurable God is!

When we forget the greatness and the power of God, we tend to submerge the mind within our own small world of selfish desires. We give prime importance to our desires, worries, and problems that confront us every day. Due to this, our mind is full of impure thoughts that give rise to anger, disappointment, lust, fear, anxiety, and tension. These feelings and emotions can also grow uncontrollably and may one day overcome us, leading to extreme grief and misery.

Close your eyes and relax your body. Take a deep breath and let it go out slowly. Concentrate on your breathing as you go deeper into a more relaxed state of mind. Now, as each action is described one by one, form a picture of the same in your mind, thinking that it is in front you, and mentally perform the actions as instructed. When the instructor says, "See this," or "Hear that," please try to do as specified, but within the realm of your mind.

Think about how unique and amazing our living world is. God's gracious and perfect actions are visible everywhere. See how soft and beautiful the morning Sun is as it appears on the horizon and slowly turns into a fireball. Observe the beautiful birds whose noisy but cheerful calls wake up all and sundry. There are some birds that make melodic sounds and attract the attention of their mates. Listen to their sounds and how perfect their calls are. See how many colorful birds God has created. Each bird has a unique body, color, and features. Parrots are green, scarlets are yellow, flamingos are pink, the crow is black, and swans are milk-white. Look at how gracefully and swiftly the swan moves across the sky. Few birds are as beautiful as a swan or a flamingo in flight is. How do they manage it? What is the secret behind such grace and poise? God has given them such powerful yet deft wings. What a sight!

Look at the peacock. It has such a long and exquisitely feathered tail, unmatched anywhere in the living world. See how he dances in the rain in front its mate! Look at its open feathered tail in iridescent green and gold. How did the peacock learn to dance so gracefully? Why did God give such a beautiful tail to a peacock and not any other bird? God has strange ways of expressing beauty.

We have all seen butterflies fluttering around in the garden. What a riot of colours they are! From flower to flower, they jump in search of the intoxicating nectar they love dearly. Watch them fold their wings and open them as they devour the nectar from the flowers. It seems like butterflies have been artistically painted from a palette of a million colors by a master artist. Their carefree flight appears to represent and celebrate God's unbound joy and happiness.

How refreshed we feel looking at the natural wonders around us. The beautiful sunrise, the soaring birds in the horizon, the beautiful meadows with rich grass for the cattle to feed on, the mountains covered with forests as far as the eyes can see, snow laden peaks piercing the clouds to kiss the sky, and gentle streams merging with eachother to create mighty rivers that unite with the ocean. What a natural wonder God has created for us to enjoy!

Now, look at the green trees in the orchard and how huge and protective they are! They are souls who are standing upside down with their heads down and legs up in the air! They stand there for years together, providing shelter for the ones who seek protection under their mighty branches. These life-giving trees consume dirty air and produce fresh oxygen for us to breathe. What a selfless service they perform and we do not even realize it. We use and abuse them, yet they stand there silently tolerating us. We surely have something to learn from the selfless benevolence of these trees.

Look at the vast oceans of the world. Endless waves are born that lash the shores, day and night. So mighty and strong, yet they are so contained within their boundaries. Under the turbulent waters thrives a deafening and vibrant world, full of creatures, big and small. How astonishing the underworld is! We hardly know anything about it. Imagine, how big and immeasurable the Creator, of whose this universe is, could be. The Creator of innumerable earths, Suns, and moons is within us and we still can't know Him! Astonishing! How could we even think of understanding God, Who created this universe by just wishing it! Our limited intellect is inadequate even to comprehend the aspects of this material world, then how can we attempt to comprehend matters beyond its reach. To know God, we will need His grace and mercy. Only then can we begin to understand everything related with creation and beyond.

God has given each living creature a special gift and a unique quality. A dog is so faithful and it can even sacrifice its life for its master. The honeybees work tirelessly day and night to fill jars of honey for us humans to consume. Cows are known for their soft and calm nature. Horses have tremendous power and can run for miles with a heavy weight behind them. God has created each animal with a lot of thought so that they can be of some use to us. We humans are forever indebted to God for the countless instances of grace He has showered on us, yet we remain unfaithful and forgetful of His greatness.

Human life is an opportunity and a priceless gift. It is not a burden or a chance to think negatively, feel depressed, discouraged, or develop bad feelings within ourselves. It has been given to us with a special purpose and we must utilize every moment of our lives for the fulfilment of that purpose and nothing else. The Vedas say, "O! Humans, Arise and Awake, do not fall down and squander this chance but move ahead and accomplish your goal. Seek the mercy and grace of a God-realized Saint and learn about the absolute truth."

4. Increasing Longing for God

Principle

In search of happiness, we humans create countless desires that we think will satisfy our senses and mind. Yet, we do not seem to have attained the ever-elusive happiness that eternally overcomes all the sadness and suffering in our lives. The state of our inner and private world has remained the same, for we constantly harbour desires, anger, disappointment, greed, jealousy, anxiety, lust, and other mental ailments. Yet, we remain optimistic that one day, peace and happiness will arrive on a magic carpet, ready to sweep us away to a world of fulfilled desires and never ending material comforts. Amazing!

To develop an appreciation for the true meaning of happiness and the way to attain it, let us start by diverting our material desires toward God. Let us begin by desiring things associated with God and the people related to Him. By associating our mind in Him frequently, our mind will slowly get attached to Him. Practicing this regularly will help us fix our mind on

Him firmly. The more we attach our mind on God, the more we get detached from the material world and our hearts will also be cleansed to the same proportion.

या अनुरागी चित्तकी गति समझे नहीं कोय।
ज्यों ज्यों डूबे श्याम रंग त्यों त्यों उज्जवल होय॥

yā anurāgī chittakī gati samujhe nahīñ koya
jyoñ jyoñ ḍūbe śhyāma raṅga tyoñ tyoñ ujjavala hoya

God has gifted us five senses (eyes, ears, mouth, nose, and skin) in their physical as well as subtle forms. The eyes can see, but vision is something more subtle and internal to us. In the same way, ears can hear but listening is a subtle faculty. The ability to recognize taste, the sense of feeling (touch), and smell are the other capabilities that we possess in the subtle form. The great thing about them is that all the five senses also reside within our minds. What else can explain the phenomenon of being able to see, hear, smell, and touch various objects in our dreams? When we are asleep, all the five sense organs also go to rest. We are unable to see or hear anything. But, in our dreams we perform all sorts of activities like seeing, walking, talking, hearing, and eating. How is this possible? It is due to the presence of the five senses in their subtle form in the mind. This is known as cognizance in the scientific world. We will now learn to divert these subtle senses in our mind toward God, by concentrating our mind on the aspects associated with God.

Meditation

Imagine that you have just arrived in the Divine Abode of Vrindavan. Create a picture in your mind of all the beautiful things that you would like to see in Vrindavan. The lush greenery, the huge eucalyptus and banyan trees, cows grazing on the meadows far and wide, birds chirping, the peacocks calling, and a waterstream flowing lethargically like a well-fed snake. As this is the Divine abode, everything here has a special significance. The warm fragrance of the Divine trees brushes your nostrils and elevates your senses to a new level. Start walking in the lane lined by trees. Watch the branches gently sway to the tunes of the Divine breeze. The nearby woods provide plenty of fresh air to breathe.

As you take a stroll, your ears are instantly captivated by a hypnotic melody being played over the hills, far away. Deeply attracted and mesmerized by the Divine tunes, imagine yourselves being magically transported in the direction of the tantalizing notes. You wonder who could be playing such a wonderful instrument and realize that this Divine music is being played by none other than your soul beloved Shree Krishna. You are now running in the direction of the music, stumbling over mounds, wading through ankle deep water and across the green meadows, disturbing the cattle's peaceful grazing and throwing their rhythm out of gear.

Unmindful of this, your senses are now firmly attached to the harmony still flowing curiously across the lowly hills. The tunes get closer and sweeter, your heart beats faster but you still can't see Him. You plead Him to reveal a glimpse of His true self. His Divine melody has all but captured your breath.

At that very instant, you think of your beloved Guru and beg Him to show you a glimpse of Shree Krishna. You pray at his lotus feet to shower his grace upon you so that you can meet your soul beloved.

Your Guru agrees to your prayers and offers his re-assuring hands, which you gladly hold on to as if your life depends on it. Slowly you gather yourself and follow your Guru in the direction of the soothing notes. Accompanying the melodic flute is the graceful tune, emanating from the anklets of Shree Krishna. Unable to comprehend or digest the sweetness of this Divine music, you resist the urge to ask your Guru to go faster. Your Guru smiles at your thoughts and comes to a stop.

Your eyes scan the horizon as your eyes fall upon the mighty and Divine River Yamuna, flowing silently across the fields of maize, corn, and wheat. The crystal clear water attracts your attention but you remain unmoved. Your revered Guru gestures at you as your gaze reaches the Divine *Kadamb* tree on the banks of the river. Nearby, standing on the tender grass, wearing a silken, yellow cloth, *Pītāmbar*, and holding the flute in both His hands, is your soul beloved Shree Krishna.

Your eyes cannot believe that Shree Krishna is indeed in front of you, playing the most attractive melodies. Shree Krishna gestures at your Guru to bring you closer to Him. As your Guru steps toward you with his arms wide open, look at yourself fall at His feet and then embrace Him. Tears roll down your eyes in humble submission toward your revered Guru with Whose grace this auspicious moment has arrived. He then hands you over to your Beloved Lord, Shree Krishna, Who waits patiently for you to step forward.

Leaving your Guru's shadow, you are drawn closer to Shree Krishna like a moth is to limelight. Behold the Lord with all your eyes for this is the ultimate moment of your life. You have been blessed and graced with the greatest of all boons and the most priceless of all treasures there is or will ever be. The most awaited day of your entire existence has now arrived, for you have a private audience with the Lord Himself!

You and your Guru are now witness to Shree Krishna's *Roop Mādhurī*, or the Nectar flowing from His Divine Form, due to which the Lord of lords appears the most beautiful and handsome. As you lift your head and look into His eyes pouring with love, Shree Krishna's gaze pierces your heart with a thousand arrows, resulting in the tears of joy cascading down your cheeks. Your voice is choked, throat dry, and unable to utter much. Your eyes now fall upon His admirable crown made of peacock feathers, perched perfectly on His tender head. The feathers fluttering in the gentle breeze appear to fan His soft and curly hair. Your eyes are drawn toward His perfectly carved eyes that resemble that of a peacock. You are now looking at the prominent *tilak* on His forehead placed so expertly.

Shree Krishna is wearing a *Vaijayantī Mālā* (Divine garland made of the choicest of Divine flowers) whose fragrance fills the air around. Every flower in the garland seems to reach out toward Shree Krishna's nostrils, trying to impress Him with their exotic fragrnace. Decked in the choicest of jewellery and the exquisite *Kaustubh Maṇi*, Shree Krishna looks extremely attractive. His trunk is partially covered in the softest of silk *dupaṭṭās* that seem to gently kiss

His skin so as not to pain His soft and delicate body. He is robed in yellow clothes, held in its place around His slender waist by a gold band. Your Beloved wears a silver anklet that sings as He steps toward you. The sound of the anklets rings in your ears like a symphony of a hundred musicians, elevating your joy to unknown heights.

Shree Krishna now plays the flute, drowning you deeper in the bliss of Divine love for your Beloved. Slowly and steadily, you and your Guru move toward Shree Krishna's feet, where you take your rightful place.

As He stands tall, you watch the grass gently support His tender feet, and go head over heels to massage them. Every object and living being that you see around Him is doing its best to be of service to Shree Krishna. Your concentration is now on His feet as you thank Him and your Guru profusely for this most fortunate event of your life. Pray to Shree Krishna to grace you in such a way that your permanent place will remain at His lotus feet in eternal service for His happiness alone. Realize you are to be the humblest of all souls and a sinner beyond redemption. Shed tears of repentance for His happiness and wash His feet lovingly for His comfort.

Think of yourself to be the most fallen soul and beg for His forgiveness. Break the chains of your heart and fill it with love for Shree Krishna. Seeing that His devotee has truly surrendered himself, Shree Krishna now lifts you with both His arms and embraces you with all His heart. When you thought that the ultimate joy had been attained, your Beloved now fills your heart with more Divine love and bliss that is countless times higher than what you received earlier. Shree Krishna Himself is very pleased with your selfless love and showers more of His Divine love upon you. The tears in yours eyes have now formed a constant stream and cleansed your heart forever.

Shree Krishna now instructs your Guru to take you back to the earth and asks you if you will continue to love Him more than ever. Reluctantly, you leave His arms and again prostrate at His lotus feet. Shree Krishna again flashes His bewitching smile and says, "I shall never leave you even for a moment. I am always with you and in you. Think of Me at all times and you shall be eternally blissful."

With these words, Shree Krishna bids adieu. Your lovelorn eyes are still filled with tears as you request the Lord for His permission to leave. Shree Krishna sends you off with His blessings as you and your Guru slowly make your way out of Vrindavan. Everything looks pale and lifeless without your Soul-Beloved, but His reassuring words lift your spirits.

Open your eyes and bring yourself back home.

5. Gratitude

There is a great importance attached with our thoughts and their related actions. Our thinking shapes the personality we are known for. If we develop and harbour negative or bad thoughts, it stops the flow of Divine grace and restricts our mind. Our mental and physical health is bound to suffer if we are filled with anger, hatred, jealousy, or any type of bad thoughts. Eventually, we are affected by some misfortune due to our negative personality and thinking.

To help change our thinking and bring about good, positive thoughts, we should develop gratitude in our hearts. We all have so many good things around us but we fail to see them and recognize their importance. By learning to appreciate even the smallest things as gifts from God, our heart will automatically feel for it and begin to appreciate the importance of God, and the feeling of gratitude slowly increases. We will now try and meditate by concentrating the heart and mind toward increasing the feeling of gratitude.

Close your eyes and begin to relax. Take a deep breath and let it out slowly. Concentrate on your breathing as you go deeper into a more relaxed state of mind. Now, as each action is described, please form a picture of the same in your mind, and think that it is in front of you and perform the same. When the instructor says, "See this" or "Hear that," please try to do that but within your mind.

Observe your breathing and how naturally it occurs. The air that we breathe in and out is a gift of God. Try and realize the fact that you are actually breathing the grace of the Lord and thank Him for that with all your heart. Think of what would happen without the air and without His grace.

Think of mother earth and bring her into your conscious mind. God has created this huge planet for our well-being. He created the fertile land, the mountains, and rivers. The food that we all get to consume is again a gift from God. Due to His grace, we have water, rice, wheat, maize, scores of vegetables, fruits, oils, and an endless variety of eatables to keep us healthy and nourished. What we eat nourishes our body, creates fresh blood, bones, and muscles. God again graces us through this wonderful creation.

You are now watching the Sun rising in the east. The bright rays vanquish the darkness of the night and illuminate the world around us. Birds begin their morning flight and chirping at the very sight of light. The Sun gives us light every day without fail. Concentrate your mind on the Sun rays and feel that it is God's grace being showered in the form of Sun rays all around us. You are standing in brilliant sunshine with the Sun rays drenching your whole body. Feel the grace of God flowing into you. If it were not for the Sun, we would never have known what is light. Thank God for this life-giving form of grace.

Now look at your own body. This was also created by God Himself. When you were an embryo in your mother's womb and curled with feet up and head down, it was God Himself who ensured your safety and protection. Today, you are a grown up person and it is due to God's grace that you are able to perform all types of actions in your daily life. Observe your tireless heart. It beats nearly 100,000 times a day. It pumps blood to every nook and corner of your body. The veins and blood vessels that carry blood span nearly 100,000 Kilometres inside your body! Is it not astonishing!

See your body from above. It has so many organs like the liver, the kidney, the lungs, the digestive system, and many more. All these work in perfect harmony to ensure that you live a healthy life. They all work like tireless servants to make sure that the body stays in good shape all the time. This is another example of God's causeless grace. You have been gifted with eyes and vision, you have been given ears and hearing, you have a mouth and the ability to speak.

"If there is any trace of goodness in me, that is due to Your grace and mercy. Not a leaf moves without Your grace! Then how is it possible for me to have any good characteristic without Your grace? In fact, I cannot do anything without Your causeless grace and even the impossible can be made possible with Your grace. Oh! Giver of life, please have mercy on this insignificant fallen soul and grace me with Your Divine love and Divine vision. I beg You for a drop of the nectar of Divine love that You hold so dearly."

7. *Karm Yog Dhyan*

Jagadguru Shree Kripaluji Maharaj has revealed this special form of *dhyan* (meditation) to facilitate the process of God-realization for every soul. It is a very flexible form of meditation that can be practiced in almost every situation. Normally, people associate God with a temple or a place of worship. But the Vedas declare that God resides in every atom in this Universe. Hence, it is not necessary that God must live only in a temple, a church, or a mosque. He is everywhere and in every being, living or dead. We will now practice to meditate on the fact that God and your Guru are always with you, everywhere.

There are many benefits from this type of meditation, and one can progress very fast toward God by practicing it. Our aspirations, attachments, and desires bind us to this material world. Our mind continuously thinks of something dearer or closer to our hearts. For example, one person may like money, another likes his wife or husband, whereas another person wants fame and so on. The minds of these people are constantly engaged in thinking about their subject of interest and attachment. With some sincere effort, a person can concentrate his or her mind on another subject thereby removing his or her mind away from the things he or she is so dearly attached to.

Karm Yog meditation helps you fix your mind on God. With this type of meditation, God's power and grace will always remain in your coscinsouness. When you feel the presence of God all the time, your conscience will remain alert and you will stop yourself from performing sinful or harmful actions. If you begin to realize that God is protecting you, then all the fears and inhibitions in your mind will slowly vanish.

Performing *Karm Yog* meditation will require patience and persistence. We have to reach a stage where the remembrance of God in all aspects of our daily life becomes very easy and a natural part of ourselves. In the beginning, we have to put in a lot of effort to concentrate and fix our mind on God and things related to Him. Slowly but steadily, we will progress and move forward. With continuous practice, meditation will become easier and more enjoyable. Sincere practice is the key. Just like the way we learnt to ride the bicycle or swim, we have to put in our best efforts and leave the rest to God. He will definitely help us come closer to Him, if we sincerely follow His path.

Close your eyes and relax. Take a deep breath and let it out slowly. Concentrate on your breathing as you go into a more relaxed state of mind. When the instructor says, "See this," or "Hear that," please form a picture of the same in your mind and think that it is in front you and perform the same. When it says, "See this," or "Hear that," please try to do that but within your mind.

You are now seated comfortably in your living room. Feel the presence of God next to you. There is no need to visualize His form but a firm feeling in your heart that He is next to you and watching you. Touch His feet and seek His grace such that you will always remember Him and that you shall live your life in His presence at all times. In your mind, perform the *Ārati* of God.

Now think that God is standing behind you and watching your every move. He is in fact your Protector. Imagine Him—the Creator and Protector of unlimited galaxies and this Universe is actually your Protector too! So, what are you worried about? Leave all your negative thoughts and worries with Him and revel in the fact that you are protected by none other than God.

God is now standing next to you and smiling at you. He holds your hand as a symbol of His friendship. Imagine in your mind that you too are holding His hand and consider Him as your best friend. As your closest associate, you will now share every moment with Him and perform every task in His presence and dedicate it to Him. You shall only perform the task and the Lord shall give the fruit of each action.

Feel that God is now next to you, and watching your actions. Feel His grace and presence. He has now placed His Divine hands on your head as if blessing you. Your heart leaps with joy and at the same time you feel very grateful to the Lord for His benevolence and grace.

You are now inviting God to grace your house and spend some time with you in leisure. Your Lord readily agrees to your request and you lead Him toward your house. You have Him seated on your sofa and you are sitting on the ground, close to His feet. Soon, you begin to take His advice on matters related to your worldly life and dealings. The Lord replies, "I will not as yet answer questions in person. When you call upon me with a sincere heart and in isolation, I shall lead you in the right way and I shall illuminate your intellect, which will guide you on the right path."

It is a very hot day and you proceed to take a shower. You also ask God if He would like to take a shower and freshen Himself. God readily agrees to your request like a child wanting to play in a pond. In the shower room, you are hesitant with your clothes and uncertain of what to do next. The Lord smiles and says, "My dear friend, I live in every atom of your body and I live in your heart. I am everywhere you see and cannot. Why this hesitation? There is nothing I do not know or cannot see. I have declared in the Bhagavad Geeta that remember Me and think of Me everywhere. In the temple, at work, while cooking, resting, and also in your shower! Hearing these words, your mind and intellect has been cleared of a great flaw and redeemed of a silly inhibition. You feel very humbled with His words.

Finishing your shower, you slowly walk toward your living room again accompanied by your Beloved Friend and Lord. Every step you take, He watches you. He knows every breath you take and every move of yours. He is watching you closely and endlessly. You realize this fact and your feeling of loneliness is gone! You now begin to believe that He had said earlier. "I am always with you. You belong to me. I am your father and you are My son."

With these words, your spirit feels free as a bird. You fall at His lotus feet and begin to pray. "Dear Lord, the reason for all problems in my life is because I had forgotten You and was thinking only of matters in the material world. I had turned my back toward You. Now, due to Your grace, I have learnt that only You are mine. I want to make this life successful by surrendering myself completely to You. I shall now attempt to perform every task by remembering You all the time. I shall aim to consider every task as Your *Sevā* (service) and to dedicate every action for Your benefit and comfort only. Dear Lord, I beg You to grace me and have mercy on me. Please grace me with Your Divine love and service."

XII. The Science of Healthy Diet*

Health is the basis of all other assets and has a meaning only if it is in good shape. You cannot get good health by visiting the doctor or eating supplements. You create it by your habits, and can change it by mending your ways. Today, we do not have any shortage of food. A majority of the people who visit doctors are the ones who have eaten too much, or eaten the wrong kind of food, or in the wrong way. Half of what we eat feeds us and the rest breeds diseases and feeds doctors and drug stores.

Among the various factors affecting health, the single most important is food. And it can be easily controlled and corrected with rewarding results. The following aspects should be known about the food that we eat:

Diet: The contents of the different nutrients in the foods.

Digestion: The process of breaking down of the food into simpler parts, so that it can be absorbed in the blood and circulated throughout the whole body.

Nutrition: What is going to nourish us toward better health? How does food influence our body after it gets absorbed?

Knowledge of diet, digestive process, and nutrition lead to a new way of life, by making us conscious of our eating habits.

Diet

Food has two primary constituents: Calories and Nutrients.

1. Calories

This is the energy content of food. Calories are required by the body to carry out all kinds of activities. This energy is measured in kilocalories (simply called calories). Calorie requirements vary with age, sex, and activity level. Roughly, men need 2450 calories and women 1800 calories a day.

At present many people in different countries are worried about their daily diet. Despite this, the list of food that they consume daily must have the required calories to adjust with the standard of life. The amount of food they consume must have the amount of good calorie that is needed for a hale and hearty body.

2. Nutrients

Nutrition or nourishment is the provision to different cells and organisms of the materials necessary (in the form of food) to sustain life. Almost all health problems can be prevented by taking a healthy diet. The nourishing nutrients present in food can be categorized in two large categories: macronutrients and micronutrients. Macronutrients are those that are needed in large quantities. Micronutrients are those that are needed in small quantities. This section discusses the nutrients, proteins, fats, vitamins, minerals, and antioxidants required for a healthy body.

Carbohydrates:

Energy giving foods are called carbohydrates. They are of two types. The first are simple sugars such as sugar, honey, candy, etc. The next are complex starches like cereal, flour-bread, rice, potato, etc. The normal daily intake of carbohydrate is about 4-6gm/kg body weight.

These are a major constituent of the diet of people, worldwide. A typical Indian diet contains 70 per cent carbohydrates. They are present in three forms—sugar (honey, white sugar, etc.), starches (cereals, pulses, grams, etc.), and fibres. There are six different functions of carbohydrates:

- Supplying energy and regulation of blood glucose.
- Sparing the use of proteins for energy.
- Breaking down fatty acids and stopping ketosis.
- Helping in the biological recognition processes.
- Adding flavor and sweeteners.
- Supplying with adequate dietary fibre.

Proteins:

Body building and repairing foods such as milk, pulses, nuts, soybeans, grams, etc. are known as proteins. They are made up of very small units called amino acids. Just as bricks are used to erect a building, proteins are used by our body as building blocks.

Every cell of our body contains proteins. They are essential macromolecules without which our bodies would be unable to repair, regulate, or protect themselves. The daily requirements of proteins are 0.8-1 gram per kilogram body-weight. Their functions in the body are:

- Building and repairing of body tissues (including muscles) and replacement of worn-out parts.
- Enzymes, hormones, and many immune molecules are made up of proteins.
- Proteins as antibodies help the body by defending it from infections caused by bacteria and viruses.
- Essential body processes such as water balancing, nutrient transport, and muscle contractions require protein to function.
- It helps keep skin, hair, and nails healthy.
- It is also a source of energy.
- Like most other nutrients, it is inevitable for overall good health.

Fats:

Fats are concentrated or reserve source of energy contained in ghee, soybean oil, corn oil, etc. They also help in the absorption of certain vitamins. They are made up of fatty acids and glycerol. They are of three types:

i. Saturated fatty acids
ii. Mono-unsaturated fatty acids
iii. Poly-unsaturated fatty acids.

The body requires fats for the following functions:

- They are a concentrated form of energy.
- They increase the taste of food.
- They give shape to the body.
- They protect the bodily organs from different injuries.
- They help transportation of fat-soluble vitamins.
- They provide essential fatty acids EFA, which have vitamin like functions. They are necessary for growth in the body. They boost the immune system and ward off diseases.

There are different categories of fats, classified according to their chemical structures:

Saturated fats: These are solid at room temperature. They include all animal fats and dairy products. They are responsible for raising our blood cholesterol levels.

Unsaturated fats: They are liquid form at room temperature. These are required by the body for proper functioning. They are present in all vegetable oils and contain essential fatty acids that are vital for the body.

Omega-6 Fatty Acids: They prevent increase in blood cholesterol, lubricate the joints, create hormones, and strengthen immune cells. Excess of this fatty acid leads to blood clots. This negative aspect can be balanced by Omega-3 fatty acids.

Omega-3 fatty Acids: They ease many health challenges like heart disease, etc. They raise the "good" cholesterol level and make arteries flexible. They also regulate the production of triglycerides in the body and help regulate blood pressure and blood clotting. Thus, they balance the negative aspect of Omega-6 fatty acids. Unfortunately, Omega-3 fatty acids are not abundant in our diet. The common cooking oils do not contain it. It is present in walnuts, flaxseed, and soybean oil.

Cholesterol: Cholesterol is exclusively present in animal foods, but not at all in vegetables foods. It is also the raw material for many hormones. Again, if consumed in excess quantity, it can clog the arteries, leading to heart diseases. If it can be kept in control, youthfulness may be prolonged and old age kept at bay.

Vitamins

Vitamins are mainly body-protecting foods that are necessary for normal functioning of all organs. They are of various kinds—A, B, C, D, E, and K. We can categorize them into two types—Fat soluble vitamins like vitamins A, D, E, and K—especially found in butter, cream, and ghee; and Water soluble vitamins like vitamin B-complex and vitamin C found in fruits and vegetables.

They are important for the proper functioning of the body. They are required in minute quantities and are present in minute quantities in food. They act as catalysts and hasten metabolic activities. They influence growth and development, improve health—thus protecting us against diseases.

Vitamins have various organic functions such as hormone-like functions, e.g., vitamin D—regulating metabolism of minerals, or vitamin A—regulating cell and tissue growth. Other vitamins (like vitamin E and even vitamin C) function as antioxidants. The vitamin with several numbers, B complex vitamin, helps enzymes in their work. The deficiency of different vitamins in the body means the probability of different problems—bleeding, diathesis, rickets, night-blindness, beriberi, and so many other diseases in the human body.

Minerals:

Minerals are inorganic substances that are more or less required in small quantities. So, they make up about 4% of body weight. They are vital for health and are needed for various body functions.

There are 16 various minerals required by the human body. They can be categorized into macrominerals, or minerals that are needed in relatively huge quantities, and microminerals that are needed in smaller quantities, and trace elements, which our body requires in minute quantities; nonetheless they are still vital for the body's proper functioning. The macromineral group contains calcium, phosphorus, magnesium, sodium, potassium, chloride, and sulphur, which are found in dark green vegetables, cereals, grain, etc. Trace minerals like zinc, copper, iodine, manganese, etc. are required in small quantities.

Both—macrominerals and microminerals—are required for growth of the bones and teeth. Calcium is also important in regulating blood clotting, muscle tone, and nerve function. Phosphorous helps in providing energy to work. Potassium and sodium help both—in osmoregulation, and contraction and relaxation of the muscles. However, potassium also assists in the regulating the heartbeat. Chlorine is a part of hydrochloric acid—thus important for digesting protein in the stomach. Sulphur is one of the vital constituents of all proteins. The human body needs the following trace elements; their functions are given below:

Iron - transport of oxygen in the blood
Manganese - bones
Iodine - regulates rate of metabolism
Copper - facilitates absorption and function of iron
Flourine - decreases tooth decay
Zinc - important regulator
Cobalt - a part of Vitamin B12
Chromium - regulates glucose metabolism

Like vitamins, minerals help your body grow and develop properly. The body uses minerals to do several functions—from building strong bones to transmitting nerve impulses. Some minerals are even used to make hormones or maintain a normal heartbeat.

Antioxidants

Free radicals are naturally produced in the body as a result of various metabolic processes, including breathing and digestion. In the process of utilizing oxygen during normal metabolism in the cells for producing energy, free oxygen radicals are created. These are unstable and have an electric charge. To neutralize the charge, they try to get an electron from any molecule or substance in their vicinity. This oxidation causes damage to cells, the vessel walls, or even genes and DNA in the nuclei of cells.

This can be prevented with the help of antioxidants. They are the anti-ageing and disease-fighting. They prevent or reduce the formation of damaging chemicals called free oxygen radicals.

Conditions promoting formation of free radicals:

- Excessive emotional and mental stress.
- Poor exercise habits or strenuous exercise.
- Pollutants in the air, food, and water.
- High fat diet (saturated fats).
- Cigarettes and alcohol.
- Medications and radiation, especially anti-cancer chemotherapeutic drugs.
- Fast-paced and pressure packed lifestyle.

Our body produces some antioxidants but cannot produce all the ones we need in the face of increasing free-radical formation, thanks to present day lifestyle and environment. So, the rest of the protective antioxidants must come from food. Fruits and vegetables, followed by nuts, seeds, and whole-grain foods are rich sources of antioxidants. The more colorful the fruits and vegetables, the richer they are in antioxidants.

Some commonly used food items and the antioxidants present in them are:

Turmeric – Curcuminoids
Green tea – Catechins
Grape seeds – Cynidins
Reishi mushrooms – Triterpenes

Digestion – The Journey of food

Understanding the digestive process helps us understand the need for good food habits, and the need to eat at the proper times.

Digestion in the Mouth

As you chew food in your mouth, the food is broken into smaller pieces and mixed with saliva. Saliva contains an enzyme—salivary amylase or ptyalin—that changes the insoluble starches into simpler soluble forms.

For effective digestion, keep the following points in mind.

- Chew the food properly. This will break it down into smaller pieces, increasing the surface area and contact with the saliva.
- Avoid very sour items (sour curds, lime, etc.) in combination with rice and chapatis. The acids in sour foods will not permit digestion in the mouth, as saliva needs an alkaline medium to work. This is especially true for people with poor digestion, who experience belching and sour liquids in the mouth after meals.

- Avoid pasty or watery foods. One tends to just swallow them, leading to poor salivary digestion. Follow the dictum—"Drink the solids, eat the liquids."

Digestion in the Stomach

The stomach is a living bag, continuously contracting and expanding so that food in it gets thoroughly churned up. While food stays in the mouth only for a few seconds, it spends more time in the stomach, between two to three hours. The digestion of proteins commences in the stomach, to be finally completed in the intestines along with carbohydrates and fats.

In the digestive process, the stomach secretes pepsin, which breaks down the long protein chains into smaller units, called peptones that are soluble in water. It also secretes Hydrochloric Acid, which does many important jobs in the stomach. It provides the acidic medium in which pepsin can work. It also kills bacteria that enters the stomach with the food.

Digestion in the Small Intestine

The third phase in digestion takes place in the small intestine, a very long tubular structure, about 5 or 6 times the body height, 20 feet in length, cleverly folded up and tucked into the abdomen behind the navel region. The pancreas and the gall bladder pour out their digestive enzymes at the beginning of the small intestine. These enzyme-rich juices digest the semi-digested proteins, starches, and sugars. Fats are digested into simpler substances with the help of enzymes. The bile secreted by the gall bladder converts simple fats into globules.

Finally the simpler units of proteins, fats, and carbohydrates are absorbed into the bloodstream, across the lining of the small intestine. The vitamins and minerals are also simply absorbed into the blood. In normal healthy state, it takes 4 to 6 hours for food to pass through the small intestine.

Digestion in the Large Intestine

It follows the small intestine. It looks like a bicycle tube and goes around the abdomen like the letter U placed upside down. As digested food passes along the large intestine, water gets absorbed along with the vitamins and minerals. The food remains become harder and finally reach the outlet called anus and pass out as stools.

Acidity

When a log of wood is burnt, it leaves behind some ash. When any food is digested, absorbed and metabolized (burnt up), it also leaves some residue in the cells of the body. This can be acidic or alkaline. This is measured on pH scale from 1 to 14, in which 7 is the neutral value. The pH value of our blood is 7.4 alkaline. Optimal health is in a mildly alkaline body. All the fluids in the body, with the exception of the stomach, are or should be alkaline.

The average 21st century lifestyle, diet, and environment produce far more acid in the body than is necessary. 90% of the population is too acidic. The results of this are:

- Connective tissues are weakened and facial skin and hair lose their tone.
- Sleep pattern gets disturbed. Relaxing, deep sleep is reduced.
- Physical and mental exhaustion by mid-afternoon.

- Colds infections, headache, and flu are common.
- Friendly bacterial in the intestines die and the immune system gets impaired.
- Vitamins and minerals from food are not absorbed well.
- Free radical oxidation occurs with a great ease.
- Digestion is impaired and flatulence and bloating is more frequent.

Thus, the number of calories we consume means nothing unless they come from proper food. We must consume both—alkali and acidic ash foods daily, since both are necessary. In general, fruits and vegetables yield an alkali ash, whereas meat, milk products, oils, nuts, etc. yield an acidic ash. Grains yield an acidic ash. Pulses and beans yield an acidic ash, but when sprouted they yield on alkali ash. Coffee, alcohol, tobacco, sauces, vinegar yield an acidic ash. Honey, ginger, herbal teas yield an alkali ash. We should eat a diet that is 75 per cent alkali ashes formation and 25 per cent acidic ashes. Our present day diet is the reverse of this.

To maintain the proper proportion of acidic and alkali ash in the body, follow the general guidelines:

- Eat some fresh fruit every day and include salads in each meal.
- Include fresh sprouts in your diet, either raw or conservatively cooked.
- Substitute in-between snacks with fresh fruits and nuts.
- Develop the habit of enjoying freshly squeezed lime in one glass of water daily, a minimum of one lime a day. Lime and other citrus fruits taste acidic and are acidic for the first hour in the body, but leave an alkaline effect on the body after being assimilated.
- Minimize fried foods, packaged foods, processed, and stale foods. Eat freshly cooked food, do not cook and store in the refrigerator.
- Reduce consumption of pasteurized milk products.
- Calm the mind through *Yog*, music, prayer, etc. React to others with love and compassion. Moderate exercise, walking in fresh air, *Yogic* stretches, and *pranayam* are all conducive to reducing the acidic ash formation in the body.

Food Groups – How to Get Maximum Benefit?

a. Vegetables – The Nutritional Powerhouse

Vegetables are the main source of good quality food like vitamins, minerals, fibre, proteins, and carbohydrates. Many vegetables can be eaten raw. They can be consumed in different ways, such as a part of main meals or as snacks. Despite all the vegetables contain slight proportion of protein or fat, and fluctuating proportions of vitamins, dietary minerals, fibres, and carbohydrates, the nutritional content of vegetables differs significantly.

Daily diet should consist of adequate quantities of fruits and vegetables as they help prevent the danger of heart diseases and diabetes. They even safeguard us against different cancers and bone-related problems. One of the minerals, potassium is found in the fruits and the vegetables—surely assists us by avoiding the risk of the stones formation in the kidney.

Healthier Ways of Cooking Vegetables:

- Buy fresh, tender vegetables and cook them as soon as possible. Do not overstock your fridge.

- Wash the vegetables in running water properly before cutting them. Vegetables used in salads should be soaked in salted water for an hour and then washed in drinking water, before they are cut and consumed. This will neutralize the pesticides used in farming.
- Cut vegetables just before consuming them. Do not cut and store in the refrigerator, or buy pre-cut vegetables from the supermarket.
- The water in which vegetables are boiled should not be discarded as it contains the essential vitamins and minerals.
- Always cover the vessel with a lid while cooking. This will reduce the loss of vitamins due to evaporation.
- Do not overheat the oil to smoking point before adding the vegetables, as this destroys their inherent nutrients.
- Cook in minimum water. Adding excess water and then cooking with the pan uncovered until water evaporates, destroys all the vitamins.
- Do not overcook the vegetables.
- When cooking green vegetables, add them to the cooking pan at the end, and add vegetables that take longer to cook, such as potatoes, in the beginning. After adding the green vegetable, stir for a few seconds and turn off the flame. This preserves the vitamins and enhances the green color and taste.
- Add salt at the end to gain more chances of preserving vitamins in the vegetables.

In the Western countries, meals are preceded by soups. They are easy to cook and easy to digest. Soups are a good source of vitamins and minerals. They cause no strain on digestion.

Carrot is the king of raw vegetables, containing the two most important antioxidants: vitamin A and C. Two or three medium-sized carrots meet our daily requirement of vitamin A.

b. Fresh Fruits – the Complete Food

They are easy to digest and metabolize, and are rich in vitamins and minerals. They are alkalizing and cooling to the body. They clean the digestive tract too.

When and How to Eat Fruits?

- Wash the fruit thoroughly before cutting or eating. This is important given the excessive use of pesticides on our farms.
- Eat fruit with the skin when possible, as the part inside the skin is rich in vitamins.
- Do not wash fruit after they have been cut. Vitamin C being water-soluble gets washed off.
- Ideally, fruit should be eaten 30-60 minutes before a meal, not after. This ensures timely digestion and passage from the stomach. If consumed after a big meal, it stays in the stomach for more than two or three hours until the other food is digested, causing a traffic jam. This causes the fruit to putrefy in the stomach, leading to flatulence, gas, and indigestion.
- Eat seasonal fruits. Fruits left to ripen on the tree with sunlight are best, rather than fruits taken from the cold storage plants.

Many people believe that citrus fruits increase acidity. Citrus fruits do contain acids, but when these are assimilated and burnt in the body, they produce alkaline ash.

Āmlā or Indian Goosebery (Phyllanthus emblica) requires special mention because it is the richest source of vitamin C. It contains twenty times more Vitamin C than a similar quantity of orange. One *Āmlā* can meet the daily requirements of vitamin C of four adults.

c. Nuts and Seeds – Source of Good Fats

The term "dry fruits" is used to indicate the commonly eaten nuts, like almonds, cashews, pistachios, dates (khajoor), raisins (kishmish), figs (anjeer), apricots, and currants. These are a good source of minerals like iron, calcium, and copper.

Many people shun nuts and seeds because they are rich in fats, containing up to 40 per cent of fats. However, they contain the good fats that are required by the body.

The benefits of consuming nuts and seeds are:

- Nuts, seeds, and cashews are totally free from cholesterol, which is a risk factor associated with fats of animal origin. However, cashews contain high percentage of fat (upto 47%). So, consumers should not confuse fat with cholesterol.
- They have a blend of essential fatty acids and vitamin E. Walnuts have a special place, being the only ones in this category to have the much-needed Omega-3 fatty acids.
- They have a healthy percentage of essential minerals like magnesium and copper.
- They are a source of good quality proteins.

How to Eat Nuts, Seeds, and Dry Fruits?

- Wash them two or three times in water before eating. Before being packed they are subjected to fumigation with SO_2. The fruit also absorbs this SO_2. The only sweet dry fruit that is free from this contamination is dates.
- Frying or roasting leads to deterioration in the quality of fats and proteins. Excess roasting leads to the formation of toxins.
- Soak for about 4-5 hours in water, to soften the fibre and render nutrients.
- Eat them in limited quantity only. They are a dense source of nutrients.
- Vegetarians can easily get essential fatty acids and amino acids simply by eating a handful of raw nuts and seeds every day.

d. Oils and Fats: Good and Bad

Depending upon the saturation of the bonds in the carbon atom, oils and fats are of two types:

Unsaturated fats: These are fats that are liquid at room temperature. Fats obtained from the plant kingdom are predominantly unsaturated fats. They reduce the harmful L.D.L. (Low Density Lipoprotein) cholesterol in the blood and are health-promoting by nature.

Saturated fats: These are fats that are solid at room temperature. They are obtained from meats and dairy products. They increase the harmful L.D.L. cholesterol level.

Dietary Measures to Reduce Blood Cholesterol

- Reduce the intake of foods rich in cholesterol and saturated fats.
- Increase fibre intake in the form of vegetables, fruits, beans, whole cereals, oats, etc. Fibre reduces the absorption of cholesterol from the gut.
- Reduce sugars and sweets as they get converted to triglycerides (the form in which fats are stored in the body).
- Reduce alcohol as it increases triglycerides.
- Increase intake of Omega-3 fatty acid.
- Chinese green tea contains chemicals called catechins, which lowers harmful cholesterol and increases good cholesterol H.D.L. (High Density Lipoprotein) levels.

Myths about Fats

1. All fats are bad for health. Incorrect! Saturated fats have to be restricted, but sufficient unsaturated fats need to be consumed.

2. Refined oils are better than unrefined oils. No, Refining robs the oilseeds of vital nutrients, particularly essential fatty acids and vitamin E.

3. We hardly consume vanaspati ghee. No. Most Indian bakery products—cakes, pastries, buns, rolls, biscuits, cookies, may be even farsans, namkeen, and sweets like gulab jamun—are made from vanaspati. Unknowingly we are consuming vanaspati ghee, which has to be controlled.

4. Fried foods are OK in refined oil. No. Frying kills the nutrients. Food exposed to high temperatures loses most vitamins and dietary proteins.

5. A zero fat diet is best. No. It cuts the essential fatty acids that are required for vibrant health. Their absence affects the immune system, making one prone to infection, auto-immune disorders, and poor mental functioning.

Tips on Fat Consumption

- **Cooking oils:** Instead of depending on sunflower oil, welcome other cooking oils also—filtered groundnut oil, til (sesame) oil, and olive oil, the latter especially for western cooking. Mustard oil contains uric acid, which is bad for health. Include foods containing Omega-3 fatty acids in your diet—flaxseed, walnuts, and soybean oil.
- Avoid hydrogenated vegetable oils and avoid bakery-cooked items.
- Reduce the intake of saturated fats by preferring skimmed milk to whole milk.
- Avoid fried foods, especially when not made at home. You can eat fried foods for psychological satisfaction but in small quantities.

e. Pulses and Beans – Rich in Proteins

They are a good source of proteins in a diet without animal proteins. They are of two kinds:

1. Pulses: *Arahar/tuvar* dal (red gram), *chanā* (Bengal gram), *uḍad* (black gram), *mūñg* (green gram), *masūr* (lentils), *maṭar* (peas), etc.

2. Beans: *Rājamā* (Kidney bean), *chholā* (chickpeas), *lobiā* (cow pea), *sem* (field beans), *maṭkī* (moth beans), soybean, etc.

Make pulses easy to digest. Follow these guidelines for their consumption:

- Soak them in water for a minimum of three hours before cooking. Soak whole beans and pulses longer, preferably overnight. Change the water several times during the soaking process, and cook them in fresh water.
- Cook them properly and fully. Indigestion is more due to partial cooking.
- Add ginger while coking to make digestion easier.
- Mint and coriander leaves also help digestion.
- Germinate them. This makes them easier to digest, and increases their nutrition value too. Some can even be eaten raw after germination, like *muñg* and *matki*.
- Proteins are easily digested when combined with green leafy vegetables.
- Eat a salad before the main course to aid digestion.

Sprouting Pulses and Beans

Sprouts are the best foods we can eat. Advantages of sprouting are:

- Starches are broken down into simpler sugars—dextrose and maltose.
- Proteins are converted into amide and amino acids.
- Fats are also broken down into simpler fatty acids. So people with weak digestion can also consume them easily.
- Sprouts are a vitamin factory. The vitamins present are doubled or tripled.
- Sprouting reduces the gassy effect of pulses and beans because they become easy to digest.
- It results in better Calcium and Iron absorption. Phytates that impede the absorption of Calcium are chemically altered.
- Minimises the effect of pesticides.

f. Cereals—The Energy Boosters

They are the cheapest sources of starch and supply heat and energy to the body. They constitute the major portion of our food. We depend on them for meeting our requirements of energy, proteins, Group B vitamins, and minerals like Calcium and Phosphorous.

Tips on Cereal Consumption

Variety: Include a variety of cereals in your diet. Rice eaters should include chapati in one meal at least.

- Eat the forgotten cereals—*rāgī* (millet) and *jowar*, etc. These coarse flours can be mixed with wheat flour to make chapatis. *Rājgirā* is consumed only on *Ekādaśhī* days. But it is very healthy and its consumption should be increased.
- Whole-wheat flour ground in the chakki—flour mill—is best for health. Avoid *maidā* (Fine flour). Eat brown bread rather than white.
- Rice-eating: Unpolished and boiled rice is more nutritious—particularly for those who do not eat chapatis.
- Cooking the rice: Wash rice two or three times, then soak in clean water. Use this water

to cook the rice. You should not throw away this water, under the mistaken notion that it will reduce the fattening property of rice. On the contrary, it leads to loss of vitamins.

- Importance of chewing: Preparations made from grains can cause complications if not chewed properly. Proper chewing can take care of 50-70 per cent of the digestion of starches—thus reducing the load on the digestive tract.
- Prefer toasted bread over untoasted bread.
- Fermented preparations: *Iḍlīs*, *ḍosas*, *ḍhoklās,* etc. are made from ground and fermented rice and black gram dal. There are many advantages of fermentation. It makes digestion easier. Friendly microbes break the complex carbohydrates and proteins into more easily assimilable elements. The vitamin and enzyme content in food is increased. Fermented foods colonize the intestinal tract with friendly bacteria.

Important Points for Good Food Habits

1. Meat and Eggs – To Eat or Not to Eat?

Humans have been created by nature to be vegetarians. Human beings do not have long canine teeth and a wide jaw to tear flesh like carnivorous animals do.

Carnivores have short bowels to allow minimal transit time for the unstable and dead animal food, which putrefies and decays faster. On the contrary, humans have a longer digestive tract for the slow and better absorption of the plant food.

The intestinal micro-organisms are different in the meat-eating animals as compared to humans—to aid meat digestion.

The stomach of carnivores is more acidic than human beings—to digest raw meat.

Harmful Effects of Meat

Hormone-fed animals: Animals are fed synthetic hormones in order to accelerate their growth, increase fat deposits, and muscle mass. These are passed on to the consumers.

Cholesterol and Saturated Fats: This is high in meat, leading to hardening and narrowing of arteries, causing high blood pressure, heart disease, etc. Fat is where animals store their toxins, and that itself is passed on to the meat-eaters.

High Uric Acid: Protein from meat has high uric acid, which leads to arthritis, kidney stones, and high chances of kidney diseases.

Poor Source of Fibre: Meat does not contain a significant amount of fibre—thus leading to constipation.

Body Acidity: Meat is highly acidic, leading to acidity in body tissues and creating ground for diseases to breed.

Fear Factor: Whenever there is threat of danger, as a response to it, levels of certain chemicals and hormones increase in our body. When an animal is killed, the fear and pain releases many toxic chemicals which are ingested by us when we eat meat.

Heaviness and Lethargy: Meat-eating leads to dullness and lethargy in the body and mind too. So the scriptures say meat is tamasic food.

Meat and Cancer: There is a strong correlation between animal protein and several kinds of cancers.

Although meats may be rich in proteins, they are simply not worth the risk.

Eggs

Gone are the days when eggs from the real mother hen were available. Today, most commercially sold eggs come from hens that are packed in small cages under bright artificial light, which lay unfertilized eggs under the effect of feeds, laced with hormones and antibiotics. Eating them can cause a highly acidifying and putrefactive excess of protein apart from the harm done by these hormone-induced eggs.

2. Sugar

Refined white sugar is stripped of all nutrients, vitamins, and minerals. It is not fit for human consumption. It has always been connected with diabetes. It is the leading cause of disease of affluence—obesity, heart diseases, diabetes, acidity, indigestion, dental cancer, weakening of immune system, arthritis, etc.

The natural sugar such as fructose (fruits and honey), lactose (milk), and maltose (grains) are not harmful as refined sugar is. Actually, natural sugar contains nutritional values. Jaggery has the additional value of iron and calcium, and vitamins like B1, B2, and B3. Honey contains simple sugar (dextrose and laevulose), which is pre-digested and requires little enzymatic digestion. So honey leads to speedy absorption and release of energy. Pure honey is blessed with many medicinal and healing properties that help in developing immunities against diseases like cough and cold, breathing difficulties, and indigestion. Obese people would do well if they take a little bit of honey instead of sugar as honey mobilizes body fat. So minimize the use of white sugar and subustitue natural sugar in your diet wherever possible.

3. Fast Food

Fast food is becoming more common across the world. The taste of burgers, pizzas, chips, *samosās, kachoris, vaḍās,* soft-drinks, milk shakes, etc. tempts all of us—particularly the younger generation. Fast foods are harmful to our health for many reasons discussed below:

- Fast foods are the best source of dead or empty calories. They are rich in calories and saturated fats, but devoid of vitamins, minerals, and fibre.
- Fats used to make the buns and rolls are usually hydrogenated vegetable fats, which are indigestible.
- The excess cheese topped on these preparations promotes obesity and eventually poor health.
- Refined flour used to make breads and the pizzas lacks fibre and promotes constipation.
- These foods are high in salt content because of additional salt in the form of baking powder to bake the bread.
- Ketchups, sauces, salami, sausages, etc. contain food additives to enhance the taste and

shelf life, but they enhance disease too.

- They are usually eaten along with soft-drinks or shakes, which makes them even more difficult to digest.

4. The Not So Soft Soft-Drinks

What do Soft-Drinks contain? They contain no more than sugar, coloring agent, flavouring agent, citric acid, caffeine, and sodium bicarbonate. All these are harmful to the body. On top of it, they contain gas CO_2 mixed under pressure, which gives a fizz.

CO_2 is the end product of metabolism that the body throws out. How can we possibly remain healthy by ingesting this gas? A good fraction of it gets ingested in the blood, making it acidic.

Harmful effects of soft-drinks:

- They are extremely acidic. Our body fluids have a pH value of around 7.4. These drinks, due to the presence of CO_2, citric acid, and sugars have pH ranging from 2.5 to 3.5. The liquids used for cleaning toilets have the same pH.
- They interfere with the process of digestion. They contain large amounts of sugar and caffeine, which virtually shut down the digestive process.
- They make us prone to metabolic diseases like diabetes due to a high content of sugar.
- They make our bones and teeth weak. High acid level acidifies the tissues. To balance, alkaline, minerals like calcium and magnesium are leeched out from the body reserves. Severe lack of minerals can lead to osteoporosis, etc.
- Soft-drinks weaken our immune system. The coloring and flavouring agents trigger abnormal immune responses, further weakening the system.

5. When Should You Eat?

Body rhythm and digestion: Our digestive capacity parallels the Sun's presence. In the southern hemisphere (the tropics and equatorial regions), the Sun is at its peak from 10 am onwards. Hence our digestion is at its best from 10 am to 6 pm. After 8-9 pm, the process of assimilation or utilization of nutrients starts to pick up. It is intense when we are sleeping. During that time, the nutrients are extracted from the food and utilized. The eliminative activity peaks in the early morning hours. That is why there is an intense urge to pass stools on waking up in the morning. The process goes on—digestion, assimilation, and elimination. The more we are in tune with the natural cycle, the healthier we shall be.

Breakfast: A heavy breakfast diverts the life forces. To ensure health, we should allow the elimination cycle to function freely and not thwart it in any way. You should enjoy your breakfast with adequate exercise.

Lunch: The digestive fire is at the peak. Do not skip it for tea as many working people normally do.

Dinner: It should be light, half the quantity of lunch. Particularly, it should be taken after 7-8 pm.

6. Water Habits

Water consumed during a meal dilutes the digestive juices and hampers digestion. Cold drinks with meals are harmful. The coolness of the drink hampers the fire of digestion in the stomach.

Drink water 30 minutes before a meal or two hours after it. This is easy if you avoid too much chilli and salt in the food.

A glass of warm water on getting up in the morning stimulates the gastro colic reflex—thus initiating bowel movement and relieving constipation.

7. Daily Dietary Check

To ensure you are in tune with the Science of Healthy Diet, ensure you are following checkpoints in your diet:

- Two servings of fresh seasonal fruit. One serving is approximately 100 grams or one moderate fruit.
- Four servings of vegetables—freshly cooked or as a salad.
- A handful of sprouts.
- A lemon a day—as an early morning drink with warm water or squeezed over salads.
- A bowl of curd or buttermilk.
- Vary your choice of cereals. Replace the wheat roti at least three-four times a week.
- Vegetarians should eat one bowl of dal every day for the proteins.
- A fistful of nuts and dry fruits.
- Strict vegetarians should eat flaxseed or also for the Omega-3 fatty acid content.
- Drink water at the right time.
- Avoid cold drinks and iced preparations with meals.
- Try to eat when you are in a relaxed state of mind.
- Do not overeat. Get up from the table when you are still hungry.
- Rest a while after lunch.
- Take a comfortable stroll after dinner.

* Source "The Ultimate Indian Diet Book" by Dr. Renu Mahtani, published by Macmillan.

XIII. Therapeutic / Curative Index for Different Syndromes and Body Parts

Jagadguru Kripaluji Yog

The table below provides an easy and simple guide to *Yogic* practices, which help in promoting the health of particular parts of the body and the prevention of common diseases. Various *asans*, *pranayams*, *mudras*, *shatkarmas*, and *bandhas* are identified for different syndromes. It is advisable that the practitioners should seek the guidance of a *Yog* expert and adopt them as per their capacity, flexibility, and structure of the body.

Sn.	Syndromes / Body Parts	Asans	Pranayams	Shatkarmas	Others
1	Abdomen	Supt Vajrasan, Shashankasan, Trikonasan, Ardh Matsyendrasan, Nauka Sanchalanasan, Halasan, Drut Halasan, Naukasan, Backward and Forward Bending *Asans*, Yog Mudrasan, Matsyasan, Ushtrasan, Meru Dandasan, Hansasan, Mayurasan, Niralamb Pashchimottanasan, Brahmacharyasan	Bhastrika, Kapalbhati	Agnisar Kriyā, *Nauli*, Kunjal, Shankh Prakshalan	Uddiyan Bandh
2	Acidity	Vajrasan for more than 10 minutes after every meal, Pashchimottanasan, Parshwa Konasan, Veerabhadrasan, Ardh Chandrasan, Padangushthasan, Pada Hastasan, Ardh Matsyendrasan, Shalabhasan, Dhanurasan, Bhujangasan, Relaxing *Asans* for soothing the stressful mind	Anulom Vilom, Bhramari, Bhastrika, Shyam Uchcharan	Kunjal, Agnisar Kriyā	Subtle Body Relaxation, *Roop Dhyan* Meditation
3	Adenoids (enlargement)	Singhasan, Surya Namaskār	Ujjayi with Khechari Mudra	*Neti*, Kunjal	
4	Adrenal glands (toning)	Surya Namaskār, Marjari Asan, Shashank Bhujangasan, Ushtrasan, Trikonasan, Dhanurasan, Bhujangasan, Shalabhasan, Pashchimottanasan, Chakrasan, Pada Hastasan, Ardh Matsyendrasan, Halasan, Meru Dandasan, Hansasan, Mayurasan	Bhastrika	*Nauli*, Agnisar Kriyā	Pashinee Mudra, Uddiyan Bandh

No.	Condition	Asans	Pranayama	Kriya	Mudras / Bandh / Relaxation
5	**Anaemia**	Surya Namaskár, Bhujangsan, Shalabhasan, Sarvangasan, Halasan, Matsyasan, Pashchimottanasan, Shirsasan, Shavasan (10 -15 minutes)	Sheetali, Sheetkari, Kapalbhati, Ujjayi		Subtle Body Relaxation
6	**Anger**	Shashankasan, Yog Mudrasan, Pashchimottanasan, Pada Hastasan, Kurmasan, Shavasan, Balasan, Matsya Kreedasan, Makarasan, Garbhasan	Jai Radhey Pranayam, Anulom Vilom, Bhramari, Shyam Uchcharan, Sheetali, Sheetkari, Ujjayi, Kapalbhati		*Bandh:* Mool Bandh, Maha Bandh *Mudras:* Pran, Bhoochari, Yoni, Pashinee Mudras *Roop Dhyan* Meditation, and different relaxation practices.
7	**Angina Pectoris (pain in the chest)**	Subtle Exercises, Shavasan, Makarasan, Akarna Dhanurasan, Hasta Urthanasan	Anulom Vilom, Ujjayi, Bhramari		Yog Mudra, Subtle Body Relaxation, *Roop Dhyan* Meditation.
8	**Anxiety (and nervous tension)**	Subtle Exercises, Surya Namaskár, Shashankasan, Yog Mudrasan, Ananda Madirasan, Pashchimottanasan, Bhujangasan, Shalabhasan, Sarvangasan, Halasan, Shavasan, Kurmasan	Anulom Vilom, Bhramari, Shyam Uchcharan, Sheetali, Sheetkari, Ujjayi	*Bhagwad Swaroop Darśhan (Trāṭak),* Jal Neti, Kunjal	*Mudras:* Pashinee, Shambhavi, Bhoochari, Pran, Yoni Mudras. Subtle Body Relaxation, *Roop Dhyan* Meditation
9	**Appetite**	Forward and Backward Bending *Asans,* Surya Namaskár	All Radhey Krishna Pranayams	*Nauli,* Agnisar Kriyā	Uddiyan Bandh
10	**Arms**	Surya Namaskár, Dhanurakarshanasan, Gomukhasan, Mayurasan, Lolasan, Baka Dhyanasan, Dwi Hasta Bhujangasan, Santolanasan			Subtle Body Relaxation, *Roop Dhyan* Meditation
11	**Arthritis**	Subtle Exercises and All Comfortable *Asans*	Jai Radhey Pranayam, Anulom Vilom, Jagadguru Kripaluji Pranayam, Bhastrika, Kapalbhati	*Neti,* Kunjal, Laghu Shankh Prakshalan	
12	**Asthma**	Supt Vajrasan, Bhujangasan, Shashankasan, Konasan, Shalabhasan, Sarvangasan, Marjari Asan, Ushtrasan, Matsyasan, Pada Hastasan, Backward Bending *Asans,* Janu Shirasan, Pashchimottanasan, Dhanurasan, Uttana Padasan, Setu Bandh Asan, Ardh Matsyendrasan	Ujjayi, Jai Radhey Pranayam, Anulom Vilom, Jagadguru Kripaluji Pranayam, Bhastrika, Kapalbhati	Jal Neti, Kunjal, Shankh Prakshalan, Vastra Dhauti	Deep Abdominal Breathing, Subtle Body Relaxation, *Roop Dhyan* Meditation. All Relaxation Techniques

		Asans	Pranayams	Cleansing / Other	Relaxation & Meditation
13	**Backache**	Supt Vajrasan, Shalabhasan, Konasan, Shashankasan, Marjari Asan, Makarasan, Sarpasan, Dhanurasan, Kandharsan, Tiryak Tadasan, Kati Chakrasan, Shirshasan, Sarvangasan, Ushtrasan, Shalabhasan, Meru Prishthasan, Baithak Merudandasan, Sphinx Asan, Bhujangasan, Ardh Matsyendrasan, All Bending *Asans*	Ujjayi, Bhramari		
14	**Baldness**	Shashankasan, Inverted *Asans*	All *Pranayams*		Subtle Body Relaxation, *Roop Dhyan* Meditation
15	**Blood Pressure (High)**	Subtle Exercises, Ananda Madirasan, Siddhasan, All Relaxation Poses, Backward Bending *Asans*, Padmasan, Halasan, Ardh Baddh Padmasan, Shavasan	Anulom Vilom, Ujjayi, Bhramari, Shyam Uchcharan, Bhramari, Sheetali, Sheetkari		
16	**Blood Pressure (Low)**	Dynamic *Asans*, Fast rounds of Surya Namaskār	All *Pranayams* (especially Bhastrika and Jagadguru Kripaluji Pranayam)		All four *Bandhas*
17	**Brain**	Shirshasan, Sarvangasan, Pashchimottanasan, Kurmasan, Shavasan	All *Pranayams*		
18	**Bronchitis**	Supt Vajrasan, Bhujangasan, Shashankasan, Konasan, Shalabhasan, Sarvangasan, Marjari Asan, Ushtrasan, Matsyasan, Pada Hastasan, Backward Bending *Asans*, Janu Shirasan, Pashchimottanasan, Dhanurasan, Uttana Padasan, Setu Bandh Asan, Ardh Matsyendrasan	Ujjayi, Jai Radhey Pranayam, Anulom Vilom, Jagadguru Kripaluji Pranayam, Bhastrika, Kapalbhati	*Neti*, Kunjal, Laghu Shankh Prakshalan	Deep Abdominal Breathing, Subtle Body Relaxation, *Roop Dhyan* Meditation, All Relaxation Techniques
19	**Cancer**	Subtle Exercises, Surya Namaskār	All *Pranayams*—particularly Bhramari and Ujjayi	*Bhagwad Swaroop Darśhan (Trāṭak)*	Subtle Body Relaxation, *Roop Dhyan* Meditation
20	**Chest (toning)**	Surya Namaskār, Subtle Exercises, Supt Vajrasan, Ushtrasan, All Standing *Asans*, Matsyasan, Lolasan, All Backward Bending *Asans*—especially Chakrasan and Dhanurasan, Topsy-turvy *Asans*, Baddh Padmasan, Baddh Konasan, Natarajasan, Gomukhasan, Kukkutasan, Baka Dhyanasan	Jai Radhey Pranayam, Ujjayi, Anulom Vilom		

#	Condition	Asans	Pranayam	Kriya	Notes
21	**Cold and Cough**	Regular practice of Surya Namaskār and other comfortable *Asans* (particularly Singhasan) Precautions: During cold one should practice Relaxing *Asans*	Anulom Vilom, Ujjayi, Bhramari, Bhastrika	*Neti*, Kunjal, Laghu Shankh Prakshalan	Avoid mucus producing foods such as milk, milk products, pickle, and non-veg foods
22	**Concentration**	All comfortable *Asans* with awareness (especially Inverted and Balancing *Asans*)	Anulom Vilom, Bhramari, Shyam Uchcharan, Bhastrika, Jagadguru Kripaluji Pranayam, Ujjayi	*Bhagwad Swaroop Darshan (Trāṭak)*	All *Mudras* mentioned in JKYog. Subtle Body Relaxation, *Roop Dhyan* Meditation
23	**Constipation**	Tadasan, Tiryak Tadasan, Kati Chakrasan, Surya Namaskār, Supt Vajrasan, Shashankasan, Ushtrasan, Trikonasan, Yog Mudrasan, Matsyasan, All Backward and Forward Bending *Asans*, All Spinal Twisting *Asans*, Shirshasan, Pashchimottanasan, Halasan, Drut Halasan, Sarvangasan	Anulom Vilom	Shankh Prakshalan, *Nauli* Agnisar Kriyā	*Bandhas:* Uddiyan and Maha Bandh Subtle Body Relaxation
24	**Coronary thrombosis**	Same as in Blood Pressure			
25	**Deafness** Precautions: Do not practice during inflamed and discharging conditions.	Singhasan, All Topsy-turvy *Asans*	Bhramari and Shyam Uchcharan with earholes and eyes closed.	*Neti*	
26	**Depression**	Surya Namaskār, Dynamic *Asans*, All Backward Bending *Asans*, Standing, and Twisting *Asans*	Jagadguru Kripaluji Pranayam in slow speed, Bhastrika, Kapalbhati, Abdominal Breathing	Kunjal, *Neti*, Laghu Shankh Prakshalan	Precautions: Omit Subtle Body Relaxation and Bhramari
27	**Diabetes**	Tadasan, Shashankasan, Bhujangasan, Pashchimottanasan, Janu Shirasan, Dhanurasan, Mayurasan, Hansasan, Shavasan, Supt Vajrasan, Sarvangasan, Halasan, Ardh Matsyendrasan, Gomukhasan, Yog Mudrasan, Matsyasan, Surya Namaskār	Anulom Vilom, Ujjayi, Bhramari, Bhastrika, Shyam Uchcharan	Kunjal, *Neti*, Laghu Shankh Prakshalan	Subtle Body Relaxation. Diet: Food restrictions should be followed

No.	Condition	Asans	Pranayam	Kriya	Other
28	**Diarrhea**	Shirshasan, Sarvangasan, Surya Namaskār, Shavasan	Anulom Vilom, Bhramari, Sheetali, Sheetkari		Diet: *Mūṅg* dal, *khichaḍī*, Yogurt, and Buttermilk
29	**Dysentery**	Shirshasan, Janu Shirasan, Sarvangasan Precautions: Omit all the Inverted and Dynamic *Asans*	Jai Radhey Pranayam	Laghu Shankh Prakshalan Precautions: Omit *Nauli*.	
30	**Dyspesia (Chronic indigestion)**	Same as in Acidity			
31	**Epilepsy**	Shashankasan, Bhujangasan, Ardh Matsyendrasan, Tadasan, Halasan, Shirshasan, Pashchimottanasan, All Relaxing *Asans*	Jai Radhey Pranayam, Ujjayi, Sheetali Precautions: Omit hyperventilating practices like Bhastrika and Kapalbhati.	*Neti* Precautions: Avoid *Trāṭak*	
32	**Eyes**	Shirshasan, Sarvangasan, Pashchimotanasan, Shavasan, Eye Exercises from Subtle Exercises along with Palming and Massaging of the eyes	Anulom Vilom, Sheetali, Jai Radhey Pranayam	*Bhagwad Swaroop Darśhan (Trāṭak)*	
33	**Face**	Surya Namaskār, Singhasan, Sarvangasan, Halasan, Karnapidasan, Shirshasan, Mayurasan	Jai Radhey Pranayam, Kapalbhati, Jagadguru Kripaluji Pranayam, Shyam Uchcharan	*Neti*, Kunjal, Laghu Shankh Prakshalan	Diet: Fasting once a week
34	**Fatigue**	All Subtle Exercises, Tadasan, Bhujangasan, Ushtrasan, Chakrasan, Dhanurasan, Surya Namaskār, Halasan, Pashchimottanasan, Ardh Matsyendrasan, Shavasan	Anulom Vilom, Bhramari, Jagadguru Kripaluji Pranayam		Subtle Body Relaxation *Bandhas:* Uddiyan and Mool Bandh
35	**Flat Foot**	All Subtle Exercises, All the Standing *Asans*, Shirshasan, Sarvangasan, Baddh Padmasan, Baddh Konasan, Gomukhasan, All Comfortable Inverted *Asans*	Jagadguru Kripaluji Pranayam		
36	**Flatulence**	All Standing *Asans*, Shirshasan, Sarvangasan, Padangushthasan, Janu Shirasan, Ardh Baddh Padma Pashchimottanasan, Ardh Matsyendrasan, Chakrasan, Yog Mudrasan, Kurmasan, Shalabhasan, Dhanurasan, Mayurasan	All *Pranayams* mentioned in JKYog	*Nauli*	Subtle Body Relaxation, Uddiyan Bandh

No.	Condition	Asans	Pranayam	Shatkarma	Relaxation / Other
37	Gall Bladder and Liver	Same *Asans* as that of Acidity, Dyspepsia, and Flatulence	Jagadguru Kriplauji Bhastrika, Kapalbhati, Shyam Uchcharan	*Nauli*	Subtle Body Relaxation
38	Gastric	Same as in Flatulence	All *Pranayams*	*Nauli*	
39	Giddiness	Shirshasan, Sarvangasan, Halasan, Pashchimottanasan, Shavasan, Balasan, Jyeshthikasan	Jai Radhey Pranayam, Chandra Anulom Vilom, Surya Anulom Vilom		Subtle Body Relaxation
40	Halitosis (Bad Breath)	Shirshasan, Sarvangasan, Pashchimottanasan, Singhasan	Ujjayi, Jai Radhey Pranayam, Chandra Anulom Vilom, Surya Anulom Vilom, Sheetali Pranayam Note: Application of Kaki Mudra while doing these *Pranayams* yields better results	Laghu Shankh Prakshalan	Breathing exercises: Dog Breathing, Rabbit Breathing, and Mukh Dhauti
41	Hamstring Muscles	All Standing *Asans*, Shirshasan, Sarvangasan, Anantasan, Pashchimottanasan, Baddh Konasan, Upvishth Konasan, Akarna Dhanurasan, Kurmasan, Ushtrasan, Shalabhasan, Dhanurasan, Ardh Matsyendrasan, Samakonasan	Anulom Vilom, Jagadguru Kripaluji Pranayam		Subtle Body Relaxation
42	Hay Fever	Surya Namaskar, Singhasan	Bhastrika, Kapalbhati	Laghu Shankh Prakshalan, Kunjal, *Neti*	Subtle Body Relaxation
43	Headache (Also Migraine)	Tadasan, Shashankasan, Halasan, Karnapidasan, All Relaxing *Asans*, Sarvangasan, All Eye Exercises from Subtle Exercises (especially Palming and Massaging)	Anulom Vilom, Ujjayi, Bhramari, Shyam Uchcharan	*Neti*, (Kunjal for migraine), *Bhagwad Swaroop Darshan (Trāṭak)*	Subtle Body Relaxation, Splashing the eyes frequently with cold water.
44	Heart Trouble	Subtle Exercises, Ananda Madirasan, Siddhasan, All Relaxing Poses, Backward Bending *Asans*, Padmasan, Halasan, Ardh Baddh Padmasan, Shavasan	Ujjayi, Anulom Vilom, Bhramari, Shyam Uchcharan		Subtle Body Relaxation
45	Heart Burn	Same as in Acidity			
46	Heels (Pain or Spurs)	Shirshasan, Sarvangasan, Konasan, Baddh Konasan, Ardh Matsyendrasan, Gomukhasan	Kapalbhati, Anulom Vilom		Frequently giving Acupressure

#	Condition	Asanas	Pranayam		Other
47	**Hernia (Umbilical)**	Shirshasan, Sarvangasan, Baddh Konasan, Upvishth Konasan, Pashchimottanasan, Pada Hastasan, Kurmasan, Mandukasan	Kapalbhati, Anulom Vilom, Jagadguru Kripaluji Pranayam		Subtle Body Relaxation
48	**Hernia (Inguinal)**	Shirshasan, Sarvangasan, Baddh Konasan, Samakonasan, Pashchimottanasan	Kapalbhati, Anulom Vilom, Jagadguru Kripaluji Pranayam		Subtle Body Relaxation
49	**HIV+**	Subtle Exercises, Halasan, Sarvangasan, Matsyasan, Kandharasan, Supt Vajrasan, All Backward Bending *Asans*	Anulom Vilom, Bhramari, Bhastrika, Shyam Uchcharan	Laghu Shankh Prakshalan	Subtle Body Relaxation
50	**Hunched-Back**	All the Standing *Asans*, Shalabhasan, Makarasan, Dhanurasan, Ushtrasan, Bhujangasan, Janu Shirasan, Upvishth Konasan, Gomukhasan, Parvatasan, Baddh Padmasan, Ardh Matsyendrasan			
51	**Hydrocele**	Slow rounds of Surya Namaskar, Vajrasan (for at least 10-15 minutes), All Inverted *Asans*, Garudasan, Brahmacharyasan, Baddh Konasan, Upvishth Konasan, Pashchimottanasan, Samakonasan	Kapalbhati, Jagadguru Kripaluji Pranayam, Bhastrika	*Nauli*	Mool Bandh and Uddiyan Bandh
52	**Impotency**	Surya Namaskar, Shirshasan, Sarvangasan, Halasan, Pashchimottanasan, Baddh Konasan, Ardh Matsyendrasan	Anulom Vilom, Bhastrika, Ujjayi		Mool Bandh, Uddiyan Bandh
53	**Impure Blood**	Surya Namaskar until sweating heavily, Dynamic *Asans*	Anulom Vilom, Kapalbhati	Laghu Shakh Prakshalan	Diet: Eat Fruits and Vegetables without salt.
54	**Indigestion**	All Standing *Asans*, Shirshasan, Sarvangasan, Shalabhasan, Dhanurasan, Pashchimottanasan, Ardh Matsyendrasan	Bhastrika, Jagadguru Kripaluji Pranayam	*Nauli*	Uddiyan Bandh
55	**Insomnia**	Subtle Exercises, Shashankasan, Shirshasan, Sarvangasan, Pashchimottanasan, Shalabhasan	Jai Radhey Pranayam (before going to bed), Anulom Vilom, Bhastrika, Bhramari, Ujjayi, Shyam Uchcharan	*Bhagwad Swaroop Darshan (Trāṭak)*	Subtle Body Relaxation (before going to bed)

No.	Category	Asanas / Exercises	Pranayama	Shatkarma	Other
56	**Kidneys (toning)**	Surya Namaskār, Supt Vajrasan, Shashankasan, Marjari Asan, Shashank Bhujangasan, Vyaghrasan, Trikonasan, Matsyasan, All Backward Bending *Asans*, Pashchimottanasan, Ardh Matsyendrasan, Halasan, Gomukhasan, Ushtrasan, Merudandasan, Hansasan, Mayurasan, Koormasan	Bhastrika	Laghu Shankh Prakshalan, *Nauli*, Agnisar Kriyā	Uddiyan Bandh Diet: Control the intake of salt and increase water intake
57	**Knees (toning)**	All Standing *Asans*, Knee exercises from Subtle Exercises, Janu Shirasan, Akarna Dhanurasan, Gomukhasan, Siddhasan, Baddh Konasan, Ardh Matsyendrasan, Kurmasan			
58	**Lactation**	Subtle Exercises, Possible Inverted *Asans* Precautions: Omit Dynamic *Asans* and do not fast.	Anulom Vilom, Bhramari, Shyam Uchcharan Awareness: On Breathing while feeding the child		Subtle Body Relaxation, *Roop Dhyan* Meditation
59	**Legs (toning)**	Subtle Exercises, Surya Namaskār, Comfortable Standing *Asans*, Shalabhasan, Dhanurasan, Bhujangasan, Pashchimottanasan, Akarna Dhanurasan, Upvishth Konasan, Anantasan, Ek Pada Shirasan, Ek Pada Pranamasan, Garudasan, Natarajasan, Samakonasan, Utthanasan, Setu Asan, Ardh Chandrasan, All Forward Bending *Asans*, Bakasan, Utthit Hasta Padangushthasan, Different Jogging exercises, Legs' Joints exercises mentioned in JKYog	Bhastrika		
60	**Liver, Spleen, Pancreas, and Intestines**	Pashchimottanasan, Meru Vakrasan, Bhu-Namanasan, Ardh Matsyendrasan, Meru Dandasan, Urthit Hasta Merudandasan, Ardh Padma Padmottanasan	Bhastrika	Laghu Shankh Prakshalan, *Nauli*, Kunjal	Uddiyan Bandh Diet: Omit oily, fried foods, alcohol, tobacco, etc.
61	**Lumbago**	Same as in Backache			

62	**Lungs (toning)**	Surya Namaskár, Supt Vajrasan, Akarna Dhanurasan, Ushtrasan, Hasta Uttanasan, Utthit Lolasan, Matsyasan, Baddh Padmasan, All Backward Bending *Asans*, Sarvangasan	All *Pranayams* (Jai Radhey Krishna Pranayam in Shavasan)	Subtle Body Relaxation *Bandhas:* Uddiyan and Mool Bandh
63	**Menopause**	Ardh Matsyendrasan, Surya Namaskár, Nauka Sanchalan, Chakki Chalan, Pada Vrittasan, Dhanurasan, Udarkarshanasan, Supt Udarkarshan, Padasanchalan, Supt Pawanmuktasan, Bhujangasan, Dhanurasan, Shirshasan, Sarvangasan, Halasan, Matsyasan, Pashchimottanasan, Baddh Padmasan, Upvishth Konasan, Baddh Konasan, Yog Mudrasan, Parvatasan, Kurmasan	Light practice of all Radhey Krishna Pranayams	
64	**Menstrual Disorders**	Naukasan, Kandharasan, Chakrasan, Sarvangasan, Halasan, Inverted *Asans*, Baddh Padmasan, Upvishth Konasan, Baddh Konasan, Yog Mudrasan, Parvatasan, Kurmasan Precautions: Do not attempt difficult and inverted *Asans*.	Abdominal Breathing, Anulom Vilom, Ujjayi, Bhramari, Shyam Uchcharan	Precautions: Omit *Nauli* while menstruating	*Bandhas:* Jalandhar, Mool, Maha Bandh. Subtle Body Relaxation
65	**Muscular Dystrophy**	Subtle Exercises	Anulom Vilom, Bhramari, Shyam Uchcharan		Subtle Body Relaxation
66	**Nasal Catarrh**	Shirshasan, Sarvangasan, Pashchimottansan	Anulom Vilom, Ujjayi, Bhastrika	*Neti* (both—Jal and Sutra Neti)	Diet: Take lemon water with a pinch of salt
67	**Neck (for toning, weakness, aches, and nerve stimulation)**	Neck and Shoulder exercises from Subtle Exercises, Jyeshthikasan, Makarasan, Greeva Sanchalan, Kandharasan, All Spinal Twisting *Asans*	Ujjayi, Clavicular Breathing		Precautions: Reduce deskwork and also avoid thick pillows
68	**Nerves (toning)**	All comfortable *Asans*, Surya Namaskár	Anulom Vilom, Bhastrika, Kapalbhati		Pran Mudra
69	**Nervous Debility**	Shirshasan, Sarvangasan, Pashchimottansan, Singha Garjan Asan	Anulom Vilom, Ujjayi, Bhastrika, Bhramari, Shyam Uchcharan		Subtle Body Relaxation and *Roop Dhyan* Meditation

		Asans	Pranayam	Shatkarma / Kriyā	
70	**Obesity**	All Warm-up exercises (especially On-spot Jogging), Subtle Exercises, Pada Sanchalan, Pada Vrittasan, Utthanapadasan, Matsyasan, Surya Namaskār, Dynamic Pada Hastasan, Drut Halasan, Vipareet Karani Asan, Vajrasan, All Abdominal and Dynamic *Asans*	All Radhey Krishna Pranayams—especially Bhastrika and Jagadguru Kripaluji Pranayam		Diet: Avoid fatty, starchy, sweet foods. Take a very light dinner. If possible, do fasting once or twice a week
71	**Palpitation**	Shirshasan, Halasan, Pashchimottanasan, Shavasan	Jai Radhey Pranayam, Anulom Vilom, Ujjayi		Subtle Body Relaxation and *Roop Dhyan* Meditation
72	**Piles**	Sarvangasan and Vipareet Karani Asan for longer periods, Tadasan, Tiryak Tadasan, Kati Chakrasan, Shashankasan, Shashank Bhujangasan, Supt Vajrasan, Ushtrasan, Matsyasan, Pashchimottanasan	Kapalbhati, Bhastrika	Laghu Shankh Prakshalan, Ganesh Kriyā (Mool Shodhan)	Mool Bandh Diet: Light and easily digestible foods with adequate fibre and nutrients
73	**Pregnancy (antenatal)**	1-3 months: See Reproductive Organ 4-6 months: Subtle Exercises, Tadasan, Tiryak Tadasan, Kati Chakrasan, Vajrasan, Hasta Utthanasan, Marjari Asan, Matsya Kridasan, Meditative *Asans*, Meru Vakrasan 7-9 months: Only Subtle Exercises	Jai Radhey Pranayam, Anulom Vilom, Bhramari, Ujjayi, Light Bhastrika, Shyam Chanting Precautions: Omit the practice of Bhastrika after the first trimester	In the first trimester: Kunjal, Laghu Shankh Prakshalan Later: *Neti*	Mool Bandh, Subtle Body Relaxation, *Roop Dhyan* Meditation Precautions: Omit Uddiyan Bandh, Agnisar Kriyā, *Nauli*
74	**Pregnancy (Post-natal)**	1st week: Only Relaxing *Asans* 2nd week: Subtle Exercises, Relaxing *Asans* 3rd week: Subtle Exercises, Relaxing *Asans*, comfortable Standing *Asans*, Backward Bending *Asans*, Spinal Twisting 4th week: Slow Surya Namaskār and Urthanasan, Different Relaxing *Asans*	After 2nd week: Jai Radhey Pranayam, Anulom Vilom, Bhramari, Shyam Uchcharan, Ujjayi, Bhastrika (gently)		After 1st week: Subtle Body Relaxation, *Roop Dhyan* Meditation After 3rd week: Mool Bandh
75	**Prostate Gland**	Siddhasan, Shirshasan, Sarvangasan, Shalabhasan, Dhanurasan, Janu Shirasan, Baddh Konasan, Padmasan, Kurmasan, Ardh Matsyendrasan, Samakonasan	Anulom Vilom, Ujjayi, Light practice of Kapalbhati		Uddiyan Bandh, Mool Bandh, and Maha Bandh

No.	Condition	Asanas / Exercises	Pranayams	Kriyas	Diet / Others
76	**Pyorrhea**		All Radhey Krishna Pranayams (particularly Sheetali and Sheetkari)		Diet: Take sour fruits like Lemon, *Āmlā*, Plum, etc.
77	**Reproductive Organs (for toning)**	Subtle Exercises, Surya Namaskār, Shashankasan, Marjari Asan, Shashank Bhujangasan, Ushtrasan, Vyaghrasan, Kati Chakrasan, Tadasan, Meru Prishthasan, Utthanasan, Trikonasan, Yog Mudrasan, Matsyasan, All Backward Bending *Asans*, Ardh Matsyendrasan, All Inverted *Asans*, Kandharasan, Garudasan, Pada Angusthasan, Mayurasan, Brahmacharyasan	All Radhey Krishna Pranayams	Agnisar Kriyā, *Nauli*	Bandhas: Mool, Maha Bandh / Others: Subtle Body Relaxation and *Roop Dhyan* Meditation
78	**Rheumatism**	Same as in Arthritis			
79	**Sciatica**	Same as in Slipped-disc and Backache			
80	**Sinusitis**	Same as in Cold or Cough			
81	**Skin problems (like eczema, acne, dermatitis, etc.)**	Surya Namaskār (as many rounds as possible without strain), Sarvangasan, Halasan, Mayurasan	All Radhey Krishna Pranayams	Laghu Shankh Prakshalan	Diet: Avoid tea, coffee, spicy items, fried and oily foods.
82	**Slipped-disc**	Advasan, Jyeshthikasan, Makarasan or Matsya Kridasan or Balasan for an extended period of time, Sphinx Asan, Tadasan, Vajrasan / Also the *Asans* mentioned in Backache (Slow practice) / Precautions: Omit all the Forward Bending *Asans*.	Ujjayi		Subtle Body Relaxation / Precautions: Use hard bed while resting in Prone Pose.
83	**Stammering and Stuttering**	Subtle Exercises, Singh Asan, Matsyasan, Supt Vajrasan, Naukasan, All Balancing *Asans*, Mayurasan	Bhramari, Ujjayi, Sheetali, Sheetkari, Shyam Uchcharan	*Neti*, Kunjal	Subtle Body Relaxation, *Roop Dhyan* Meditation
84	**Sterility**	Shirshansan, Sarvangasan, Pashchimottanasan, Baddh Konasan	Anulom Vilom, Ujjayi		Mool Bandh
85	**Stress and Strain**	Same as in Anxiety			
86	**Stroke**	Subtle Exercises	Jai Radhey Pranayam in Shavasan		Subtle Body Relaxation

#	Ailment	Asans	Pranayam	Shatkarma	Bandh/Mudra
87	**Throat (removal of ailments and irritations)**	Subtle Exercises, Singha Garjan Asan, All Inverted Asans, Supt Vajrasan, Matsyasan, All Backward Bending Asans	Ujjayi, Sheetali, Sheetkari, Bhramari, Shyam Uchcharan	*Neti*, Kunjal	Jalandhar Bandh
88	**Thyroid and Parathyroid (toning)**	Surya Namaskār, Subtle Exercises, Sarvangasan, Yog Mudrasan, Vipareet Karani Asan, Halasan, Karna Pidasan, Greeva Sanchalan, All Backward Bending Asans, Also see: Throat	All *Pranayams* (especially Ujjayi, Bhramari, and Bhastrika with three *Bandhas*)	*Neti*, Kunjal	Jalandhar Bandh and Subtle Body Relaxation
89	**Tonsillitis**	Shirshasan, Sarvangasan, Padmasan, Standing *Asans*, Ushtrasan, Dhanurasan, Ardh Matsyendrasan, Pashchimottanasan	Ujjayi, Anulom Vilom, Bhastrika		Uddiyan Bandh
90	**Tuberculosis**	After medical treatment, resume *Yogic* exercises, after due guidance of a competent *Yog* instructor			
91	**Tumor of the Stomach (only in the beginning phase)**	Shirshasan, Sarvangasan, All Comfortable Standing *Asans*, Janu Shirasan, Parvatasan, Pashchimottanasan, Baithak Merudandasan, Matsyasan	Anulom Vilom, Ujjayi		Uddiyan Bandh
92	**Ulcer (Peptic and Duodenal)**	All Relaxing *Asans*, Subtle Exercises, Ananda Madirasan, Bhadrasan, Singha Garjan Asan, Veerasan, Marjari Asan, Vyaghrasan, Shashankasan, Shashank Bhujangasan, Pranamasan, Ushtrasan, Supt Vajrasan, Janu Shirasan, Pashchimottanasan, Kurmasan, Ardh Matsyendrasan	Anulom Vilom, Ujjayi, Sheetali, Sheetkari, Bhramari, Shyam Uchcharan	Precautions: Kunjal should not be practiced.	Yoni Mudra, Uddiyan Bandh, and Subtle Body Relaxation
93	**Urine (dribbling or excessive)**	Shirshansan, Sarvangasan, Matsyasan, Singhasan, Baddh Konasan	Anulom Vilom		Uddiyan Bandh
94	**Varicose Veins**	All Topsy-turvy *Asans*, Subtle Exercises, Veerasan			
95	**Vertigo (dizziness)**	All Balancing *Asans*, Shashankasan	Bhramari, Shyam Uchcharan	*Bhagwad Swaroop Darshan (Trāṭak)*, Jal Neti	Subtle Body Relaxation

96	Wind (removal from intestine)	Shashankasan, Supt Vajrasan, Shashank Bhujangasan, Kati Chakrasan, Yog Mudrasan, Matsyasan, All Forward Bending *Asans*, Halasan, Drut Halasan, Hansasan, Mayurasan, Urthan Prishthasan, Mandukasan and Vajrasan (Sit in this *Asan* for at least 10-15 minutes after meals.)	Bhastrika, Kapalbhati	Agnisar Kriyā, *Nauli*, Laghu Shankh Prakshalan, Kunjal	Uddiyan Bandh
97	Worms (removal)	Naukasan	Kapalbhati		Laghu Shankh Prakshalan

GLOSSARY

A

Abhiniveśh—The fear of death.

Āchārya—An enlightened spiritual teacher.

Āgyā Chakra—Sixth primary *chakra*.

Ahankār—Ego.

Apān—One of the five vital airs in the body that moves in the sphere of the lower abdomen and controls the function of elimination of urine and faeces.

Ārati—Ceremony of lights, in which a lamp is waved around the deity of God (Radha Krishna or a Saint) with great faith and reverence.

Ārogya—Good health.

Āsans/Yogāsans—*Yogic* exercise/posture for health and well-being.

Āshram—Spiritual centre for learning and devotion.

Aṣhṭāṅg Yog—The eight limbs of *Yog* described by Patanjali.

Asmitā—Pride due to identification with the designations of the body.

Avidyā—Lack of knowledge.

Ayurvedic—Of or pertaining to Ayurveda (the Indian medicinal system; medicinal science).

B

Bandha—An act of contraction or squeezing of different muscles—practiced traditionally to lock the *prāṇic* energy and enhance the effect of the accompanying pose or *pranayam*.

Bankey Bihari—A name for Shree Krishna, meaning "He Who stands crooked in His three-fold bending form."

Basti—One of the *Ṣhaṭkarmas*, a process to cleanse the colon tract through enema.

Bhagavad Geeta—A popular Vedic scripture. It contains the dialogue between Shree Krishna and Arjun in 700 verses, on the battlefield of Kurukshetra.

Bhagavān—Supreme Soul.

Bhagawad Swaroop Darśhan—Devotional form of *Trāṭak*, on the form of God.

Bhagirathi—A name of the holy river Ganga.

Bhakti—Devotion, Divine Love.

Bhaktiyog Rasāvatār—Descention of the Bliss of Divine Love (title conferred on Jagadguru Shree Kripaluji Maharaj by the *Kāśhī Vidvat Pariṣhat*)

Bindu—A dot or a point. At the top part of your head where Hindus grow a small tuft of hair, is a point known as *bindu*. This is the point where semen is produced.

Brahm—The formless all-pervading aspect of God.

Braj—The land in Mathura, India, where Shree Krishna performed His childhood pastimes 5000 years ago. It includes many holy places like Vrindavan, Goverdhan, Barsana, Nandgaon, and Gokul.

Buddhi—Intellect.

C

Chakras—Psychic energy centres along the channel of the spine.

Charaṇāmṛit—Holy water that is obtained after washing out the Lotus Feet of Saints.

Chirāyu—Longevity.

Chir Ghat—The place in Vrindavan where Shree Krishna stole the clothes of the *Gopīs* while they were bathing in the river Yamuna.

Chīr Haraṇ—One of the *leelas* of Shree Krishna in which Shree Krishna hid the clothes of *Gopīs*, when they were taking a bath in the pond of Vrindavan.

Chitta—Mind.

D

Devanāgarī—It is the script used to write Sanskrit, many North-Indian languages, and Nepali.

Devatā—Celestial gods who governs some particular affair of the material world from the higher abodes.

Devī Bhāgavat—One of the eighteen ancient Hindu mythological scriptures.

Dharm Kāyā—Truth Body.

Dhāraṇā—Concentration.

Dhātu—Element.

Dhauti—One of the *Ṣhaṭkarmas*, a process to cleanse the digestive tract.

Ḍhoklā—A Gujarati snack, usually made by fermenting batter of one or more lentils.

Ḍholak—A small drum.

Diyā—The symbolic flame.

Ḍosā—A South Indian cuisine, usually large round pancakes made of fermented black lentils and rice.

Doṣhas—Humors of the body. According to Ayurveda, the three components which control our whole body function.

Dupaṭṭās—A shawl of double materials which *Gopīs* used to wear in Braj.

Dveṣh—Dislike for objects and persons.

E

Ekādaśhī—In Vedic Caldendar, a month is divided into two phases of the moon, i.e. waxing and waning phases of the moon. Each phase consists of fifteen days. *Ekādaśhī* is the eleventh day of the moon, occurring twice a month.

G

Garuḍ Purāṇa—One of the eighteen ancient Hindu mythological scriptures.

Gopīs—The village maidens who resided in Braj, when Shree Krishna displayed His *leelas* there 5000 years ago.

Gorakhnath—One of the famous *Yogīs* in history.

Granthis—Glands.

Guṇa—The three characteristics or qualities of the illusive energy Maya, which is manifested in the form of universe. They are *sattva guṇa, tamo guṇa,* and *rajo guṇa.*

Guru/Gurudev—A God-realized teacher of spirituality who illumines people with the knowledge of God.

Gyān—Knowledge.

Gyānī—One who follows the path of *Gyān Yog.*

H

Haṭha Yog—The way toward realization through rigorous disciplines.

Haṭha Yog Pradīpikā—A celebrated text on *Haṭha Yog* written by Swatmarama.

I

Iḍā—A *nāḍī,* a channel of energy starting from the left nostril, then moving to the crown of the head and then descending to the base of the spine. In its course it conveys lunar energy and so is called *chandra nāḍī* (channel of the lunar energy).

Iḍlī—A South Indian cuisine, usually round shaped cakes, cooked by steaming batter made of fermented black lentils and rice.

Iṣhṭa Dev—The form of God chosen by the devotee for his or her personal devotion.

J

Jaggery—Coarse brown sugar, extracted from sugarcane.

Jagadguru—Spiritual Master of the world. Equivalent to the Pope in Christianity.

Jagadguru Shankaracharya—He came to the earth planet about 2000 years ago. He re-established the greatness of Vedic *Sanātan Dharm* (eternal religion mentioned in Vedas) in India. His philosophy is known as *Advait-vād* or Non-dualism.

Jaṭharāgni—Fire of digestion in the stomach, gastric juices.

Ji—Suffix added after someone's name as a mark of respect.

Jīva—An individual soul.

K

Kachoris—An Indian snack, made from flour and deep-fried in oil.

Kadamb—A native, abundantly flowering tree of Braj, having golf ball size and shape yellow flowers with rich perfume.

Kali/Kaliyug—The name of the present era on the planet earth. This was preceded by Dwāpar Yug, Tretā Yug, and Satya Yug.

Kalia—Name of a ferocious serpent who was badly beaten by Lord Shree Krishna for his poisoning the lake in Vrindavan.

Kapālbhāti—One of the *Shaṭkarmas*, a process to cleanse the respiratory passage—especially cranial sinuses.

Kaph—Phlegm, one of the three components in the body controlling its health.

Karm—Work in accordance with the prescribed rules of the Vedas.

Karm Yog—The path of attaining God while doing one's *Karm*.

Kaśhī Vidvat Parishat—The supreme body of Vedic Scholars in the city of Kashi (highest seat of Vedic learning).

Kaustubh maṇi—A ruby-like large Divine jewel with marvelous faceting, which is worn by the supreme God (Krishna, Ram, and Vishnu) in His necklace.

Khichaḍī—A type of Indian food in which rice and dal (pulse or lentil) are cooked with water until it is soft.

Kīrtan—Devotional song or chanting, which is sung as a supplication to God, or in glorification of His Names, Forms, Virtues, and Pastimes.

Kirti—Mother of Shree Radha.

Kriyā—A cleaning process.

L

Leelas—A Divine pastime enacted by God in His personal form.

Lokas—*Lok* is another name for the world. According to Hindu Mythology there are 14 *lokas* (six above the earth and seven below).

M

Mahābhāv—The topmost state of absorption in the Bliss of Divine Love, which manifests in devotional Saints of the highest calibre.

Mahārās—The Divine dance performed by Shree Krishna with the *Gopīs*, filled with the Bliss of Divine Love.

Mahārās Leela—It is very special *leela* that happened in Vrindavan in Braj. It was the descension of the true Vrindavan Bliss on the earth planet when the grace of Krishna established Divine Vrindavan on the soils of Braj, and in that Divine space, Shree *Raseshwari* Radha Rani, Who is the life essence of Krishna's all greatness, revealed the most intimate Divine Bliss to all the *Gopīs*, on the *Śharat Pūrṇimā* night. On that particular night, Radha, Krishna, and all the *Gopīs* sang, danced, and played together in an extremely elevated Divine state, which is only seen in Divine Vrindavan.

Mālā—Rosary beads.

Maṇipūr Chakra—Third primary *chakra*.

Mathura—Holy place where Shree Krishna appeared 5000 years go; currently situated in the Uttar Pradesh State of India.

Maya—It is the illusiory power of God comprising of three modes—*sattva guṇa* (goodness), *Rajo guṇa* (passion), and *Tamo guṇa* (ignorance). Souls who have turned their backs towards God are overcome by Maya, which covers them in ignorance and makes them rotate in the cycle of life and death.

Mudrā—Postures of the hand that seal and control the energy of the body.

Mūlādhār Chakra—First of the seven *chakras* in the body according to Hindu Tantrism.

Mūñg—A kind of lentil.

Murali Manohar—One of the Names of Shree Krishna, "He Who plays the flute melodiously."

N

Nāḍīs—Literally, meaning tubes or pipes; they are the subtle channels in the body through which *prāṇic* energy flows.

Nārad Bhakti Darśhan—A holy scripture on *Bhakti* (devotion) composed by Saint Narad.

Namaskār—The act of paying Namaste with folded hands.

Nauli—One of the *Ṣhaṭkarmas*, a process to cleanse the abdominal region, especially digestive organs and small intestines by messaging internal belly organs.

Neti—One of the *Ṣhaṭkarmas*, a process to cleanse the nasal passage.

Nidhivan—The place in Vrindavan where Radha and Krishna would take rest at night, during their Divine pastimes.

Nirmāṇ Kāyā—Special body that accomplished *Yogīs* create for themselves through their austerities.

O

Oṁ—The sound representation for the formless aspect of God.

Oṁ Namaḥ Shivaya—A popular phrase chanted by the devotees of Lord Shiv, literally meaning, "I offer my obeisances to Lord Shiv."

P

Pada—A devotional song composed in a traditional style that has been commonly used by many *Bhakti* Saints such as Soordas, Meerabai, Tulsidas, Guru Nanak, Kabir etc.

Pān—Beetle nut and leaf.

Pañchadaśhī— It is an introductory work of *Advait Vedānt*, written by Swami Vidyaranya.

Paramātmā—The aspect of God that resides in the hearts of all living beings.

Parvati—A goddess, consort of Shiv, daughter of Himalaya.

Patañjali Yog—The system of *Yog* propounded by Sage Patanjali.

Patañjali Yog Sūtra—Ancient Sanskrit text on *Ashṭāṅg Yog* written by Patanjali.

Piṅgalā—A *nāḍī* or channel of energy, starting from the right nostril, then moving toward the base of the spine. As the solar energy flows through it, it is also regarded as the Surya *nāḍī*. *Piṅgalā* means tawny or reddish color.

Pītāmbar—A saffron color silk material. It is worn by draping it over shoulders/putting it on the shoulders and leaving it hanging down. It has a delicate, thin, and fancy edge and fancy wide border at the ends. It is also worn on the lower part of the body from the waist and down to heels. When it is worn on the upper part, it is called shawl and it is 2.5 yards in length, and when on the lower part, it is called *dhoti* and it is 5 yards in length. A common name for both is *Pītāmbar*. It is worn by Krishna, Radha, and also Vishnu.

Pitta—Bile, one of the three components in the body controlling its health.

Prāṇ—Life-giving energy that is subtler than air, and present everywhere.

Pranayam—Breathing exercise for controlling the breath and assimilating *prāṇic* energy.

Prāṇic—Pertaining to *prāṇ*.

Prasād—Something that is offered to God as part of religious worship.

Pratyāhār—Withdrawal of the senses, the fifth stage among the eight stages of Patanjali's *Aṣhṭāṅg Yog*.

Pūjā—An act of worshipping God with flowers, water, offerings, etc.

Pūrak—Inhalation.

Purāṇas—These are scriptures, full of philosophic knowledge, that discuss the creation of the universe, its annihilation and recreation, and the history of humankind. There are eighteen *Purāṇas*, all written by Ved Vyas.

R

Radha Rani—God takes on two forms in His Divine pastimes—Krishna (the Energetic) and Radha Rani (His Divine Energy). Radha is also called the Divine Mother of the Universe, to whom all the other energies of God are subservient.

Rāg—Attachment towards material objects or personalities.

Rajas—Mode of ignorance, one of the three modes of material nature.

Rajgirā—A less commonly used cereal, that is usually eaten on days of fasting such as *Ekādaśhī* (eleventh day of the moon).

Rās—The Divine dance of Shree Krishna with the *Gopīs* in Braj, in which He bestowed the highest Bliss of Divine Love.

Raseshwar—One of the names of Shree Krishna, meaning one who performed the Divine dance (*Mahārās*) with the *Gopīs*.

Rechak—Exhalation.

Ṛiṣhis and Munis—Saints and hermits who do meditation in the solitary places like jungle, mountains, caves, etc.

Roop Dhyan—Meditation upon the Form of God.

Roop Mādhurī—The nectar emanating from the beauty of the Personal form of God.

S

Sādhanā—A kind of spiritual practice or quest.

Sahasrār—Seventh primary *chakra*.

Samān—One of the vital airs, whose function is to assist in digestion.

Sambhog Kāyā—The body in which the soul engages in worldly enjoyment.

Samosās—It is a triangular shaped patty, stuffed with vegetables, fried in ghee or oil.

Sanyāsī—A person in the renounced order of life, who has taken a vow of celibacy and detachment.

Satsaṅg—A gathering where the Names, Virtues, and Pastimes of God and Guru are recited, sung, and remembered.

Sattva guṇa—The mode of goodness; one of the three modes of material nature.

Sāttvic—Having the quality of *sattva guṇa*.

Sevā—To serve, the act of service.

Seva Kunj—The place where Shree Krishna performed His Divine *Rās* dance with the *Gopīs*.

Śhakti—Power.

Śharat Pūrṇimā—The full-moon night (usually falling on Sept/Oct) in which Shree Krishna did the *Rās* dance.

Shaṭkarmas—It is a six fold purificatory process, consisting of *Neti*, *Dhauti*, *Nauli*, *Basti*, *Kapālbhāti*, and *Trāṭak*—developed by ancient *Yogīs* for removing unwanted substances from the body.

Shiv—Name of the third God of the Hindu Trinity, Who is entrusted with the task of destruction.

Shree—A title given to a respectable personality.

Shree Krishna—God takes on two forms in His Divine pastimes—Krishna (the Energetic) and Radha Rani (His Divine Energy). Krishna is also called the Complete Brahm (Absolute God) of the Universe, to whom all the other forms of God are subservient.

Shreemad Bhagavatam—The most important of the eighteen *Purāṇas* written by Ved Vyas. It consists of 18,000 verses, full of philosophical knowledge and the descriptions of the Names, Forms, Virtues, and Pastimes of the various Avatars of God.

Shyam Sundar—One of the nicknames of Shree Krishna among infinite Names.

Sushumṇā—The main channel situated inside the spinal column.

Swami Swatmarama—The writer of the famous book, *Haṭha Yog Pradīpikā*.

Swar varṇa—Hindi vowels.

T

Tamas—Mode of ignorance, one of the three modes of material nature.

Tapas—A burning effort which involves purification, self-discipline, and austerity.

Tilak—A religious (or decorative) mark on the forehead made by certain thin paste or color in a particular style according to one's religious tradition.

Trāṭak—A method of meditation that involves concentration on a single point, such as a flame or a dot.

Tribhangilal—"Tribhangi" is one of the standing poses of Krishna when His body is elegantly bent from the three places: neck, waist, and ankle. Hence, He has got the nickname Tribhangilal.

Triphalā—A mixture of three myrobalans, viz. chebulic myrobalan *(Haḍ)*, belleric myrobalan *(Baheḍa)*, and emblic myrobalan *(Āmlā)*.

U

Udān—One of the five *prāṇs* in the body.

Upanishads—Philosophical portions of the Vedas, dealing with the nature of man and the universe and the union of individual soul or self with the universal soul—God.

Upanishadic—Of the Upanishads.

V

Vaḍā—A ball or doughnut shaped fried delicacy made of fermented flour of various lentils.

Vaijayantī Mālā—A garland made out of the seeds of the *Vaijayantī* plant.

Vairāgya—Detachment from the world.

Vamshivat—"*Vaṭ*" means tree and "*Vaṁshī*" means flute. *Vamshivat* is the tree under which Shree Krishna stood and played His flute, while beckoning the *Gopīs* for the *Rās* dance.

Vanaspati Ghee—It is a kind of processed oil, made by hydrogenating various fatty oils, e.g. vegetable oil, animal fats, etc., under pressure.

Vasishth—Teacher of Lord Shree Ram, Lakshman, Bharat, and Shatrughna.

Vāt—Air, one of the three components in the body controlling its health.

Vāyu—The wind, the vital airs.

Vedas—The eternal knowledge of God that He manifested at the beginning of creation, which was passed down from master to disciple through hearing, and finally divided and written in four books—Ṛig Veda, Yajur Veda, Sāma Veda, Atharva Veda.

Vedāntic—Pertaining to the Vedas.

Vedic—Of Vedas.

Viśhuddhi Chakra—The fifth of the seven primary *chakras* in the body.

Vrindavan—The place in Mathura district (India) where Shree Krishna performed many sweet pastimes 5000 years ago.

Vyān—One of five *prāṇs* in the body.

Y

Yāgyavalkya Sanhitā—A *Yog* treatise by Saint Yagyavalkya.

Yāgyavalkya Smriti—One of three most important *Smritis* of Hindu Philosophy.

Yamuna—Name of a holy river that flows through the land of Braj, and on the banks of which, Shree Krishna performed several blissful pastimes.

Yashoda and Nand—"Yashoda" is the mother and "Nand" is the father of Krishna from Gokul.

Yog—Union of *jīva* (soul) with the Supreme Soul.

Yogī—One who follows the path of *Yog*; a "*Yoginī*" is the female equivalent to a practicing male "*Yogī*" (Plural—"*Yogīs/Yoginīs*").

Yog Nidrā—A kind of *Yogic* sleep, in which one consciously and alertly diverts his mind according to the given instruction.

Yog Vāsishṭha—It is a scripture traditionally attributed to the Sage Valmiki, recounting a dialogue between him and Lord Ram.

Yugal Sarkar—Yugal refers to both. Hence, by the terms Yugal Sarkar, both Radha Krishna are understood.

Index

A

B

E

F

G

H

J

R

S

T

U

V

Y

Other Publications by Jagadguru Kripaluji Yog

1. Healthy Body Healthy Mind - Yoga for Children

2. Inspiring Stories for Children Volume 1

3. Inspiring Stories for Children Volume 2

4. Inspiring Stories for Children Volume 3

5. Inspiring Stories for Children Volume 4

6. Saints of India

7. Festivals of India

8. Bal-Mukund Wisdom Book

9. Bal-Mukund Painting Book

10. Essence of Hinduism

11. Spiritual Dialectics

12. Bhagavad Gita - The Song of God

13. Mahabharat - The Story of Virtue and Dharma